Neutrophilic Dermatoses

Daniel Wallach
Marie-Dominique Vignon-Pennamen
Angelo Valerio Marzano
Editors

Neutrophilic Dermatoses

Springer

Editors
Daniel Wallach
Physician (Hon.) of Paris Hospitals
Paris
France

Angelo Valerio Marzano
Dipartimento di Fisiopatologia Medico-Chirurgica e dei Trapianti
Universita' degli Studi di Milano
Unita' Operativa di Dermatologia
IRCCS Fondazione Ca' Granda
Ospedale Maggiore Policlinico
Milano
Italy

Marie-Dominique Vignon-Pennamen
Pathology Department
APHP Hôpital Saint Louis
Paris
France

ISBN 978-3-030-10244-9 ISBN 978-3-319-72649-6 (eBook)
https://doi.org/10.1007/978-3-319-72649-6

Printed on acid-free paper

This Springer imprint is published by the registered company Springer International Publishing AG, part of Springer Nature.
The registered company address is: Gewerbestrasse 11, 6330 Cham, Switzerland

Contents

Contributors

Christine S. Ahn Department of Dermatology, Wake Forest University School of Medicine, Winston-Salem, NC, USA

Marc André Université Clermont Auvergne, CHU Clermont-Ferrand, Service de Médecine Interne, Hôpital Gabriel Montpied, Inserm U1071, Clermont-Ferrand, France

Maxime Battistella Pathology Department, APHP Hôpital Saint Louis, INSERM UMR_S1165, Université Paris Diderot, Paris, France

Didier Bessis Department of Dermatology, St Eloi Hospital, Montpellier, France

Sébastien Buche Service de Dermatologie, Hôpital Nord, Marseille, France

Alessandro Borghi Dipartimento di Scienze Mediche, Sezione di Dermatologia e Malattie Infettive, Università degli Studi di Ferrara, Ferrara, Italy

Luca Borradori Department of Dermatology, Inselspital, Bern University Hospital, University of Bern, Bern, Switzerland

Jeffrey P. Callen Division of Dermatology, University of Louisville School of Medicine, Louisville, KY, USA

Emmanuel Contassot Department of Dermatology, University Hospital Zurich, Zurich, Switzerland

Antonio Costanzo Department of Biomedical Sciences, Humanitas University and Skin Pathology Laboratory Humanitas Research Hospital, Milan, Italy

Massimo Cugno Dipartimento di Fisiopatologia Medico-Chirurgica e dei Trapianti, Università degli Studi di Milano, Medicina Interna, IRCCS Fondazione Ca' Granda, Ospedale Maggiore Policlinico, Milano, Italy

Giovanni Damiani Dipartimento di Fisiopatologia Medico-Chirurgica e dei Trapianti, Universita' degli Studi di Milano, Unita' Operativa di Dermatologia, IRCCS Fondazione Ca' Granda, Ospedale Maggiore Policlinico, Milano, Italy

Emmanuel Delaporte Service de Dermatologie, Hôpital Nord, Marseille, France

Lauryn M. Falcone West Virginia University School of Medicine, Morgantown, WV, USA

Laurence Feldmeyer Department of Dermatology, Inselspital, Bern University Hospital, University of Bern, Bern, Switzerland

Lars E. French Department of Dermatology, University Hospital Zurich, Zurich, Switzerland

Roberta Gualtierotti Divisione e Cattedra di Reumatologia, Dipartimento di Scienze Cliniche e di Comunità, Università degli Studi di Milano, Milan, Italy

Laurence Gusdorf Service de Dermatologie, Hôpitaux Universitaires de Strasbourg, Strasbourg, France

Takashi Hashimoto Department of Dermatology, Osaka City University Graduate School of Medicine, Osaka, Japan

William W. Huang Department of Dermatology, Wake Forest University School of Medicine, Winston-Salem, NC, USA

Andrew Johnston Department of Dermatology, University of Michigan, Ann Arbor, MI, USA

Joseph L. Jorizzo Department of Dermatology, Weill Cornell Medicine, New York, NY, USA

Riccardo Lazzari Dipartimento di Fisiopatologia Medico-Chirurgica e dei Trapianti, Università degli Studi di Milano, Unità Operativa di Dermatologia, IRCCS Fondazione Ca' Granda, Ospedale Maggiore Policlinico, Milano, Italy

Unità Operativa di Dermatologia, IRCCS Fondazione Ca' Granda, Ospedale Maggiore Policlinico, Milano, Italy

Ramtin Lichtenberger Department of Dermatology, University Hospital Zurich, Zurich, Switzerland

Dan Lipsker Service de Dermatologie, Hôpitaux Universitaires de Strasbourg, Strasbourg, France

Angelo Valerio Marzano Dipartimento di Fisiopatologia Medico-Chirurgica e dei Trapianti, Università degli Studi di Milano, Unità Operativa di Dermatologia, IRCCS Fondazione Ca' Granda, Ospedale Maggiore Policlinico, Milano, Italy

Alessandra Narcisi Department of Biomedical Sciences, Humanitas University and Skin Pathology Laboratory Humanitas Research Hospital, Milan, Italy

Alexander A. Navarini Department of Dermatology, University Hospital Zurich, Zurich, Switzerland

Courtney R. Schadt Division of Dermatology, University of Louisville School of Medicine, Louisville, KY, USA

Jean-Luc Schmutz Dermatology and Allergology Department, CHRU Nancy–Brabois, Vandœuvre-lès-Nancy, France

Robert A. Schwartz Dermatology, Rutgers-New Jersey Medical School, Newark, NJ, USA

Rutgers School of Public Affairs and Administration, Newark, NJ, USA

Rivka C. Stone Dermatology, Rutgers-New Jersey Medical School, Newark, NJ, USA

Anh N. Tran Department of Dermatology, Weill Cornell Medicine, New York, NY, USA

Marie-Dominique Vignon-Pennamen, M.D. Pathology Department, APHP Hôpital Saint Louis, Paris, France

Daniel Wallach Physician (Hon.) of Paris Hospitals, Paris, France

Introduction

1

Daniel Wallach, Marie-Dominique Vignon-Pennamen, and Angelo Valerio Marzano

The goal of this book is to present the current knowledge about a group of skin conditions collectively known as the Neutrophilic Dermatoses. It is rather unusual for dermatologists to name cutaneous diseases according to the main cellular type found in the lesions. In doing so, and not bringing to the foreground the clinical appearance of the lesions, one could expect a wide variety of clinical aspects. Indeed, some neutrophilic dermatoses are pustular, others are papular, nodular, ulcerative, and the diversity of their appearance gave rise to a great number of denominations when distinct clinical entities were described by twentieth century dermatologists.

The first clue towards a grouping of these seemingly disparate entities came from a reflection on the fact that in spite of different clinical aspects, some skin conditions shared many common characteristics. This led us to propose criteria for inclusion into a group, or a spectrum, of neutrophilic dermatoses [1, 2].

Two criteria appear of crucial importance: the first one, obviously, is the afflux of polymorphonuclear leukocytes, or neutrophils, into the skin. Neutrophils are the main effector cells of the innate immune system, and their physiological role is to phagocyte microbes. But neutrophilic dermatoses are sterile and neutrophils are not attracted by pathogens, they accumulate due to complex, non infectious mechanisms.

D. Wallach (✉)
Physician (Hon.) of Paris Hospitals, Paris, France

M.-D. Vignon-Pennamen, M.D.
Pathology Department, APHP Hôpital Saint Louis, Paris, France
e-mail: dominique.vignon-pennamen@wanadoo.fr

A. V. Marzano (✉)
Dipartimento di Fisiopatologia Medico-Chirurgica e dei Trapianti, Universita' degli Studi di Milano, Unita' Operativa di Dermatologia, IRCCS Fondazione Ca' Granda, Ospedale Maggiore Policlinico, Milano, Italy

D. Wallach et al. (eds.), *Neutrophilic Dermatoses*,
https://doi.org/10.1007/978-3-319-72649-6_1

The second main feature of the neutrophilic dermatoses is their belonging to internal medicine. The fact that a great number of patients with a neutrophilic dermatosis suffer from a multisystemic condition (mainly blood malignancy, digestive inflammation, joint disorder) attracted much medical attention and could even be considered as a publication bias. Another systemic dimension is less well appreciated: in some cases, the neutrophilic inflammation is not limited to the skin but also involves other organs [3]. We proposed to name Neutrophilic disease [4] this cutaneous and non-cutaneous neutrophilic autoinflammation. The diagnosis of extracutaneous aseptic neutrophilic inflammation can be very difficult, especially when it precedes the cutaneous involvement, or in the absence of such an involvement. A practical consequence is that patients with the neutrophilic disease are managed by non-dermatologists, physicians of all medical and surgical specialties, who should be familiar with this aseptic inflammation.

The neutrophilic inflammation which is not secondary to a microbial invasion is called autoinflammation [5]. Discovered and studied only recently, autoinflammation is the pathophysiological explanation of many monogenic systemic diseases. It now appears that it is also the explanation of many polygenic or complex diseases, including the neutrophilic dermatoses [6].

This book is divided in two parts: in the first part, the main neutrophilic dermatoses are described. The chapters are arranged following the classification we proposed in 2006, based on the main localization of the neutrophilic infiltrate in the skin [7]. According to this classification, the group of the neutrophilic dermatoses can be divided in three subgroups. The first one encompasses superficial, epidermal, pustular diseases such as Sneddon-Wilkinson's disease and other pustuloses; the second one is centered around Sweet's syndrome, characterized by a dermal infiltrate, papules and plaques; the third group includes deep dermatoses, inducing abscesses or ulcerations, the prototype of these ulcerations being pyoderma gangrenosum (Fig. 1.1). It is very important to understand that the three conditions named above may be regarded as arbitrary points on a wide spectrum. These conditions present as typical or atypical forms, and associations, transitions, overlaps are not rare in clinical practice. As a consequence, whether we deal with many different conditions, three subgroups or only one group, is a question that is presently not solved, but belongs more to the academic discussions than to medical practice.

In the second part, pathology, internal involvement, pathophysiology and therapy will be exposed.

All the authors are experts in the field and wrote comprehensive, updated reviews of their topic. In such a work, redundancies and overlaps are unavoidable and we did not try to avoid them. They are an expression of the complexity of such a domain, and also allow to better understand the diversity of approaches.

The field of the neutrophilic dermatoses is in constant evolution. The existence itself of this group has not been easily acknowledged. The progress in the understanding of innate immunity and autoinflammation, the discovery of the precise role of each of the numerous cytokines involved and of the efficacy of targeted

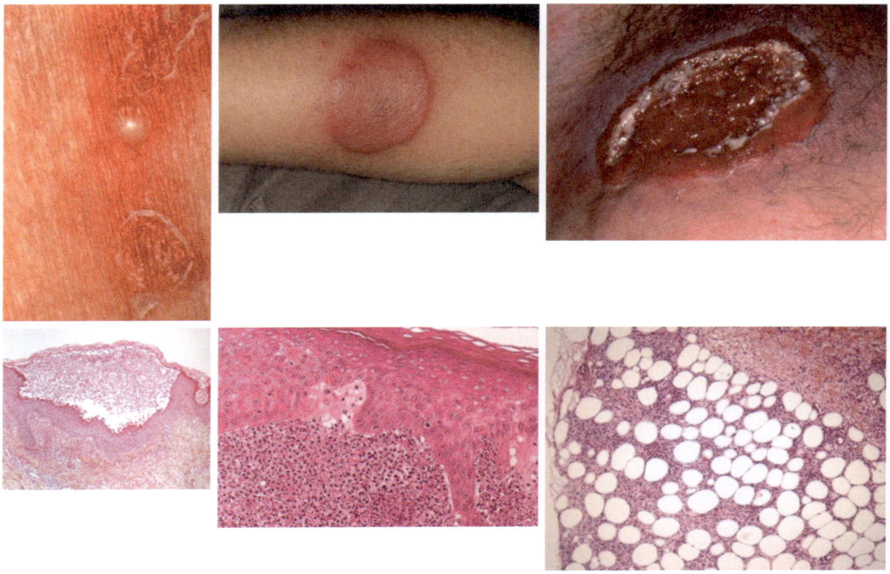

Fig. 1.1 These images illustrate typical clinical and histopathological figures of the prototypic conditions of the three main groups of neutrophilic dermatoses. On the left, subcorneal pustular dermatosis (Sneddon-Wilkinson disease); in the middle, Sweet syndrome; on the right, pyoderma gangrenosum (Coll D Wallach and MD Vignon-Pennamen)

therapeutic agents, will improve our ability to adequately manage patients suffering from a neutrophilic dermatosis.

We would like to express our gratitude and thanks to Mr. Grant Weston and to Ms. Rajeswari Balachandran, from Springer, and to the authors who devoted their efforts to the completion of this book. We hope dermatologists, internal medicine specialists and clinical immunologists will find here the essentials of to-day's knowledge, and the basis for future progress.

References

1. Wallach D. Les dermatoses neutrophiliques. Presse Med. 1991;20:105–7.
2. Wallach D. Neutrophilic dermatoses: an overview. Clin Dermatol. 2000;18:229–31.
3. Vignon-Pennamen MD. The extracutaneous involvement in the neutrophilic dermatoses. Clin Dermatol. 2000;18:339–47.
4. Vignon-Pennamen MD, Wallach D. Cutaneous manifestations of neutrophilic disease. A study of seven cases. Dermatologica. 1991;183:255–64.
5. Abramovits W, Oquendo M. Introduction to autoinflammatory syndromes and diseases. Dermatol Clin. 2013;31:363–85.
6. Marzano AV, Borghi A, Meroni PL, Cugno M. Pyoderma gangrenosum and its syndromic forms: evidence for a link with autoinflammation. Br J Dermatol. 2016;175:882–91.
7. Wallach D, Vignon-Pennamen MD. From acute febrile neutrophilic dermatosis to neutrophilic disease: forty years of clinical research. J Am Acad Dermatol. 2006;55:1066–71.

2 Neutrophilic Dermatoses: An Overview

Daniel Wallach

Neutrophilic Dermatoses (ND) appeared in the medical literature in 1964, when RD Sweet coined this term to name a previously undescribed skin condition characterized by a non-infectious acute, febrile "cutaneous and systemic neutrophilic reaction" [1]. Sweet discussed the differential diagnosis in citing erythema multiforme, erythema elevatum diutinum and erythema nodosum. One of Sweet's first eight patients had ulcerative colitis and some pustular, acneiform lesions, but pyoderma gangrenosum is only cited to be ruled out, because "the clinical picture was quite unlike".

The occurrence of what had been soon called Sweet's syndrome in patients with acute leukemia [2] attracted much attention to this rare condition. In the ante-1964 literature, non-specific cutaneous manifestations of leukemia, also called leukemids, can be considered as precursors of Sweet's syndrome [3].

The association with leukemia or related blood malignancies was also the main motive for establishing a link between Sweet's syndrome and pyoderma gangrenosum [4]. In 1983, Caughman, Stern and Haynes described a "neutrophilic dermatosis of myeloproliferative disorders" as a continuum or overlap between Sweet's syndrome, the acute febrile neutrophilic dermatosis, and pyoderma gangrenosum, described earlier as a completely different condition [5].

Personal observations as well as a review of the literature led me to propose, in 1991 [6], that some skin diseases could be clustered in a group, or spectrum, of neutrophilic dermatoses. In addition to Sweet's syndrome and pyoderma gangrenosum, this group included subcorneal pustular dermatosis and erythema elevatum diutinum.

The criteria for inclusion in this group of the neutrophilic dermatoses were:

1. Skin disorders characterized by an infiltration of the skin by normal neutrophils;
2. No infectious cause;

D. Wallach
Physician (Hon.) of Paris Hospitals, Paris, France

D. Wallach et al. (eds.), *Neutrophilic Dermatoses*,
https://doi.org/10.1007/978-3-319-72649-6_2

3. Diverse cutaneous features (pustules, plaques, nodules, ulcerations), with associations, overlaps and transitional forms;
4. Extracutaneous symptoms (lung, joints, others);
5. Association with systemic disorders (blood malignancies, inflammatory bowel diseases, arthritis, others);
6. Sensitivity to steroids and other anti-inflammatory drugs.

Although never formally validated, these criteria were widely accepted and in the following years, other conditions were added to this group.

In 2006, Dr. Vignon-Pennamen and I proposed a simple classification of the numerous ND. This classification is based on the localization of the neutrophilic infiltrate in the epidermis, the superficial dermis or the deep dermis/subcutis [7] (Table 2.1). The clinical-pathological classification of diseases is very familiar to dermatologists and this proposal was well received. The plan of this book is based on this classification. In examining this classification however it is important to remember the frequent existence of associations, transitions, overlaps, between the typical entities.

The neutrophilic dermatoses are part of internal medicine. Two situations must be distinguished here:

Table 2.1 Classification of the neutrophilic dermatoses (adapted and updated from [7])

Superficial (epidermal, pustular) ND
Sneddon-Wilkinson disease (Subcorneal pustular dermatosis)
Amicrobial pustulosis of the folds
Pustular vasculitis
Bowel-associated dermatosis-arthritis syndrome
Pyodermatitis/Pyostomatitis vegetans
Pustular psoriasis
Palmoplantar pustuloses
SAPHO syndrome
Behçet disease
Acne fulminans
Drug-induced pustuloses (Acute generalized exanthematous pustulosis)
Infantile acropustulosis
Dermal (en plaques) ND
Sweet syndrome (Acute febrile neutrophilic dermatosis)
Neutrophilic eccrine hidradenitis
Erythema elevatum diutinum
Vegetative (granulomatous) pyoderma gangrenosum
Neutrophilic urticarial dermatitis
Schnitzler syndrome
Neutrophilic lupus erythematosus
Deep ND
Pyoderma gangrenosum
PAPA and related syndromes (Syndromic PG)
Neutrophilic panniculitis
Aseptic abscesses
Hidradenitis suppurativa

1. The neutrophilic dermatoses are often associated with a multisystemic disease. Sweet's syndrome, pyoderma gangrenosum, and all the typical and atypical neutrophilic dermatoses often occur in the setting of a blood disorder as mentioned above, but as well of an inflammatory bowel disease, a chronic arthritis, or many other multisystemic conditions. Drug intake may now be added to these situations.
2. The neutrophilic dermatoses are characterized by the afflux of neutrophils into the skin in the absence of any infection. But the skin is not the only organ targeted by activated neutrophils. In fact, all the organs of the body may suffer from a similar sterile inflammation. We proposed to name this condition "The neutrophilic disease" [8]. Internal neutrophilic aseptic infiltrates pose serious diagnostic challenges to physicians confronted with such patients. Clinical symptoms are variable and non-specific. If the cutaneous counterpart is delayed or absent, the diagnosis can be extremely difficult. Internists, surgeons, physicians of all specialties should be familiar with the neutrophilic disease and its protean manifestations. It is one of the goals of this book.

The pathophysiology of the neutrophilic dermatoses has long been elusive. The morphology and the function of the infiltrating leukocytes has been investigated without significant results.

As soon as 1987, Going suggested that interleukin-1, the master cytokine of inflammation, was involved in the pathogeny of Sweet's syndrome [9]. This proved to be the right track, and in recent years research has focused on the identification of cytokines responsible for the inflammation in the ND. Angelo Valerio Marzano and his group [10] are the main contributors in this research, as will be seen in many chapters of this book.

Neutrophils are the main effector cells of the innate immune system. They are responsible for the inflammation required to eliminate many bacterial pathogens. In the ND however, the neutrophilic inflammation is not caused by external pathogens, but by internal stimulis. This is known as autoinflammation, a concept proposed in 1999 to explain monogenic diseases characterized by spontaneous bouts of cutaneous, articular, and systemic inflammation [11].

Although the concept of autoinflammation initially referred to mendelian diseases, many arguments suggest that non monogenic, complex diseases, could also be due to autoinflammation.

One of the most convincing of these arguments is the fact that cutaneous lesions pertaining to the three subgroups of the ND spectrum are present in many monogenic autoinflammatory diseases. Deficiencies of IL-1 and IL-36 receptor antagonists, known as the DIRA and DITRA syndromes, are severe autosomal recessive disorders which present with pustular eruptions of early onset [12, 13]. Familial Mediterranean Fever, or periodic disease, a prototype of monogenic autoinflammatory diseases, is well known for erysipelas-like erythemas, very similar to Sweet syndrome; other ND, such as neutrophilic panniculitis, may as well be found in this disease [14]. PAPA syndrome and related conditions are syndromic, genetic variants of pyoderma gangrenosum [15].

Table 2.2 Timeline of ideas on the neutrophilic dermatoses

Date	Emerging concept	References
1964	Acute febrile neutrophilic dermatosis (Sweet's syndrome)	[1]
1983	Neutrophilic dermatosis of myeloproliferative disorders	[5]
1991	A group of neutrophilic dermatoses	[6]
1991	The neutrophilic, multisystemic disease	[8]
2006	A classification of the neutrophilic dermatoses	[7]
2016	The neutrophilic dermatoses are autoinflammatory disorders	[18]

In conclusion, three stages may be individualized in the recent history of our conceptions about the neutrophilic dermatoses: in a first stage, starting in 1908 with Brocq's description of geometrical phagedenism [16], clinician dermatologists described many skin conditions caused by a cutaneous invasion by neutrophils, in the absence of infection. In a second stage, it was recognized that these numerous, clinically distinct, skin conditions, could be grouped in a unified spectrum, later subdivised in three subgroups. It was also acknowledged that these neutrophilic dermatoses represent the most obvious component of a wider condition, the neutrophilic disease. Recently, these aseptic neutrophilic dermatoses and disease were included in the spectrum of the autoinflammatory diseases. In the classification of immunological diseases proposed in 2006 by McGonagle and McDermott [17], the neutrophilic dermatoses/disease can be included in the group of the polygenic (or complex) autoinflammatory diseases.

This progress in our understanding of the neutrophilic dermatoses leads to therapeutic consequences. Until now, therapy of the ND relies on non-specific anti-inflammatory drugs, such as corticosteroids and immunosuppressives. The accumulation of many case reports suggests that therapy targeting IL-1, or in the future other operative cytokines, will improve the management of all autoinflammatory diseases, whether monogenic or polygenic [18]. Table 2.2 summarizes the history of ideas from Sweet's original description to modern concepts.

References

1. Sweet RD. An acute febrile neutrophilic dermatosis. Br J Dermatol. 1964;76:349–56.
2. Matta M, Malak J, Tabet E, Kurban AK. Sweet's syndrome: systemic associations. Cutis. 1973;12:561.
3. Costello MJ, Canizeres O, Montague M, Buncke CM. Cutaneous manifestations of myelogenous leukemia. AMA Arch Derm. 1955;71:605–14.
4. Burton JL. Sweet's syndrome, pyoderma gangrenosum and acute leukaemia. Br J Dermatol. 1980;102:239.
5. Caughman W, Stern R, Haynes H. Neutrophilic dermatosis of myeloproliferative disorders. Atypical forms of pyoderma gangrenosum and Sweet's syndrome associated with myeloproliferative disorders. J Am Acad Dermatol. 1983;9:751–8.
6. Wallach D. Les dermatoses neutrophiliques. Presse Med. 1991;20:105–7.
7. Wallach D, Vignon-Pennamen MD. From acute febrile neutrophilic dermatosis to neutrophilic disease: forty years of clinical research. J Am Acad Dermatol. 2006;55:1066–71.

8. Vignon-Pennamen MD, Wallach D. Cutaneous manifestations of neutrophilic disease. A study of seven cases. Dermatologica. 1991;183:255–64.
9. Going JJ. Is the pathogenesis of Sweet's syndrome mediated by interleukin-1? Br J Dermatol. 1987;116:282–3.
10. Marzano AV, Fanoni D, Antiga E, et al. Expression of cytokines, chemokines and other effector molecules in two prototypic autoinflammatory skin diseases, pyoderma gangrenosum and Sweet's syndrome. Clin Exp Immunol. 2014;178:48–56.
11. McDermott MF, Aksentijevich I, Galon J, et al. Germline mutations in the extracellular domains of the 55 kDa TNF receptor, TNFR1, define a family of dominantly inherited autoinflammatory syndromes. Cell. 1999;97:133–44.
12. Aksentijevich I, Masters SL, Ferguson PJ, et al. An autoinflammatory disease with deficiency of the interleukin-1-receptor antagonist. N Engl J Med. 2009;360:2426–37.
13. Marrakchi S, Guigue P, Renshaw BR, et al. Interleukin-36-receptor antagonist deficiency and generalized pustular psoriasis. N Engl J Med. 2011;365:620–8.
14. Leiva-Salinas M, Betlloch I, Arribas MP, Francés L, Pascual JC. Neutrophilic lobular panniculitis as an expression of a widened spectrum of familial mediterranean fever. JAMA Dermatol. 2014;150:213–4.
15. Marzano AV, Borghi A, Meroni PL, Cugno M. Pyoderma gangrenosum and its syndromic forms: evidence for a link with autoinflammation. Br J Dermatol. 2016;175:882–91.
16. Brocq L, Simon CL. Contribution à l'étude du phagédénisme. Bull Soc Méd Hôp Paris 3eme série. 1908;25:290–307.
17. McGonagle D, McDermott MF. A proposed classification of the immunological diseases. PLoS Med. 2006;8:e297.
18. Satoh TK, Mellett M, Contassot E, French LE. Are neutrophilic dermatoses autoinflammatory disorders? Br J Dermatol. 2016 Nov 30. https://doi.org/10.1111/bjd.15105.

Part I

The Skin Conditions of the ND Spectrum

3 Sweet's Syndrome

Marie-Dominique Vignon-Pennamen

Sweet's syndrome (SS) is the prototypic neutrophilic dermatosis, first reported in 1964 by Robert Douglas Sweet who describes eight female patients with a new dermatosis entitled an "acute febrile neutrophilic dermatosis" [1]. It consists of acute onset of multiple tender, red, cutaneous plaques, often accompanied by fever and neutrophilic leukocytosis. Cutaneous biopsy contains dermal infiltrates of mature neutrophils. Response to systemic steroids is dramatic. Originally known as Gomm-Button disease (in reference to the first two patients), the condition rapidly acquired the well-established eponym "Sweet's syndrome" (SS).

Although a definitive mechanism of pathogenesis for the development of SS still remains to be determined, the role of interleukin-1 and tumor necrosis factor (TNF) alpha, in the immunopathogenesis of this condition supports its classification as an autoinflammatory disease [2]. In malignancy-associated SS, the role of the malignant clone in myeloid neoplasms can also be underlined [3, 4].

Many excellent reviews on SS have been published describing all presentations of this syndrome and associated disorders [5–10].

History

During the 15 year period from 1949 to 1964, Robert Douglas Sweet encountered eight women with "a distinctive and fairly severe illness". He authored a paper entitled "An Acute Febrile Neutrophilic Dermatosis" in order to "draw a composite picture of the condition and behaviour of these patients and to describe briefly their variations". The cardinal features were "fever, neutrophil polymorphonuclear leukocytosis of the blood, raised painful plaques of the limbs, face and neck, and histologically a dense dermal

M.-D. Vignon-Pennamen, M.D.
Pathology Department, APHP Hôpital Saint Louis, Paris, France
e-mail: dominique.vignon-pennamen@wanadoo.fr

D. Wallach et al. (eds.), *Neutrophilic Dermatoses*,
https://doi.org/10.1007/978-3-319-72649-6_3

infiltration with mature neutrophils polymorphs". The other important features were the absence of any evidence of infection, the dramatic response to corticosteroids and the absence of scarring. In 1955, prior to Sweet's original publication, Costello et al., had described in an article entitled "Cutaneous Manifestations of Myelogeneous Leukemia", the case of 16-year old girl with acute myelogeneous leukemia who had recurrent cutaneous lesions [11]. This case can be retrospectively considered as the initial description of a patient with SS associated with leukemia. In 1973, Matta et al., report five cases of SS [12]. They underline the possible associaton with acute leukemia revealed by cutaneous lesions in two patients. Moreover, four of their patients had urinary abnormalities with kidney involvement on biopsy and one of them, with acute leukemia, had neutrophilic infiltrates of the portal triad on liver biopsy. They suggest the possibility that the lesions in SS may not be limited to the skin but involve other organs as well.

Epidemiology

SS has a worldwide distribution and no racial predilection. Limited data are available about the incidence and prevalence of SS. In Scotland, the annual incidence is 2.7 cases for one million [13]. In Switzerland, the variability of incidence suggests the role of infectious agents [14]. In a retrospective German study, between 1985 and 1993, 38 cases of SS have been observed with peaks of onset in spring and autumn [7]. SS predominantly affects women between 30 and 60 years of age. However, the sex ratio is variable according to the published series [7, 13–24]. The condition can affect younger adults and children [25]. The condition presents in four clinical settings: classic (or idiopathic) SS, malignancy-associated SS, parainflammatory SS and drug-induced SS.

Clinical Features

Symptoms

The systemic symptoms that characteristically accompany the skin eruption are fever and leukocytosis and patients with SS may appear dramatically ill. Fever is described in 40–80% of patients. It may precede the skin disease by several days or weeks or be present concurrently during the dermatosis. However its presence should not be considered a requirement for diagnosis. Other symptoms include, to variing degrees, arthralgia, general malaise, headache and myalgia. Classically an upper respiratory tract viral infection precedes the skin disease. However less usual infections are also noted [24].

Cutaneous Lesions

Classical Sweet's Syndrome

Typically, the skin lesions of SS appear as tender, often painful red or purple-red papules or nodules. They most frequently occur on the upper extremities, face and neck (Fig. 3.1). They also develop on the trunk and lower extremities where they may mimic those of erythema nodosum. The eruption may present with either a single lesion or multiple (often asymetrically distributed) with a widespread localization. The lesions may have a mamillated appearance with pseudovesiculation secondary to the pronounced edema in the upper dermis, sometimes compared to a profile relief of a montain. Partial central clearing may accentuate the deeper red and more actively, sometimes pustular, advancing marginal mountain range. The lesions enlarge over a period of days to weeks. They coalesce and form irregular, sharply bordered plaques (Fig. 3.2). The size is usually a few centimeters, but large plaques up to 10 × 20 cm in diameter may develop. They usually resolve, spontaneously or after treatment without scarring.

Skin hypersensitivity, also referred to as cutaneous pathergy may be present, with lesions occuring at the site of biopsies, vaccination, cat scratches, IV catheter placement, radiation therapy, sunburn and venipuncture. Occasionally, lesions have been photodistributed, located on the arm affected by postmastectomy lymphedema or have devopped after surgery [26, 27].

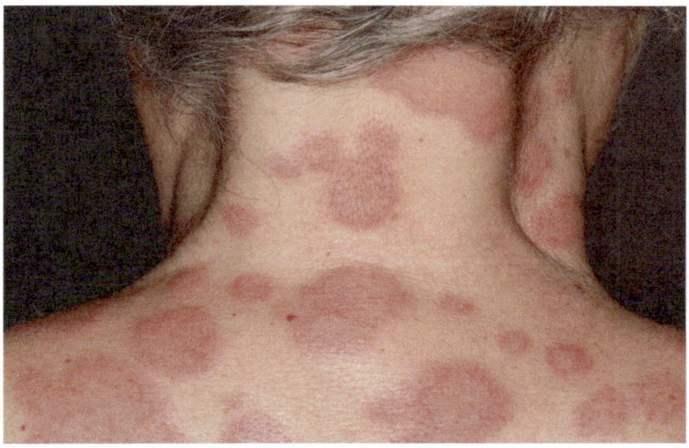

Fig. 3.1 Classic lesions of Sweet's syndrome

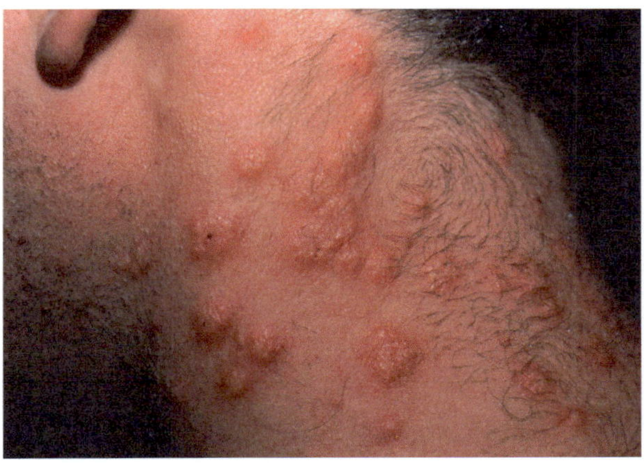

Fig. 3.2 Plaques and papules with a vesicle-like appearance

Oral mucosal involvement is uncommon in idiopathic SS. However, oral or genital ulcers or pustules may occur more frequently in patients with hematologic disorders [6].

Clinical Variants of Sweet's Syndrome

Bullous Sweet's syndrome. In rare instances, severe blistering may occur. Blisters develop on erythematous plaques, enlarge, and break leaving a superficial ulceration (Fig. 3.3). This variant overlaps with bullous pyoderma gangrenosum. Initially identified in patients with hematologic malignancies [28, 29], bullous SS is observed in classic, idiopathic SS as well [18, 20, 24].

Pustular Sweet's syndrome. SS can present as a pustular dermatosis. This clinical variant includes patients with neutrophilic dermatosis of the dorsal hands. The term "pustular vasculitis of the dorsal hands" was initially proposed in 1995 to describe a peculiar cutaneous eruption limited to the dorsa of the hands and fingers [30]. Clinical presentation is quite similar to classical SS with leukocytoclastic vasculitis on biopsy (Fig. 3.4). However, patients may have lesions located on either the arm, leg, back, face and oral mucosa and necrotizing vasculitis is not a constant feature [31, 32]. Neutrophilic dermatosis of the dorsal hands is now considered as a

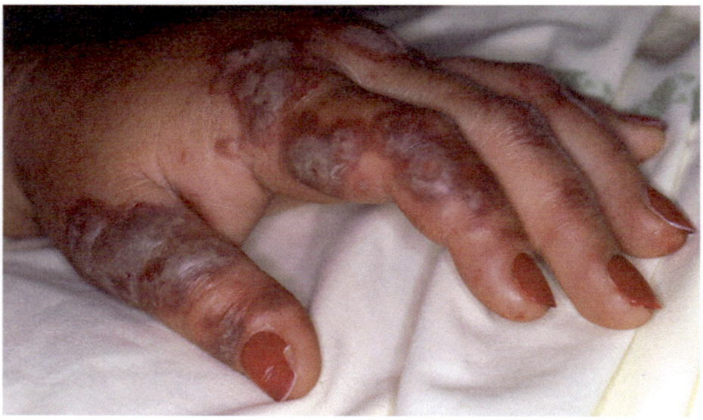

Fig. 3.3 Hemorrhagic and necrotic bullae in a case without associated disease

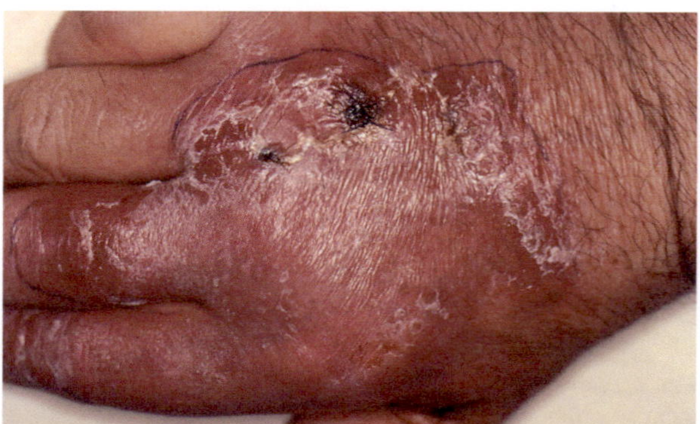

Fig. 3.4 Sweet's syndrome located on the dorsal hands

localized variant of SS in which the lesions are predominantly restricted to the dorsal hands and pathologic changes are interpretated to represent a secondary leukocytoclastic vasculitis [33].

Some patients present with a pustular eruption characterized by painful tender pustules occurring on erythematous purpuric bases. They accompany ulcerative colitis or hematologic malignancy [34–36].

Subcutaneous Sweet's syndrome. Subcutaneous SS and neutrophilic panniculitis can be considered as the same condition [37]. The cutaneous lesions often present as erythematous inflammatory painful nodules on the extremities [38]. They may mimic erythema nodosum when they are located on the legs (Fig. 3.5). Skin biopsy shows a neutrophilic inflammation that involves only the adipose tissue. However in many patients, the neutrophilic infiltrate invades both the dermis and the subcutaneous fat [39]. This clinical variant is frequently observed in patients with myelodysplastic syndromes [40].

Cellulitic and necrotizing Sweet's syndrome. Some patients may have a severe febrile dermatosis especially located on the face simulating erysipela or infectious cellulitis (Fig. 3.6). This subset is especially observed in the setting of myeloid leukemia [41, 42]. More recently, a new variant of neutrophilic dermatosis mimicking necrotizing fasciitis has been described [43]. Three immunocompromised patients

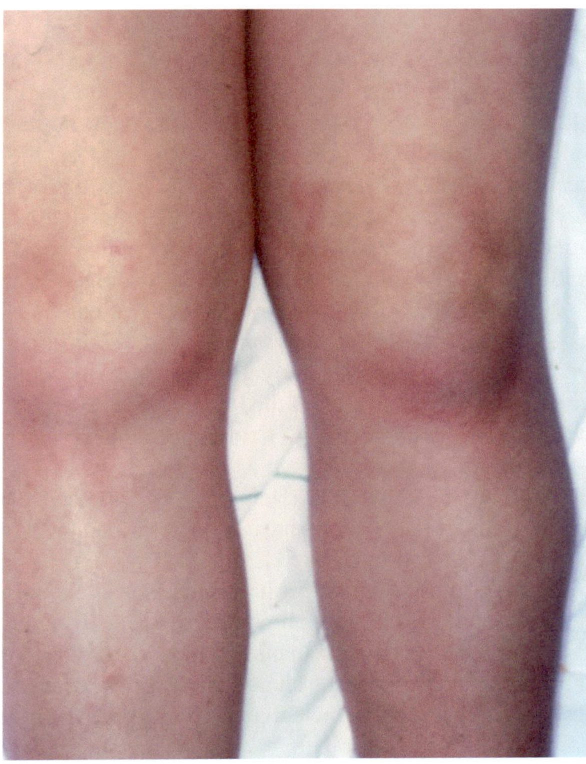

Fig. 3.5 Subcutaneous Sweet's syndrome in a patient with myelodysplastic syndrome

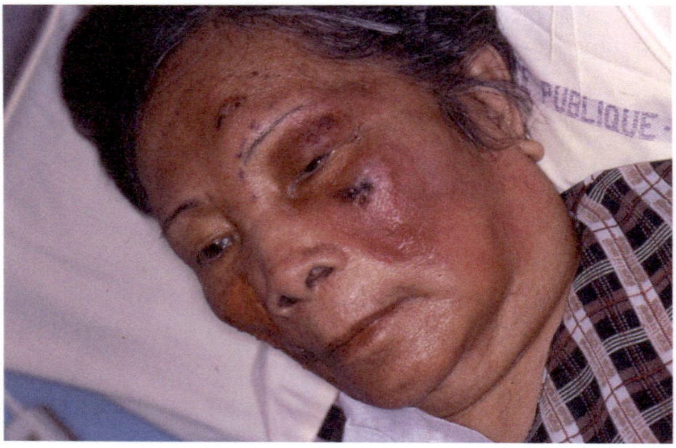

Fig. 3.6 Cellulitic Sweet's syndrome in a woman with acute myeloid leukemia

developed a progressive erythematous edematous inflammation with deep-tissue neutrophilic infiltration and soft tissue necrosis including myonecrosis in the absence of infectious cause. Finally, cases of giant cellulitis-like Sweet's syndrome have been recently reported [44].

Extracutaneous Manifestations

The possible occurrence of extracutaneous aseptic infiltrates in SS has been suggested few years after the first description of the syndrome, in 1973 by Matta et al. [12]. It is one of the characteristics of the neutrophilic dermatoses that are now be called the neutrophilic disease [45]. They can affect the lungs, the bones, the central nervous system, the eyes, the joints, the liver, the bronchi, the intestines, the kidneys, the muscles, the heart, potentially all the organs [46]. They constitute a very important chapter that is exposed in detail in this book, concerning not only dermatologists but also all physicians of all specialities.

Arthralgias or arthritis occur in 30–60% of patients. Joint involvement manifests as polyarthritis and affects asymmetrically, wrists, ankles, knees and shoulders [46].

In children, sterile osteomyelitis has been reported [47]. Focal aseptic osteitis underlying a lesional site on the lower leg has been published in a 25-year old man with deep SS associated with Crohn disease [48].

Ocular manifestations such as conjonctivitis and episcleritis may be present in 30–75% of patients. Less commonly conjonctival hemorrhage, glaucoma, iritis, limbal nodules and scleritis have been described [49]. Peripheral ulcerative keratitis has also been reported [50, 51].

Myalgias are present in up to half of the patients and sometimes a more severe involvement with myositis has been reported in patients with myeloid disorders [52, 53].

Among extracutaneous manifestations, the pulmonary involvement is one of the most important to know and clinicians need to be aware of the possibility of these manifestations because of the potential development of severe respiratory compromise. The eruption of SS can occur before, concomitantly or after the pulmonary symptoms [54,

55]. It is frequently associated with an hematologic malignancy [46]. Diagnosis is difficult requiring an extensive work up to excude an infection. Some rare cases of systemic inflammatory response syndrome have been described in the setting of SS [56].

Neuro-Sweet's disease is a rare occurrence that can affect regions of the central nervous system causing a large variety of neurological symptoms [57].

Rare extracutaneous manifestations of SS with aseptic abscesses in the liver, the spleen, the lymph nodes and cardio-vascular involvement have been reported [58, 59].

Laboratory Findings

The most consistent laboratory findings in SS are an elevated erythrocyte sedimentation rate and peripheral leukocytosis with neutrophils. While small series have reported high incidences of pyrexia, hyperleukocytosis and elevated erythrocytes sedimentation rate, these features have not been as common in larger series. Incidences between 50 and 70% are probably more representative than reviews on the subject have suggested. Anemia, a normal or low neutrophil count and/or an abnormal platelet count may be observed in malignancy-associated SS [6, 8, 9, 60]. In two recent series, the low hemoglobin level appears a significant variable among patients with SS associated with hematologic malignancies and solid tumors [20, 24]. Hepatic enzymes abnormalities, proteinuria, and less often hematuria can be observed in patients with liver and renal involvement. The presence of circulating autoantibodies against neutrophilic cytoplasm antigens is not a serologic marker for the majority of patients [61].

Pathology

The clinical diagnosis of SS needs to be confirmed by a biopsy. In most of the cases, it shows an infiltrate of mature neutrophils in the dermis, separated from the epidermis by an edema in the papillary dermis (Fig. 3.7). Swelling of the

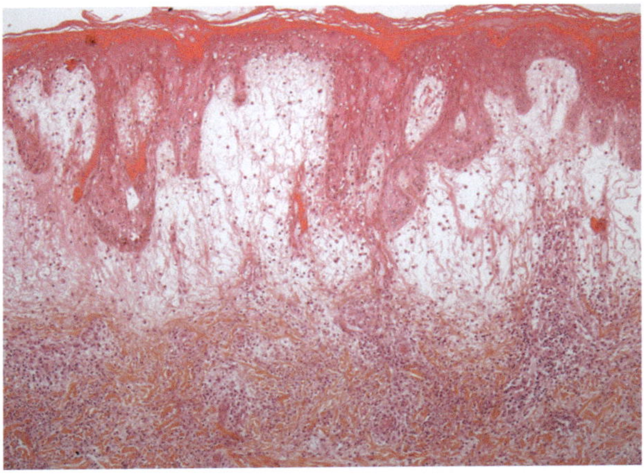

Fig. 3.7 Typical histologic features of Sweet's syndrome (HEx200)

endothelial cells, dilatation of the small blood vessels, and fragmentation of the neutrophils nuclei are also frequently observed. Usually, fibrin deposition or neutrophils are not present within the vessel wall and the overlying epidermis is normal. The infiltrate, moderate to extensive, is distributed within the upper dermis and is usually dense and diffuse, less often, around the vessels. Sometimes, there is a leukocytoclastic vasculitis that is considered as an epiphenomenon secondary to the damages caused by neutrophils [62]. In some cases, neutrophils may migrate into the epidermis to form spongiotic vesicles or intraepidermal pustules. In some patients, the infiltrates are located, either entirely or partially in the subcutaneous fat, defining the subcutaneous SS (or neutrophilic panniculitis) [39]. In these cases, the infiltrates invade the lobules, septae or both. The mature neutrophils are the typical and the most frequent inflammatory cells in SS lesions. Occasional lymphocytes and histocytes may be present as well as eosinophils [63]. Histiocytoid SS refers to an infiltrate of immature myeloid cells with a histiocytoid appearance which may be misinterpretated as histiocytes [64]. This histological variant is indicative for a myeloid malignancy, especially a myelodysplastic syndrome [4, 65]. It needs to be differenciated from leukemia cutis [66].

Clinical Course

Without treatment, the lesions of SS may persist for weeks or even several months. They then may involute without leaving scar. In some of the patients with SS associated with solid tumor, resolution of the lesions occurs following complete resection of the tumor [8]. In patients with drug-induced SS, discontinuation of the causative medication is often followed by the clearing of the lesions [67]. Under treatment, usually systemic corticosteroids, there is a prompt relief of cutaneous and systemic symptoms. Fever, general malaise, arthralgias resolve within 24–48 h and skin eruption disappears within 1–4 weeks. Despite the good initial response to therapy, the disease is characterized by frequent recurrence. The relapse rate is variable among series or reviews. It is usually estimated to be about 30% of patients [24]. One or more recurrences often develop during tapering of steroid dosage but new episodes of SS can also occur after cessation of therapy. A chronic relapsing form of SS is reported in 10–15% of patients [7]. A higher rate of relapses in SS associated with hematologic malignancies has been reported in some reviews [8] but not confirmed in more recent series [24].

Diagnosis and Differential Diagnosis

The diagnosis of SS is based on clinical, histological and biological findings. In 1986, Su and Liu have proposed criteria for the diagnosis [68]. They have been modified in 1994 by von den Driesch [7] and are widely accepted (Table 3.1). They are very useful for clinical studies on series of patients.

Table 3.1 Criteria of Sweet's syndrome initiated by Su and Liu [68] and revised by von den Driesch [7]

Major criteria	
1.	Abrupt onset of tender or painful erythematous plaques or nodules occasionally with vesicles, pustules or bullae
2.	Predominantly neutrophilic infiltration in the dermis without leukocytoclastic vasculitis
Minor criteria	
1.	Preceded by a nonspecific respiratory or gastrointestinal tract infection or vaccination or associated with:
	(a) Inflammatory diseases such as chronic autoimmune disorders, infections
	(b) Hemoproliferative disorders or solid malignant tumors
	(c) Pregnancy
2.	Accompanied by periods of general malaise and fever (>38 °C)
3.	Laboratory values during onset: ESR > 20 mm; C-reactive protein positive; segmented-nuclear neutrophils and stabs >70% in peripheral blood smear; leukocytosis >8000 (three or four of these values necessary)
4.	Excellent response to treatment with systemic corticosteroid or potassium iodide

Diagnosis requires both major criteria and at least two minor criteria

Table 3.2 The differential diagnosis of Sweet's syndrome

Classical Sweet's syndrome
Erythema multiforme
Urticaria
Drug eruptions
Insect bites
Granuloma faciale
Lupus erythematosus
Familial mediterranean fever
Classical Sweet's syndrome with systemic inflammatory response
Bacterial sepsis
Bullous Sweet's syndrome
Herpes simplex virus infection
Varicella-zoster virus infection
Impetigo contagiosum
Pustular Sweet's syndrome
Behçet's disease
Bowel bypass syndrome
Subcutaneous Swedet's syndrome
Erythema nodosum
Panniculitis
Cellulitic/necrotizing Sweet's syndrome
Erysipelas
Cellulitis

In most cases, the diagnosis may be easily made by a dermatologist and confirmed by a biopsy.

Differential diagnoses are summarized in Table 3.2. They are classified according to the clinical presentation.

Classical SS

In patients with fever, blood cultures are required to exclude a bacterial sepsis.

Erythema multiforme may mimic lesions of SS. In contrast to erythema multiforme, the assymetric distribution of the lesions, their tenderness, the usual absence of oral and genital erosions favor the diagnosis of SS. Central clearing of the plaques in SS with an infiltrated, raised inflammatory border is also quite different from the target-like lesions of erythema multiforme. Histology allows distinction of erythema multiforme from SS.

In some cases, urticaria may be confused with SS. However, pruritus is never observed in SS and the prompt resolution or fading of lesions characterize the common presentation of urticaria. When the infiltrates are composed of neutrophils rather than eosinophils, differential diagnosis is more difficult and a discussion between clinicians and pathologits is needed to exclude a neutrophilic urticarial dermatosis that is the subject of a chapter in this book [69].

Medical history of drug intakes is always indicated to exclude a drug reaction and explore the possibility of a drug-induced SS.

Insect bites can, sometimes mimic lesions of SS. The papular aspect of the lesions with central vesiculation, the distribution of the eruption and pruritus as well as a usually eosinophil rich infiltrate allow diagnosis.

It may be more difficult to exclude granuloma faciale when lesions are not exclusively located on the face. The absence of systemic symptoms, the brownish color of lesions and a very different histological aspect are indicative of granuloma faciale.

Some clinical presentations of lupus erythematosus may simulate SS and both conditions may be associated. The differential diagnosis requires a precise evaluation of clinical, histological and immunological parameters [70].

Bullous SS

In this clinical variant, infectious dermatoses are easily excluded by viral and bacterial analyses.

Pustular SS

This variant leads to discuss after exclusion of infection, Behçet's disease and bowel by-pass syndrome. Behçet's disease may be clinically similar to SS. Characteristic features like genital aphtae, recurrent uveitis, superficial thrombophlebitis, involvement of the central nervous system and a distinct HLA pattern provide criteria for differenciation [71, 72]. Bowel by-pass syndrome occurs after jejunoileal by-pass surgery or in association with inflammatory bowel disease. The diagnosis relies on the medical history.

Subcutaneous SS

Subcutaneous SS needs to be differenciated from erythema nodosum and other forms of panniculitis. Erythema nodosum can be present concurrently or sequentially in SS patients [73].

Cellulitic or Necrotizing SS

In these rare forms of SS, erysipelas or cellulitis are very difficult to exclude and a final diagnosis of non infectious neutrophilic dermatosis is usually established after many weeks or months because of absence of response to diverse antibiotics and sometimes surgical debridment.

SS and Other Neutrophilic Dermatoses

In most of reviews or series, pyoderma gangrenosum, erythema elevatum diutinum, neutrophilic eccrine hidradenitis, subcorneal pustular dermatosis, pustular eruption of colitis are discussed as differential diagnoses of SS in its typical or atypical forms. Obviously, these clinical conditions are fairly distinctive entities, but not always recognizable on histopathological grounds. In 1980 Burton, then in 1983 Caughman, Stern and Haynes underlined that pyoderma gangrenosum and SS when associated with myeloid malignancies, are closer than usually expected and they suggest that these two conditions are linked and represent the two ends of a nosological continuum [28, 74]. In the followings years, other reports have illustrated this overlapping neutrophilic dermatosis in association with bowel disorders [75, 76] as well as in patients without systemic disease [45]. In 1991, D Wallach extended this clinical spectrum [77], and proposed criteria for the inclusion of new conditions in the group of neutrophilic dermatoses:

Skin disorders characterized by an infiltrate of the skin by normal neutrophils
No infectious cause
Diverse cutaneous features (pustules, plaques, nodules, ulcerations), with associations, overlap and transitional forms
Extracutaneous symptoms
Association with systemic disorders
Sensitivity to steroids and other antiinflammatory drugs

Other entities can now be included in the group of neutrophilic dermatoses [78]. They constitute different chapters of this book. According to the classification we proposed in 2006, pyoderma gangrenosum, subcorneal pustular dermatosis, erythema elevatum diutinum and other such entities do not constitute a stricto sensu differential diagnosis of SS. They belong to the same group of diseases representing overlaps or transitions or associations. In addition to the association of SS and pyoderma gangrenosum, it is interesting to cite other reports of pyoderma gangrenosum associated with subcorneal pustular dermatosis [79], erythema elevatum diutinum [80] or of SS associated with erythema elevatum diutinum [81], neutrophilic eccrine hidradenitis or subcorneal pustular dermatosis [82].

Associated Diseases

SS can be classified into classic (idiopathic), malignancy-associated, and drug-induced, depending on the clinical setting in which the disease develops. As proposed by von den Driesch, another group of parainflammatory SS may be proposed (Table 3.4). The frequency of associated diseases is not well known for all categories. It is variable, according to origination of recruitment and publication. Moreover, some associated conditions may represent a coincidental occurrence. In about 50% of cases, SS is classic or idiopathic. Approximately 20% of cases are malignancy-associated, 10% are drug-induced and 10% are parainflammatory.

Malignancy-Associated Sweet's Syndrome

Hematologic Malignancies

They are the first significant association recognized in SS [12, 29]. Many clinical reviews have emphasized on this association and tried to identify some differences between "malignant" SS and classic SS [5, 6, 29]. Hematologic disorders are the most frequent, representing more than 80% of SS associated with malignancy, most commonly acute myeloid leukemia. In recent studies, the myelodysplastic syndromes are even more often observed [24, 83, 84]. Moreover SS can be associated more frequently in acute myeloid leukemia with myelodysplastic syndrome-related features [85]. The other hematologic disorders that can be encountered in SS are myeloproliferative disorders, essentially chronic myeloid leukemia, chronic lymphoid leukemia, monoclonal gammopathies (mainly Ig G type) and multiple myeloma. In a majority of cases, the skin lesions either appear concurrent with the discovery of hematological malignancy or precede diagnosis by up to several months or even years [84]. In the setting of acute myeloid leukemia, SS is diagnosed at the time of diagnosis of leukemia, during primary induction chemotherapy or during treatment for relapsed disease and less frequently before the development of leukemia [81]. Currently, no clinical differences are significant between classic and malignancy-associated SS [20, 24]. The response to treatment and the rate of recurrences are similar. In this group of patients, a lower mean hemoglobin level is the only biological parameter significantly reported in most of the series. Since the identification of histiocytoid SS in 2005, many studies indicate a strong correlation between this histological variant and the development of a myelodysplastic syndrome [64, 65]. Some patients having a rare chronic relapsing type of SS with lymphocytic and/or histiocytoid like infiltrate on biopsy may also develop a myelodysplastic syndrome [84, 86]. It is not well known if the clinical course and prognosis are worsened in patients with SS associated with hematologic malignancies and the literature contains conflicting results [85, 87, 88].

Solid Tumors

Albeit less commonly, SS is also reported in patients with solid tumors. The most frequent malignancies are carcinoma of the genito-urinary organs, breast and gastrointestinal tract. SS either precedes the initial diagnosis or is the harbinger of a recurrent tumor or asymptomatic metastatic tumor [6]. As in patients with hematologic malignancies, the presence of anemia is significantly observed in this group of patients [24].

Drug-Induced Sweet's Syndrome

In about 10% of cases, SS appears to have been induced by drug intake. Hundreds of case reports have been published and criteria for a drug-induced SS have been proposed (Table 3.3) [89]. In a recent systematic review of the literature, the authors have incorporated some of these criteria into an expanded Naranjo monogram, adding SS-specific criteria to the basic structure of the monogram [67]. Using these expanded criteria, they have found that causality is probable for granulocyte colony-stimulating factors and all-trans retinoic acid which are directly involved in the pathogenesis of SS [90–92]. The cases of SS-induced by all-trans retinoic acic and the new *FLT3* inhibitor might result in a differenciation syndrome [93]. The evidence implicating some vaccines [94, 95], and minocycline [96] are also convincing. Many other drugs have been implicated in reports considered as anecdotal [9]. Recently cases of drug-induced SS have been reported with the following medications: antiretroviral therapy [62], azacitidine [97], bortezomid [98], imatinib [99], ipilimumab [100], diverse antibiotics [101]. Their role needs to be confirmed. Interestingly, some of the drugs used for the treatment of SS are also observed, though rarely, to elicit the condition. These drugs include the tumor necrosis factor inhibitors [102] and lenalidomide [103]. Cases of SS induced by azathioprine, more often in the setting of Crohn's disease, are now considered as a manifestation of azathioprine hypersensibility [104, 105].

Table 3.3 Criteria of drug-induced Sweet's syndrome (from Walker and Cohen [89])

(a)	Abrupt onset of painful erythematous plaques or nodules
(b)	Histopathologic evidence of a dense neutrophilic infiltrate without evidence of leukocytoclastic vasculitis
(c)	Pyrexia >38 °C
(d)	Temporal relationship between drug ingestion and clinical presentation *or* temporally related recurrence after oral challenge
(e)	Temporally related resolution of lesions after drug withdrawal or treatment with systemic corticosteroids

Table 3.4 Sweet's syndrome and associated conditions

Cancer: hematologic malignancies (most commonly acute myeloid leukemia and myelodysplastic syndromes) and solid tumors (most commonly carcinomas of the genitourinary organs, breasts and gastrointestinal tract)
Infections: most commonly of the upper respiratory tract and the gastrointestinal tract
Inflammatory diseases: most commonly Crohn's disease and ulcerative colitis, Behçet's disease, relapsing polychondritis, rheumatoid arthritis, sarcoidosis and thyroid disease
Medications: most commonly G-CSF
Pregnancy

Parainflammatory Sweet's Syndrome

The major parainflammatory diseases are infectious, autoimmune and autoinflammatory (Table 3.4). Infections of the upper respiratory tract and the gastro-intestinal tract are more often observed in the prodromic phase of SS. Some more unusual infections have been reported [20, 24]. Pregnancy is considered by some authors as a predisposing condition for the development of SS [7].

Among the parainflammatory conditions associated with SS, inflammatory bowel diseases (Crohn's disease, ulcerative colitis) are the most common [106]. One of the patient in the initial description of the syndrome by RD Sweet had ulcerative colitis. Crohn's disease is more frequently observed than ulcerative colitis. It affects more often females and is associated with an active underlying bowel disease. Lesions of SS often follow the initial diagnosis of inflammatory bowel disease. Arthralgias or arthritis are frequent. Colonic disease is seen in 100% of cases.

Behçet's disease, erythema nodosum, relapsing polychondritis, rheumatoid arthritis, sarcoidosis, lupus erythematosus and thyroid disease are probably SS-associated conditions [107].

Pathogenesis

The pathogenesis of SS remains unknown. It is thought to be an immune-mediated hypersensitivity reaction to infectious, inflammatory, drug or tumor-cell antigens. SS can be defined as a neutrophil-mediated inflammation and understanding the pathophysiology relies mainly on the study of the mechanisms of invasion into the skin and other tissues by normally-appearing neutrophils.

Key Pathways Leading to SS

Recently, SS like other neutrophilic dermatoses has been classified within the group of autoinflammatory diseases which includes genetically determined forms caused by mutations of genes regulating innate immunity [108]. It can be observed that some of them include cutaneous symptoms which are part of the spectrum of the neutrophilic dermatoses. For example, familial mediterranean fever is well known for the occurrence of acute so-called erysipelas-like erythema which are similar to SS [109].

It has been shown that interleukin-1, interleukin-2, interferon and G-CSF are significantly elevated in the serum of patients with SS [72]. All these overexpressed cytokines amplify the inflammatory response and neutrophil recruitment. Cases of SS induced by G-CSF emphazise on the major role of this cytokine in the development of the skin lesions [90, 91].

Marzano et al. have evaluated the cytokine expression profile in the lesional skin of pyoderma gangrenosum and SS and compared with healthy skin [2]. They show that interleukin-1 beta and its receptor, interleukin-8, interleukin-17, tumor necrosis factor, the chemokines CXCL1/2/3, CXCL16 and metalloproteinases 2 and 9 are significantly overexpressed in lesional skin compared with normal skin. They also show that these cytokines and chemokines are differentially expressed in SS and pyoderma gangrenosum, which might explain the differences in tissue inflammation, destruction and clinico-pathological features.

Role of the Myeloid Lineage Leukocytes in the Immunopathogenesis

Genetic studies are essential to classify myeloid malignancies that are observed in about 20% of cases of SS. It can be hypothezised that neutrophils in the dermal infiltrate are clonally related to the underlying myeloid malignancy. The same chromosomal abnormality (20q deletion) has been identified by flow cytometry both in the skin infiltrate and in the bone marrow cells in a patient with myelodysplastic syndrome and SS [110]. A study analyzing the cytogenetic anomalies in skin-infiltrating neutrophils and in the bone marrow using fluorescent in situ hybridization revealed that in most cases, skin-infiltrating neutrophils in the context of acute lyeloid leukemia or myelodysplastic syndrome differenciate from the malignant clone [3]. Another recent study in histiocytoid SS also shows the same cytogenetic abnormality in the skin and the bone marrow in patients with hematological malignancies [4]. These clonal neutrophils showing an aberrant phenotype which promotes dermal invasion can be mature, resulting from a probable maturation and differenciation of myeloblasts, or immature in cases of histiocytoid SS, that we proposed to consider as a myelodysplasia cutis [66]. Some unknown mediators of a systemic inflammatory response could exert an influence on the maturation of myeloid cells released from the bone marrow and lead to a mature or immature tissue reaction.

Treatment

The choice of treatment depends on the severity of the dermatosis, coexistence of an associated disease and past history of the patient. A treatment algorithm for SS is indicated in Fig. 3.8. Without therapeutic intervention, SS lesions persist for weeks

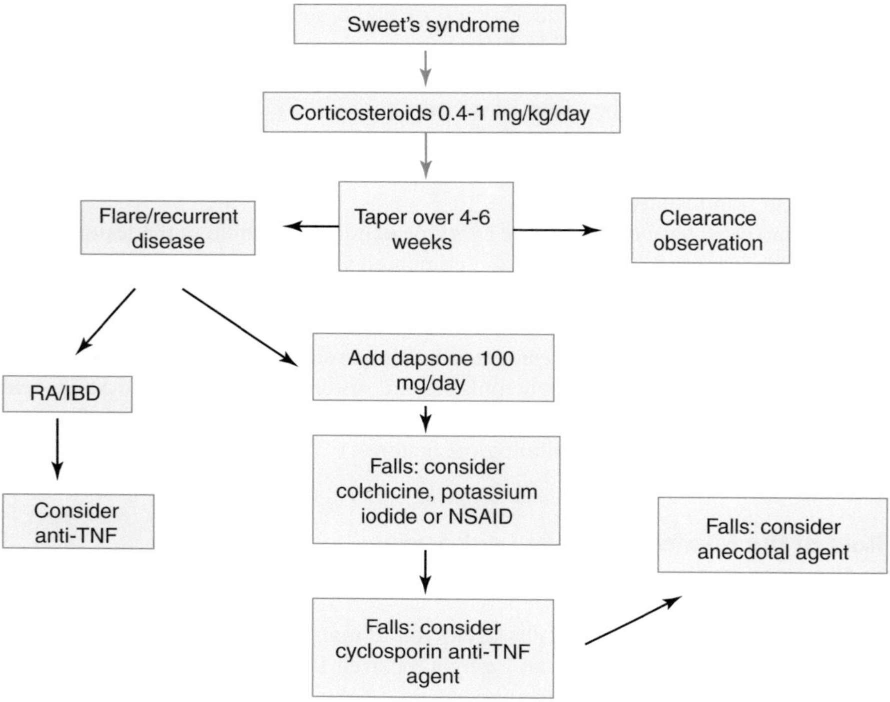

Fig. 3.8 Treatment algorithm for Sweet's syndrome [111]. *Anti-TNF* tumor necrosis factor-alpha antagonists, *IBD* inflammatory bowel disease, *NSAID* nonsteroidal anti-inflammatory drug, *RA* rheumatoid arthritis

or even several months. However, symptoms may eventually resolve spontaneously especially in the classic form of the dermatosis. Moreover improvement and clearing of the dermatosis in patients with malignancy-associated SS or drug-induced SS may occur following successful treatment of the underlying cancer or discontinuation of the causative medication [67].

First-Line Therapy

Corticosteroids. Systemic corticosteroids are first-line treatment for SS. A dose of 0.5–1 mg/kg/day usually achieves a rapid response in days to weeks and can be tapered over 4–6 weeks. In some patients, in order to suppress recurrences, daily or alternate-day treatment at lower prednisone doses of 10–30 mg may be necessary for 2 or 3 months [9, 111]. In patients with refractory disease, successful management of SS occurs after daily pulse intravenous administration of methylprednisolone for three to five consecutive days [112].

Localized SS lesions may be treated with topical high-potency corticosteroids. Alternatively, intralesional corticosteroids can be used.

Second-Line Therapy

Dapsone. Dapsone inhibits neutrophil myeloperoxydase and chemotaxis and has demonstrated some efficacy in the treatment of neutrophilic dermatoses. A small number of cases have shown efficacy as either monotherapy or as steroid-sparing agent at doses of 75–100 mg/day [113].

Colchicine. Colchicine decreases neutrophil chemotaxis, adhesion and degranulation. Some retrospective studies show its efficacy at doses of 1–1.5 mg/day, as monotherapy or in combination with potassium iodide or prednisone [114]. None of these studies have demonstrated a clear steroid-sparing effect.

Potassium iodide. Potassium iodide appears to have a similar mechanism of action as dapsone in interfering with neutrophil chemotaxis and function. Several small series and case reports have demonstrated efficacy both as monotherapy and a steroid-sparing agent at a dosage of 900 mg/day [115].

Nonsteroidal anti-inflammatory medications. They are thought to impair neutrophil function and a small number of case reports have demonstrated efficacy as monotherapy in SS. The largest study was an open trial of 18 patients treated with indomethacin 150 mg/day for 1 week. Seventeen patients responded without relapse [116]. Other case reports have shown efficacy with naproxen 750 mg/day.

Tumor necrosis factor (TNF)-alpha antagonists. Anti-TNF agents have demonstrated efficacy in a small number of case reports and most patients have an underlying inflammatory condition. Etanercept, infliximab have induced remission in patients with SS associated with rheumatoid arthritis, Crohn's disease or myelodysplastic syndromes [117]. Anti-TNF agents may be considered if patients have underlying arthritis or inflammatory bowell disease.

Cyclosporin. Multiple individual case reports have shown success with cyclosporin, in some as a steroid-sparing agent at doses ranging from 2 to 10 mg/kg/day in the treatment of SS [118].

Third-Line Therapy

Several new treatments have been proposed as a therapeutic option for SS. Intravenous immunoglobulin in conjonction with standard treatment may provide a possible therapeutic role [119]. Anakinra, an anti-interleukin-1 receptor antagonist have shown promising results in the treatment of refractory SS [120]. Isolated reports and small studies have also described other effective drugs to treat SS: chlorambucil, cyclophosphamide, danazol, etretinate, interferon alpha and thalidomide [121].

Conclusion

SS, initially described by Robert Douglas Sweet 52 years ago as an acute febrile neutrophilic dermatosis, remains a fascinating dermatological condition with regards to clinical manifestations, investigation and treatment. For the possibility of extracutaneous manifestations and the frequency of associated diseases, SS belongs to internal medecine and requires an experienced evaluation. Although the pathogenesis of SS remains to be definitively established, the role of interleukin-1 ans tumor necrosis factor alpha cytokines supports its classification as an autoinflammatory disease.

References

1. Sweet RD. An acute febrile neutrophilic dermatosis. Br J Dermatol. 1964;76:349–56.
2. Marzano AV, Fanoni D, Antiga E, Quaglino P, Caproni M, Crosti C, Meroni PL, Cugno M. Expression of cytokines, chemokines and other effector molecules in two prototypic autoinflammatory skin diseases, pyoderma gangrenosum and Sweet's syndrome. Clin Exp Immunol. 2014;178:48–56.
3. Sujobert P, Cuccuini W, Vignon-Pennamen D, Martin-Garcia N, Albertini AF, Uzunov M, Redjoul R, Dombret H, Raffoux E. Evidence of differenciation in myeloid malignancies associated neutrophilic dermatosis: a fluorescent in situ hybridization study of 14 patients. J Invest Dermatol. 2013;133:1111–4.
4. Chavan RN, Cappel MA, Ketterling RP, Wada DA, Rochet NM, Knudson R, Gibson LE. Histiocytoid Sweet syndrome may indicate leukemia cutis: a novel application of fluorescent in situ hybridization. J Am Acad Dermatol. 2014;70:1021–7.
5. Cohen PR, Talpaz M, Kurzrock R. Malignancy-associated Sweet's syndrome: review of the world literature. J Clin Oncol. 1988;6:1887–97.
6. Cohen PR, Kurzrock R. Sweet's syndrome and cancer. Clin Dermatol. 1993;11:149–57.
7. von den Driesch P. Sweet's syndrome (acute febrile neutrophilic dermatosis). J Am Acad Dermatol. 1994;31:535–56.
8. Cohen PR, Kurzrock R. Sweet's syndrome: a neutrophilic dermatosis classically associated with acute onset and fever. Clin Dermatol. 2000;18:265–82.
9. Cohen PR, Kurzrock R. Sweet's syndrome revisited: a review of disease concepts. Int J Dermatol. 2003;42:761–78.
10. Wallach D, Vignon-Pennamen MD. Pyoderma gangrenosum and Sweet syndrome: the prototypic neutrophilic dermatoses. Br J Dermatol. 2015. https://doi.org/10.1111/bjd.13955.
11. Costello MJ, Canizares O, Montague M, Buncke CM. Cutaneous manifestations of myelogenous leukemia. Arch Dermatol. 1955;71:605–14.
12. Matta M, Malak J, Tabet E, Kurban AK. Sweet's syndrome: systemic associations. Cutis. 1973;12:561–5.
13. Kemmett D, Hunter JA. Sweet's syndrome: a clinicopathologic review of twenty-nine cases. J Am Acad Dermatol. 1990;23:503–7.
14. Hommel L, Harms M, Saurat JH. The incidence of Sweet's syndrome in Geneva. Dermatology. 1993;187:303–5.
15. Sitjas D, Puig L, Cuatrecasas M, De Moragas JM. Acute febrile neutrophilic dermatosis (Sweet's syndrome). Int J Dermatol. 1993;32:261–8.
16. Chan HL, Lee YS, Kuo TT. Sweet's syndrome: clinicopathologic study of eleven cases. Int J Dermatol. 1994;33:425–32.
17. Fett DL, Gibson LE, Su WPD. Sweet's syndrome: systemic signs and symptoms and associated disorders. Mayo Clin Proc. 1995;70:234–40.
18. Bourke JF, Keohane S, Long CC, Kemmett D, Davies M, Zaki I, Graham-Brown RA. Sweet's syndrome and malignancy in the U.K. Br J Dermatol. 1997;137:609–13.
19. Cho KH, Han KH, Kim SW, Youn SW, Youn JI, Kim BK. Neutrophilic dermatoses associated with myeloid malignancy. Clin Exp Dermatol. 1997;22:269–73.
20. Neoh CY, Tan AW, Ng SK. Sweet's syndrome: a spectrum of unusual clinical presentations and associations. Br J Dermatol. 2007;156:480–5.
21. Borges da Costa J, Silva R, Soares de Almeda L, Filipe P, Marques Gomes M. Sweet's syndrome: a retrospective study of 42 admitted patients in a Portuguese hospital. Int J Dermatol. 2009;48:953–5.

22. Abbas O, Kibbi AG, Rubeiz N. Sweet's syndrome: retrospective study of clinical and histologic features of 44 cases from a tertiary care center. Int J Dermatol. 2010;49:1244–9.
23. Wojcik AS, Nishimori FS, Santamaria JR. Sweet's syndrome: a study of 23 cases. An Bras Dermatol. 2011;86:265–71.
24. Rochet NM, Chavan RN, Cappel MA, Wada DA, Gibson LE. Sweet syndrome: clinical presentation, associations and response to treatment in 77 patients. J Am Acad Dermatol. 2013;69:557–64.
25. Uilhein LC, Brandling-Bennett HA, Lio PA, Liang MG. Sweet syndrome in children. Pediatr Dermatol. 2012;29:38–44.
26. Demitsu T, Tadaki T. Atypical neutrophilic dermatosis on the upper extremitiy affected by postmastectomy lymphedema: report of 2 cases. Dermatologica. 1991;183:230–3.
27. Minocha R, Sebaratnam DF, Choi JY. Sweet's syndrome following surgery: cutaneous trauma as a possible aetiological co-factor in neutrophilic dermatoses. Australas J Dermatol. 2015;56:e74–6.
28. Caughman W, Stern R, Haynes H. Neutrophilic dermatosis of myeloproliferative disorders. Atypical forms of pyoderma gangrenosum and Sweet's syndrome associated with myeloproloferative disorders. J Am Acad Dermatol. 1983;9:751–8.
29. Cooper PH, Innes DJ, Greer KE. Acute febrile neutrophilic dermatosis (Sweet's syndrome) and myeloproliferative disorders. Cancer. 1983;51:1518–26.
30. Strutton G, Weedon D, Robertson I. Pustular vasculitis of the hands. J Am Acad Dermatol. 1995;32:192–8.
31. Galaria NA, Junkins-Hopkins JM, Kligman D, James WD. Neutrophilic dermatosis of the dorsal hands: pustular vasculitis revisited. J Am Acad Dermatol. 2000;43:870–4.
32. DiCaudo DJ, Connolly SM. Neutrophilic dermatosis (pustular vasculitis) of the dorsal hands. A report of 7 cases and review of the literature. Arch Dermatol. 2002;138:361–5.
33. Cohen PR. Skin lesions of Sweet syndrome and its dorsal hand variant contain vasculitis. An oxymoron or an epiphenomenon? Arch Dermatol. 2002;138:400–3.
34. Sarkany RP, Burrows NP, Grant JW, Pye RJ, Norris PG. The pustular eruption of ulcerative colitis: a variant of Sweet's syndrome? Br J Dermatol. 1998;138:365–6.
35. Yoon TY, Ahn GB, Yang TH, Shin HS. Sweet's syndrome with abscess-like lesions in a patient with acute myelogenous leukemia. J Dermatol. 2000;27:794–7.
36. Horiguchi Y, Lee SG, Matsumoto I, Arima N, Fugiino H, Ohnuma Y, Imamura S. Abscess-forming neutrophilic dermatosis: report of three cases associated with hemopathies. Dermatology. 1998;197:174–7.
37. Cohen PR. Subcutaneous Sweet's syndrome: a variant of acute febrile neutrophilic dermatosis that is included in the histopathologic differential diagnosis of neutrophilic panniculitis. J Am Acad Dermatol. 2005;52:927–8.
38. Sutra-Loubet C, Carlotti A, Guillemette J, Wallach D. Neutrophilic panniculitis. J Am Acad Dermatol. 2004;50:280–5.
39. Chan MP, Duncan LM, Nazarian RM. Subcutaneous Sweet syndrome in the setting of myeloid disorders: a case series and review of the literature. J Am Acad Dermatol. 2013;68:1006–15.
40. Chen HC, Kao WY, Chang DM, Gao HW, Lai WY, Lai JH. Neutrophilic panniculitis with myelodysplastic syndromes presenting as pustulosis: case report and review of the literature. Am J Hematol. 2004;76:61–5.
41. Dompmartin A, Troussard X, Lorier E, Jacobs F, Reman O, Leroy D, Leporrier M. Sweet syndrome associated with acute myelogenous leukemia. Atypical form simulating facial erysipelas. Int J Dermatol. 1991;30:644–7.
42. Khatri ML, Taha M. Sweet's syndrome associated with myelodysplastic syndrome presenting as periorbital cellulitis. Int J Dermatol. 2007;46:496–9.
43. Kroshinsky D, Alloo A, Rothschild B, Cummins J, Tan J, Montecino R, Hoang MP, Duncan L, Minh M, Sepehr A. Necrotizing Sweet syndrome: a new variant of neutrophilic dermatosis mimicking necrotizing fasciitis. J Am Acad Dermatol. 2012;67:945–54.
44. Surovy AM, Pelivani N, Hegyi I, Buettiker U, Beltraminelli H, Borradori L. Giant cellulitis-like Sweet syndrome, a new variant of neutrophilic dermatosis. JAMA Dermatol. 2013;149:79–83.

45. Vignon-Pennamen MD, Wallach D. Cutaneous manifestations of neutrophilic disease. Dermatologica. 1991;183:255–64.
46. Vignon-Pennamen MD. The extracutaneous involvement in the neutrophilic dermatoses. Clin Dermatol. 2000;18:339–47.
47. Ferguson PJ, Chen S, Tayeh MK, Ochoa L, Leal SM, Pelet A, Munnich A, Lyonnet S, Majeed HA, El-Shanti H. Homozygous mutations in *LIPN2* are responsible for the syndrome of chronic recurrent multifocal osteomyelitis and congenital dyserythropoietic anaemia (Majeed syndrome). J Med Genet. 2005;42:551–7.
48. Marie I, Boyer A, Heron F, Joly P, Levesque H, Thomine E, Courtois H. Focal aseptic osteitis underlying neutrophilic dermatosis. Br J Dermatol. 1998;139:744–5.
49. Gottlieb CC, Mishra A, Belliveau D, Green P, Heathcote JG. Ocular involvement in acute febrile neutrophilic dermatosis (Sweet syndrome): new cases and review of the literature. Surv Ophthalmol. 2008;53:219–26.
50. Wilson DM, John GR, Callen JP. Peripheral ulcerative keratitis-an extracutaneous neutrophilic disorder: report of a patient with rheumatoid arthritis, pustular vasculitis, pyoderma gangrenosum, and Sweet's syndrome with an excellent response to cyclosporine therapy. J Am Acad Dermatol. 1999;40:331–4.
51. Bilgin AB, Tavas P, Turkoglu EB, Ilhan HD, Toru S, Apaydin KC. An uncommon ocular manifestation of Sweet syndrome: peripheral ulcerative keratitis and nodular scleritis. Arq Bras Oftalmol. 2015;78:53–5.
52. Marie I, Levesque H, Joly P, Reumont G, Courville P, Baudrimont M, Baudion D, Cailleux N, Courtois H. Neutrophilic myositis as an extracutaneous manifestation of neutrophilic dermatosis. J Am Acad Dermatol. 2001;44:137–9.
53. Mosnier E, Rousset P, Hugol D, Bouscary D, Aslangul E. Neutrophilic myositis *sine* dermatitis in a neutropenic patient with myelodysplastic syndrome. Ann Hematol. 2013;92:551–2.
54. Astudillo L, Sailler L, Launay F, Josse AG, Lamant L, Couret B, Arlet-Suau E. Pulmonary involvement in Sweet's syndrome: a case report and review of the literature. Int J Dermatol. 2006;45:677–80.
55. Lawrence K, Hachem R, Wildes TM, Canizares M. A 54-year old man with a rash and pulmonary infiltrates. Chest. 2008;134:1340–3.
56. Shugarman IL, Schmit JM, Sbicca JA, Wirk B. Easily missed extracutaneous manifestation of malignancy-associated Sweet's syndrome: systemic inflammatory response syndrome. J Clin Oncol. 2011;29:e702–5.
57. Hisanaga K, Iwasaki Y, Ytoyama Y. Neuro-Sweet disease: clinical manifestations and criteria for diagnosis. Neurology. 2005;64:1756–61.
58. Fain O, Mathieu E, Feton N, Sibony M, Sitbon M, Lejeune F, Thomas M. Intestinal involvement in Sweet's syndrome. J Am Acad Dermatol. 1996;35:989–90.
59. Li B, Ma Z, Xu X, Yin J, Wang X, Ren J, Wang S, Yang J, Ma T, Zhang Q, Yu J, Yan B. Multiorgan involvement of Sweet's syndrome; a case report and literature review. Intern Med. 2015;54:339–43.
60. Aractingi S, Mallet V, Pinquier L, Chosidow O, Vignon-Pennamen MD, Degos L, Dubertret L, Dombret H. Neutrophilic dermatoses during granulocytopenia. Arch Dermatol. 1995;131:1141–5.
61. von den Driesch P, Weber MF. Are antibodies to neutrophilic cytoplasmic antigens (ANCA) a serologic marker for Sweet's syndrome. J Am Acad Dermatol. 1993;29:666.
62. Malone JC, Slone SP, Wills-Frank LA, Fearneyhough PK, Lear SC, Goldsmith LJ, Hood AF, Callen JP. Vascular inflammation (vasculitis) in Sweet syndrome: a clinicopathologic study of 28 biopsy specimens from 21 patients. Arch Dermatol. 2002;138:345–9.
63. Rochael MC, Pantaleao L, Vilar EA, Zacaron LH, Spada EQ, Xavier MH, Rodrigues KS. Sweet's syndrome: study of 73 cases, emphasizing histopathological findings. An Bras Dermatol. 2011;86:702–7.
64. Requena L, Kutzner H, Palmedo G, Pascual M, Fernandez-Herrera J, Fraga J, Garcia-Diez A, Yus ES. Histiocytoid Sweet syndrome: a dermal infiltration of immature neutrophilic granulocytes. Arch Dermatol. 2005;141:834–42.

65. Ghoufi L, Ortonne N, Ingen-Housz-Oro S, Barhoumi W, Begon E, Haioun C, Pautas C, Beckerich F, Robin C, Wolkenstein P, Cordonnier C, Chosidow O, Toma A. Histiocytoid Sweet syndrome is more frequently associated with myelodysplastic syndromes than the classical neutrophilic variant: a comparative series of 62 patients. Medicine. 2016;95:e3033.
66. Osio A, Battistella M, Feugeas JP, Cuccuini W, Noguera ME, Petrella T, Raffoux E, Janin A, Vignon Pennamen MD. Myelodysplasia cutis versus leukemia cutis. J Invest Dermatol. 2015;135:2321–4.
67. Thompson DF, Montarella KE. Drug-induced Sweet's syndrome. Ann Pharmacother. 2007;41:802–11.
68. Su WP, Liu HN. Diagnostic criteria for Sweet's syndrome. Cutis. 1986;37:167–74.
69. Kieffer C, Cribier B, Lipsker D. Neutrophilic urticarial dermatosis: a variant of neutrophilic urticaria strongly associated with systemic disease. Report of 9 new cases and review of the literature. Medicine. 2009;88:23–31.
70. Hau E, Vignon Pennamen MD, Battistella M, Saussine A, Bergis M, Cavelier-Balloy B, Janier M, Cordoliani F, Bagot M, Rybojad M, Bouaziz JD. Neutrophilic skin lesions in autoimmune connective tissue diseases: nine cases and a literature review. Medicine. 2014;93:e346.
71. Karadogan SK, Baskan EB, Alkan G, Saricaoglu H, Tunali S. Generalized Sweet syndrome lesions associated with Behçet disease: a true association or simply co-morbidity? Am J Clin Dermatol. 2009;10:331–5.
72. Kawakami T, Ohashi S, Kawa Y, Takahama H, Ito M, Soma Y, Mizoguchi M. Elevated serum granulocyte colony-stimulating factor levels in patients with active phase of Sweet syndrome and patients with active Behçet disease: implication in neutrophil apoptosis dysfunction. Arch Dermatol. 2004;140:570–4.
73. Waltz KM, Long D, Marks JG, Billingsley EM. Sweet's syndrome and erythema nodosum. The simultaneous occurrence of 2 reactive dermatoses. Arch Dermatol. 1999;135:62–6.
74. Burton JL. Sweet's syndrome, pyoderma gangrenosum and acute leukemia. Br J Dermatol. 1980;102:239.
75. Salmon P, Rademaker M, Edwards L. A continuum of neutrophilic disease occurring in a patient with ulcerative colitis. Australas J Dermatol. 1998;39:116–8.
76. Castro-Fernandez M, Sanchez-Munoz D, Ruiz-Granados E, Merchante N, Corzo J. Coexistence of pyoderma gangrenosum and Sweet's syndrome in a patient with ulcerative colitis. Am J Gastroenterol. 2007;102:2865–6.
77. Wallach D. Les dermatoses neutrophiliques. Presse Med. 1991;20:105–7.
78. Wallach D, Vignon Pennamen MD. From acute febrile neutrophilic dermatosis to neutrophilic disease: forty years of clinical research. J Am Acad Dermatol. 2006;55:1066–71.
79. Scerri L, Zaki I, Allen BR. Pyoderma gangrenosum and subcorneal pustular dermatosis without monoclonal gammopathy. Br J Dermatol. 1994;130:398–9.
80. Caucanas M, Heylen A, Rolland F, Müller G, Olemans C, Sass U, Vanhooteghem O. Associated pyoderma gangrenosum, erythema elevatum diutinum, and Sweet's syndrome: the concept of neutrophilic disease. Int J Dermatol. 2013;52:1185–8.
81. Wang T, Liu H, Wang L, Guo Z, Li L. An unusual case of Sweet syndrome in a child: overlapping presentation with erythema elevatum diutinum. Am J Dermatopathol. 2014;36:e114–6.
82. Cohen PR. Neutrophilic dermatoses occurring in oncology patients. Int J Dermatol. 2007;46:106–11.
83. Buck T, Gonzalez LM, Lambert WC, Schwartz RA. Sweet's syndrome with hematologic disorders: a review and reappraisal. Int J Dermatol. 2008;47:775–82.
84. Kulasekararaj AG, Kordasti S, Basu T, Salisbury JR, Mufti GJ, du Vivier AW. Chronic relapsing remitting Sweet syndrome—a harbinger of myelodysplastic syndrome. Br J Haematol. 2015;170:649–56.
85. Kazmi SM, Pemmaraju N, Patel KP, Cohen PR, Daver N, Tran KM, Ravandi F, Duvic M, Garcia-Manero G, Pierce S, Nazha A, Borthakur G, Kantarjian H, Cortes J. Characteristics of Sweet syndrome in patients with acute myeloid leukemia. Clin Lymphoma Myeloma Leuk. 2015;15:358–63.

86. Vignon Pennamen MD, Juillard C, Rybojad M, Wallach D, Daniel MT, Morel P, Verola O, Janin A. Chronic recurrent lymphocytic Sweet syndrome as a predictive marker of myelodysplasia. Arch Dermatol. 2006;142:1170–6.
87. Vignon Pennamen MD, Aractingi S. Sweet's syndrome and leukemia cutis: a common skin homing mechanism? Dermatology. 2003;206:81–4.
88. Lee SJ, Park JK, Lee EY, Joo SH, Jung KC, Lee EB, Song YW, Yoon SS. Certain autoimmune manifestations are associated with distinctive karyotypes and outcomes in patients with myelodysplastic syndrome. A retrospective cohort study. Medicine. 2016;95:e3091.
89. Walker DC, Cohen PR. Trimethoprim-sulfamethoxazole-associated acute febrile neutrophilic dermatosis: case report and review of drug-induced Sweet's syndrome. J Am Acad Dermatol. 1996;34:918–23.
90. Arbetter KR, Hubbard KW, Markovic SN, Gibson LE, Phyliky RL. Case of granulocyte colony-stimulating factor-induced Sweet's syndrome. Am J Hematol. 1999;61:126–9.
91. Draper BK, Robbins JB, Stricklin GP. Bullous Sweet's syndrome in congenital neutropenia: association with pegfilgrastim. J Am Acad Dermatol. 2005;52:901–5.
92. Al-Saad K, Khanani MF, Naqvi A, Krafchik B, Grant R, Pappo A. Sweet syndrome developing during treatment with all-*trans* retinoic acid in a child with acute myelogenous leukemia. J Pediatr Hematol Oncol. 2004;26:197–9.
93. Varadarajan N, Boni A, Elder DE, Bagg A, Micheletti R, Perl AE, Rosenbach M. *FLT3* inhibitor-associated neutrophilic dermatoses. JAMA Dermatol. 2016;152:480–2.
94. Jovanovic M, Poljacki M, Vujanovic L, Duran V. Acute febrile neutrophilic dermatosis (Sweet's syndrome) after influenza vaccination. J Am Acad Dermatol. 2005;52:367–8.
95. Gunawardena DA, Gunawardena KA, Ratnayaka RM, Vasanthanathan NS. The clinical spectrum of Sweet's syndrome (acute febrile neutrophilic dermatosis). A report of eighteen cases. Br J Dermatol. 1975;92:363–73.
96. Kalai C, Brand R, Yu L. Minocycline-induced Sweet's syndrome (acute febrile neutrophilic dermatosis). J Am Acad Dermatol. 2012;67:e289–91.
97. Tintle S, Patel V, Ruskin A, Halasz C. Azacitidine: a new medication associated with Sweet syndrome. J Am Acad Dermatol. 2011;64:e77–9.
98. Murase JE, Wu JJ, Theate I, Cole GW, Barr RJ, Dyson SW. Bortezomid-induced histiocytoid Sweet syndrome. J Am Acad Dermatol. 2009;60:496–7.
99. Ayirookuzhi SJ, Ma L, Ramshesh P, Mills G. Imatinib-induced Sweet syndrome in a patient with chronic myeloid leukemia. Arch Dermatol. 2005;141:368–70.
100. Gormley R, Wanat K, Elenitsas R, Giles J, McGettigan S, Schuchter L, Takeshita J. Ipilimumab-associated Sweet syndrome in a melanoma patient. J Am Acad Dermatol. 2014;71:e211–3.
101. Azfar RS, Cohn J, Schaffer A, Kim EJ. Trimethoprim-sulfamethoxazole-induced Sweet syndrome. Arch Dermatol. 2009;145:215–6.
102. Banse C, Sobocinski V, Savoye G, Avenel G, Vittecoq O. Occurrence of Sweet syndrome under anti TNF. Clin Rheumatol. 2015;34:1993–4.
103. Thieu KP, Rosenbach M, Xu X, Kist JM. Neutrophilic dermatosis complicating lenalidomide therapy. J Am Acad Dermatol. 2009;61:709–10.
104. Bidinger JJ, Sky K, Battafarano DF, Henning JS. The cutaneous and systemic manifestations of azathioprine hypersensibility syndrome. J Am Acad Dermatol. 2011;65:184–91.
105. Cyrus N, Stavert R, Mason AR, Ko CJ, Choi JN. Neutrophilic dermatosis after azathioprine exposure. JAMA Dermatol. 2013;149:592–7.
106. Marzano AV, Ishak RS, Saibeni S, Crosti C, Meroni PL, Cugno M. Autoinflammatory skin disorders in inflammatory bowel diseases, pyoderma gangrenosum and Sweet's syndrome: a comprehensive review and disease classification criteria. Clin Rev Allergy Immunol. 2013;45:202–10.
107. Anzalone CL, Cohen PR. Acute febrile neutrophilic dermatosis (Sweet's syndrome). Curr Opin Hematol. 2013;20:26–35.
108. Braun-Falco M, Ruzicka T. Skin manifestations in autoinflammatory syndromes. J Dtsch Dermatol Ges. 2011;9:232–46.

109. Oskay T, Anadolu R. Sweet's syndrome in familial mediterranean fever: possible continuum of the neutrophilic reaction as a new cutaneous feature of FMF. J Cutan Pathol. 2009;36:901–5.
110. Van Loon K, Gill RM, McMahon P, Chigurupati R, Siddiqi I, Fox L, Damon L, McCalmont TH, Jordan R, Wolf J. 20q-clonality in a case of oral Sweet syndrome and myelodysplasia. Am J Clin Pathol. 2012;137:310–5.
111. Schadt CR, Callen JP. Management of neutrophilic dermatoses. Dermatol Ther. 2012;25:158–72.
112. Case JD, Smith SZ, Callen JP. The use of pulse methylprednisolone and chlorambucil in the treatment of Sweet's syndrome. Cutis. 1989;44:125–9.
113. Inamadar AC, Anitha B. HIV-seropositive patient with Sweet's syndrome and nodular scleritis, showing dramatic response after adding dapsone to systemic corticosteroid therapy. Int J Dermatol. 2008;47:836–8.
114. Maillard H, Leclech C, Peria P, Avenel-Audran M, Verret JL. Colchicine for Sweet's syndrome. A study of 20 cases. Br J Dermatol. 1999;140:565–6.
115. Horio T, Inamura S, Danno K, Furukawa F, Ofuji S. Treatment of acute febrile neutrophilic dermatosis (Sweet's syndrome) with potassium iodide. Dermatologica. 1980;160:341–7.
116. Jeanfils S, Joly P, Young P, Le Corvaisier-Pieto C, Thomine E, Lauret P. Indomethacin treatment of eighteen patients with Sweet's syndrome. J Am Acad Dermatol. 1997;36:436–9.
117. Yamauchi PS, Turner L, Lowe NJ, Gindi V, Jackson JM. Treatment of recurrent Sweet's syndrome with coexisting rheumatoid arthritis with the tumor necrosis factor antagonist etanercept. J Am Acad Dermatol. 2006;54:S121–2.
118. von den Driesch P, Steffan C, Zobe A, Hornstein OP. Sweet's syndrome—therapy with cyclosporin. Clin Exp Dermatol. 1994;19:274–7.
119. Gill HH, Leung AY, Trendell-Smith NJ, Yeung CK, Liang R. Sweet syndrome due to myelodysplastic syndrome: possible therapeutic role of intravenous immunoglobulin in addition to standard treatment. Adv Hematol. 2010;2010:328316.
120. Kluger N, Gil-Bistes D, Guillot B, Bessis D. Efficacy of antiinterleukin-1 receptor antagonist anakinra (Kineret) in a case of refractory Sweet's syndrome. Dermatology. 2011;222:123–7.
121. Browning CE, Dixon JE, Malone JC, Callen JP. Thalidomide in the treatment of recalcitrant Sweet's syndrome associated with myelodysplasia. J Am Acad Dermatol. 2005;53:S135–8.

Erythema Elevatum Diutinum

4

Anh N. Tran and Joseph L. Jorizzo

Introduction and History

Erythema elevatum diutinum (EED) is a rare, chronic low-grade form of cutaneous leukocytoclastic vasculitis (LCV) of unknown etiology that usually presents with a relapsing course. The entity was first described in males in 1888 by Hutchinson [1] and in females in 1889 by Bury [2]. Hutchinson described a 58-year-old man with gout and purplish plaques on his legs, dorsal hands, and forearm [1]. Bury reported a 12-year-old girl with similar skin findings who had had rheumatic fever 3 years earlier [2]. Radcliffe-Crocker and Williams named the condition in 1894, dividing these persistent erythemas into a Hutchinson type occurring in elderly males and a Bury type found in young females with a history of rheumatism [3]. This distinction, however, has since been abandoned.

Epidemiology

EED is a rare condition with about 250 cases reported to date [4]. It can occur at any age with no sex or race predilection but most commonly occurs in the fourth to sixth decade of life. It may present earlier and in a more advanced form in patients with human immunodeficiency virus (HIV) [5].

A. N. Tran (✉) • J. L. Jorizzo
Department of Dermatology, Weill Cornell Medicine, New York, NY, USA
e-mail: joj9026@med.cornell.edu

D. Wallach et al. (eds.), *Neutrophilic Dermatoses*,
https://doi.org/10.1007/978-3-319-72649-6_4

Pathogenesis

The exact pathogenesis of EED remains unclear. The favored hypothesis is an immune complex-mediated vasculitis induced by chronic antigenic exposure or excess antibody levels. It is postulated that immune complex deposition occurs in post-capillary venules often secondary to infection or hematologic or autoimmune diseases. These immune complexes then activate the complement cascade as well as cytokines such as interleukin-8, which in turn attracts neutrophils containing lysozymes, collagenases, myeloperoxidase, and acid hydrolases. Release of these enzymes induces fibrin deposition within and around small dermal vessels. Repetitive damage to blood vessels results in fibrosis and appearance of cholesterol crystals and myelin figures [6]. In support of this, typical lesions have been reproduced by the intradermal injection of streptodornase [7] and streptococcal antigen in patients with EED, suggesting EED may be a circulating immune complex-mediated (Gell and Coombs Type III) reaction to bacterial antigens [5, 8, 9]. Moreover, immunofluorescent studies have demonstrated deposits of complement, immunoglobulin (Ig)G, IgA, IgM, and fibrin around damaged vessels within EED lesions [5]. Several studies in recent years have demonstrated IgA antineutrophil cytoplasmic antibody (ANCA) positivity in patients with EED, suggesting neutrophil activation through IgA ANCA may play a role in the pathogenesis, and IgA ANCA may serve as a useful clinical marker for EED [10–13].

Associations

EED has been associated with a wide range of clinical illnesses including hematologic diseases (most frequently paraproteinemias [4, 7, 14–19] and myelodysplastic syndrome [20, 21]; less frequently IgA myeloma [14, 22], multiple myeloma [23], chronic lymphocytic leukemia [24], chronic myelogenous leukemia [21], hairy cell leukemia [25], and mixed cryoglobulinemia) [26], autoimmune diseases (most frequently rheumatoid arthritis [20, 27], inflammatory bowel disease [28, 29], relapsing polychondritis [20], and celiac disease [30, 31]; less frequently dermatitis herpetiformis [32], systemic lupus erythematosus (SLE) [33], antiphosphopholipid syndrome [34], Sjogren's syndrome [11], dermatomyositis [35], ankylosing spondylitis [36], hypothyroidism [37], granulomatosis with polyangiitis [12, 16], and microscopic polyangiitis) [12, 13], recurrent bacterial and viral infections (most frequently streptococcal [7] and HIV [38–41]; less frequently human herpes virus 6) [42], and other malignancies (non-Hodgkin's lymphoma [43], B cell lymphoma [44], breast cancer [45], and verrucous carcinoma) [18]. The association between EED and paraproteinemia, particularly IgA, is well described [15, 22]. Of note is the association between EED and HIV. In the majority of cases, EED is seen in patients with low CD4 counts, i.e., <200 cells/μL. In some cases, however, EED has been reported as the first clinical manifestation of HIV infection [41]. HIV-associated

EED is often associated with extensive and nodular lesions occurring at an earlier age, palmoplantar involvement, and nonresponsiveness to dapsone [40]. The lack of response to dapsone may reflect the preponderance of fibrosis rather than neutrophils in these advanced lesions [38].

Clinical Features

EED generally follows a chronic, benign course with relapses. Some cases spontaneously remit in 5–10 years, with the longest reported duration being 39 years [5]. Lesions are initially soft, become more indurated over time, reflecting their tendency towards fibrosis, and often leave a hypo- or hyperpigmented, atrophic surface as they regress [5, 7]. Although EED typically presents as red-violaceous or red-brown papules and nodules, vesiculobullous, ulcerative, verrucous, and annular types have also been reported (Fig. 4.1) [7, 13, 15, 17, 20, 22, 23, 26, 31, 40, 45–48]. Lesions are commonly symmetrically distributed over the extensor surfaces of joints including the hands, feet, elbows, and knees. Other common locations include the ears, buttocks, and Achilles tendon [7, 15]. Unilateral presentations [27] and atypical sites including palmar, plantar, truncal, and genital lesions are also possible [17, 19, 43, 44, 49]. Lesions are generally asymptomatic,

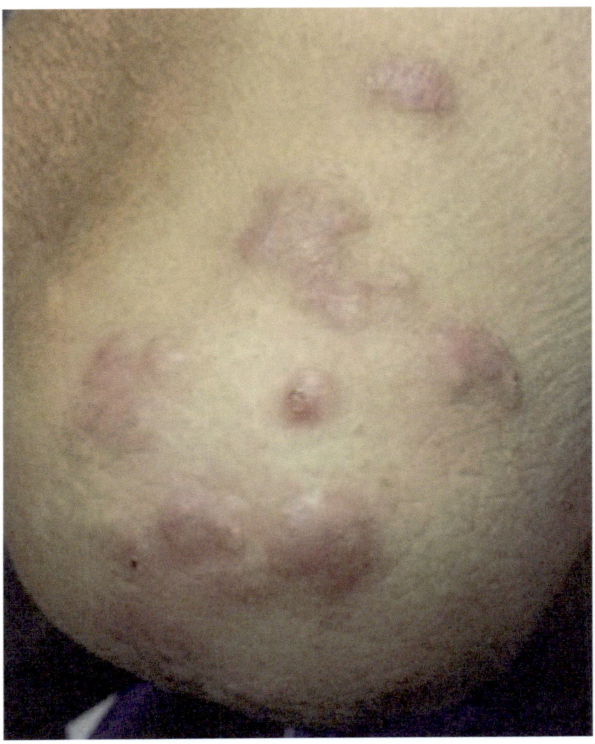

Fig. 4.1 Lesions of erythema elevatum diutinum located over the right elbow. Omar Sangueza, MD, Professor of Pathology and Dermatology, Wake Forest University School of Medicine

but some patients may complain of pruritus, burning, or pain [5–7, 23, 28, 41]. There are several reports of EED exacerbated by the cold or menses [5, 7, 26]. Systemic complications are rare, as these patients are not prone to develop systemic vasculitis. Constitutional symptoms including fever and malaise, however, are common and can be severe [6, 40]. Joint pain is the most common associated symptom [6, 18, 22, 26, 31], although there are isolated reports of ocular involvement such as peripheral ulcerative keratitis, episcleritis, nodular scleritis, and panuveitis [50].

Histopathology

Acute lesions of EED display a LCV with neutrophilic, perivascular infiltrates, fibrin deposition within and around vessel walls, endothelial expansion, and leukocytoclasis in the superficial and mid-dermis (Fig. 4.2). The overlying epidermis may be acanthotic, atrophic, or ulcerated. As the process continues, histiocytes make up a larger proportion of the infiltrate. Chronic lesions exhibit dermal fibrosis, histiocytic infiltration, lipid deposition, and vascular prominence. One of the most distinctive features is the appearance of progressive concentric perivascular fibrosis [20, 38]. Ultrastructural studies have shown that the majority of the lipid collections are intracellular within histiocytes and, to a lesser degree, within keratinocytes, mast cells, and lymphocytes, as opposed to the older nomenclature, which refers to EED as 'extracellular cholesterosis' [47].

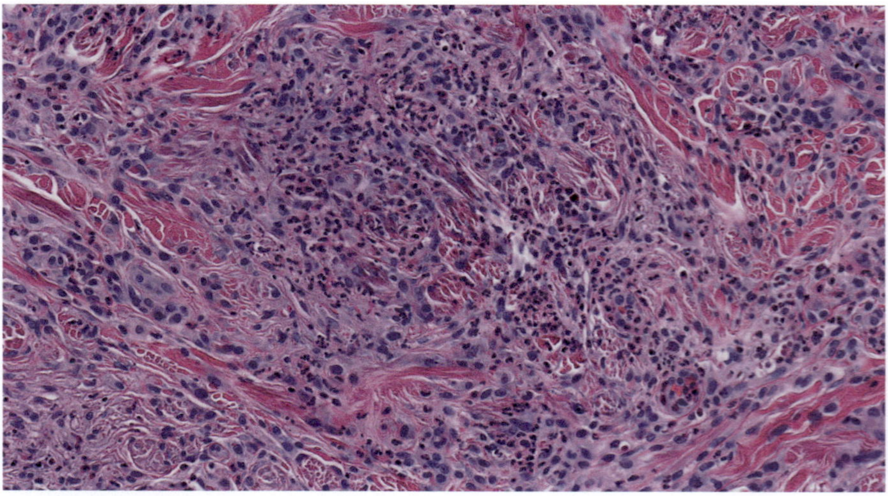

Fig. 4.2 Histology of erythema elevatum diutinum lesions with hematoxylin and eosin stain. Omar Sangueza, MD, Professor of Pathology and Dermatology, Wake Forest University School of Medicine

Diagnosis

The diagnosis of EED is established based on the characteristic clinical features and confirmatory histopathologic findings. An accurate diagnosis is important, as this can prompt the search for associated conditions that may require monitoring or treatment. In addition to a detailed systemic inquiry, serological testing including a complete blood count, electrolytes, screening for infections including HIV and streptococcal, and serum protein electrophoresis are essential. IgA ANCA may be a clinical marker of the disease. Additional testing may be appropriate in the right clinical context including a rheumatologic workup or systemic evaluation for gluten-sensitive enteropathy [51].

Differential Diagnosis

The clinical differential diagnosis of EED may include granuloma annulare, sarcoidosis, pseudolymphoma and multicentric reticulohistiocytosis. Although neutrophilic dermatoses (such as Sweet's syndrome and neutrophilic rheumatoid dermatitis) and fibrous proliferations (such as dermatofibroma and dermatofibrosarcoma protuberans) share histologic similarities with EED, the foci of LCV help to distinguish EED. At the same time, EED differs from ordinary cutaneous LCV, as individual lesions of LCV usually resolve without cutaneous sequelae while in patients with EED, acute inflammatory lesions are followed by formation of fibrous nodules. The chronic and recurrent nature of EED helps distinguish it from other entities with a similar clinical and histologic appearance.

Treatment

EED is notoriously resistant to treatment. Any number of agents and modalities have been used without consistent success. For patients with an underlying condition, treatment of these conditions has been shown to improve EED [30, 31, 43]. Otherwise, dapsone is used as the mainstay of treatment. It is thought to interfere with complement deposition within vessel walls as well as to inhibit neutrophil chemotaxis and myeloperoxidase and lysosomal activity, thereby breaking the cycle of continuing vascular damage [52]. A rapid response can be seen within 48 hours and near complete resolution has been achieved in weeks to months. A suppressive but not curative response to dapsone therapy has been reported in some but not all patients [4–8, 17, 21, 26, 28, 32, 40, 41, 44, 47, 48, 50, 53]. Advanced stage of the disease with the presence of marked fibrosis appears to be associated with lack of response to dapsone [23]. Other treatments suggested by case reports include sulfapyridine [7, 14], chloroquine [54], colchicine [36, 55], tetracycline [4, 46], niacinamide [46], cyclosporine [48], topical [40] and systemic corticosteroids [8, 21, 35, 45, 49], and surgical excision [19, 23, 53].

Marginal improvement has been observed with intralesional corticosteroids [53]. Intermittent plasma exchange in an EED patient with IgA paraproteinemia has been reported to be effective [22].

Acknowledgements We thank Omar Sangueza, MD, Professor of Pathology and Dermatology, Wake Forest University School of Medicine for photographs and histology.

References

1. Hutchinson J. On two remarkable cases of symmetrical purple congestion of the skin in patches, with induration. Br J Dermatol. 1888;1:10–5.
2. Bury JS. A case of erythema with remarkable nodular thickening and induration of the skin associated with intermittent albuminuria. Illus Med News. 1889;3:145.
3. Radcliffe-Crocker H, Williams C. Erythema elevatum diutinum. Br J Dermatol. 1894;6:1–9.
4. Patnala GP, Sunandini AP, Rayavarapu R, Yandapalli PS. Erythema elevatum diutinum in association with IgA monoclonal gammopathy: a rare case report. Indian Dermatol Online J. 2016;7(4):300–3. https://doi.org/10.4103/2229-5178.185472.
5. Wilkinson SM, English JS, Smith NP, Wilson-Jones E, Winkleman RK. Erythema elevatum diutinum: a clinicopathological study. Clin Exp Dermatol. 1992;17:87–93.
6. Grabbe J, Haas N, Möller A, Henz BM. Erythema elevatum diutinum—evidence for disease-dependent leucocyte alterations and response to dapsone. Br J Dermatol. 2000;14:415–20.
7. Katz SI, Gallin JI, Hertz KC, Fauci AS, Lawley TJ. Erythema elevatum diutinum: skin and systemic manifestations, immunologic studies, and successful treatment with dapsone. Medicine (Baltimore). 1977;56:443–55.
8. Cream JJ, Leven GM, Calnan CD. Erythema elevatum diutinum: an unusual reaction to streptococcal antigen and response to dapsone. Br J Dermatol. 1971;84:393–9.
9. Wolff HH, Scherer R, Maciejewski W, Braun-Falco O. Erythema elevatum diutinum. II. Immunoelectronmicroscopical study of leukocytoclastic vasculitis within the intracutaneous test reaction induced by streptococcal antigen. Arch Dermatol Res. 1978;261: 17–26.
10. Ayoub N, Charuel JL, Diemert MC, Barete S, André M, Fermand JP, et al. Antineutrophil cytoplasmic antibodies of IgA class in neutrophilic dermatoses with emphasis on erythema elevatum diutinum. Arch Dermatol. 2004;140:931–6.
11. Shimizu S, Nakamura Y, Togawa Y, Kamada N, Kambe N, Matsue H. Erythema elevatum diutinum with primary Sjögren syndrome associated with IgA antineutrophil cytoplasmic antibody. Br J Dermatol. 2008;159(3):733–5. https://doi.org/10.1111/j.1365-2133.2008.08676.
12. de Boysson H, Martin Silva N, de Moreuil C, Néel A, de Menthon M, Meyer O, et al. Neutrophilic dermatoses in antineutrophil cytoplasmic antibody-associated vasculitis: a French multicenter study of 17 cases and literature review. Medicine (Baltimore). 2016;95:e2957. https://doi.org/10.1097/MD.0000000000002957.
13. Adachi A, Komine M, Murata S, Tsuda H, Kawahara Y, Morimoto A, et al. Pediatric case of microscopic polyangiitis with skin manifestations resembling vesiculobullous type erythema elevatum diutinum with immunoglobulin A antineutrophil cytoplasmic antibody. J Dermatol. 2016;43(11):1377–8. https://doi.org/10.1111/1346-8138.13394.
14. Kövary PM, Dhonau H, Happle R. Paraproteinaemia in erythema elevatum diutinum. Arch Dermatol Res. 1977;260:155–8.
15. Yiannias JA, el-Azhary RA, Gibson LE. Erythema elevatum diutinum: a clinical and histopathologic study of 13 patients. J Am Acad Dermatol. 1992;26:38–44.
16. Kavanagh GM, Colaco CB, Bradfield JW, Archer CB. Erythema elevatum diutinum associated with Wegener's granulomatosis and IgA paraproteinemia. J Am Acad Dermatol. 1993;28:846–9.

17. Barzegar M, Davatchi CC, Akhyani M, Nikoo A, Daneshpazhooh M, Farsinejad K. An atypical presentation of erythema elevatum diutinum involving palms and soles. Int J Dermatol. 2009;48:73–5. https://doi.org/10.1111/j.1365-4632.2009.03867.
18. Nair SR, Viswanath V, Sonavane AD, Doshi AC, Parab MG, Torsekar RG. Erythema elevatum diutinum with verrucous carcinoma: a rare association. Indian J Dermatol Venereol Leprol. 2010;76:420–2. https://doi.org/10.4103/0378-6323.66595.
19. Thomas CL, Ffolkes L, Akhras V. A case of mistaken identity: unilateral erythema elevatum diutinum associated with IgA paraproteinaemia. Clin Exp Dermatol. 2015;40:761–4. https://doi.org/10.1111/ced.12622.
20. Wahl CE, Bouldin MB, Gibson LE. Erythema elevatum diutinum: clinical, histopathologic, and immunohistochemical characteristics of six patients. Am J Dermatopathol. 2005;27:397–400.
21. Atallah J, Garces JC, Loayza E, Carlson JA. Chronic localized fibrosing leukocytoclastic vasculitis associated with lymphedema, intralymphatic and intravascular lymphocytosis, and chronic myelogenous leukemia: a case report of unilateral erythema elevatum diutinum. Am J Dermatopathol. 2017;39(6):479–84.
22. Chow RK, Benny WB, Coupe RL, Dodd WA, Ongley RC. Erythema elevatum diutinum associated with IgA paraproteinemia successfully controlled with intermittent plasma exchange. Arch Dermatol. 1996;132:1360–4.
23. Soubeiran E, Wacker J, Hausser I, Hartschuh W. Erythema elevatum diutinum with unusual clinical appearance. J Dtsch Dermatol Ges. 2008;6:303–5. https://doi.org/10.1111/j.1610-0387.2008.06589.
24. Delaporte E, Alfandari S, Fenaux P, Piette F, Bergoend H. Erythema elevatum diutinum and chronic lymphocytic leukemia. Clin Exp Dermatol. 1994;19:188.
25. Dorsey JK, Penick GD. The association of hairy cell leukemia with unusual immunologic disorders. Arch Intern Med. 1982;142:902–3.
26. Morrison JG, Hull PR, Fourie E. Erythema elevatum diutinum, cryoglobulinaemia, and fixed urticaria on cooling. Br J Dermatol. 1977;97:99–104.
27. Collier PM, Neill SM, Branfoot AC, Staughton RC. Erythema elevatum diutinum—a solitary lesion in a patient with rheumatoid arthritis. Clin Exp Dermatol. 1990;15:394–5.
28. Walker KD, Badame AJ. Erythema elevatum diutinum in a patient with Crohn's disease. J Am Acad Dermatol. 1990;22:948–52.
29. Buahene K, Hudson M, Mowat A, Smart L, Ormerod AD. Erythema elevatum diutinum—an unusual association with ulcerative colitis. Clin Exp Dermatol. 1991;16:204–6.
30. Rodriguez-Serna M, Fortea JM, Perez A, Febrer I, Ribes C, Aliaga A. Erythema elevatum diutinum associated with celiac disease: response to a gluten-free diet. Pediatr Dermatol. 1993;10:125–8.
31. Tasanen K, Raudasoja R, Kallioinen M, Ranki A. Erythema elevatum diutinum in association with coeliac disease. Br J Dermatol. 1997;136:624–7.
32. Chandrasekaran SS, Rai R, Vedachalam S, Dorairaj L, Palaniraman S. Erythema elevatum diutinum in association with dermatitis herpetiformis. Indian Dermatol Online J. 2014;5:48–50. https://doi.org/10.4103/2229-5178.126032.
33. Bouaziz JD, Barete S, Le Pelletier F, Amoura Z, Piette JC, Francès C. Cutaneous lesions of the digits in systemic lupus erythematosus: 50 cases. Lupus. 2007;16:163–7.
34. Yamamoto T, Nakamura S, Nishioka K. Erythema elevatum diutinum associated with Hashimoto's thyroiditis and antiphospholipid antibodies. J Am Acad Dermatol. 2005;52:165–6.
35. Marie I, Courville P, Levesque H. Erythema elevatum diutinum associated with dermatomyositis. J Am Acad Dermatol. 2011;64:1000–1. https://doi.org/10.1016/j.jaad.2009.08.037.
36. Yıldız F, Karakaş T, Açıkalın A, Taş DA, Erken E. Erythema elevatum diutinum coexisting with ankylosing spondylitis. Eur J Rheumatol. 2015;2:73–5.
37. Cirvidiu DC, Elias BL, Jorge JC, Lira ML, Mandelbaum SH. Erythema elevatum diutinum and hypothyroidism: coincidence or causal relationship? An Bras Dermatol. 2015;90:561–3. https://doi.org/10.1590/abd1806-4841.20153284.
38. LeBoit PE, Cockerell CJ. Nodular lesions of erythema elevatum diutinum in patients infected with the human immunodeficiency virus. J Am Acad Dermatol. 1993;28:919–22.

39. Shanks JH, Banerjee SS, Bishop PW, Pearson JM, Eyden BP. Nodular erythema elevatum diutinum mimicking cutaneous neoplasms. Histopathology. 1997;31:91–6.
40. Smitha P, Sathish P, Mohan K, Sripathi H, Sachi G. A case of extensive erosive and bullous erythema elevatum diutinum in a patient diagnosed with human immunodeficiency virus (HIV). Int J Dermatol. 2011;50:989–91. https://doi.org/10.1111/j.1365-4632.2010.04616.
41. Jose SK, Marfatia YS. Erythema elevatum diutinum in acquired immune deficiency syndrome: can it be an immune reconstitution inflammatory syndrome? Indian J Sex Transm Dis. 2016;37:81–4. https://doi.org/10.4103/0253-7184.180287.
42. Drago F, Semino M, Rampini P, Lugani C, Rebora A. Erythema elevatum diutinum in a patient with human herpesvirus 6 infection. Acta Derm Venereol. 1999;79:91–2.
43. Hatzitolios A, Tzellos TG, Savopoulos C, Tzalokostas V, Kaiafa G, Psomas E, et al. Erythema elevatum diutinum with rare distribution as a first clinical sign of non-Hodgkin's lymphoma: a novel association? J Dermatol. 2008;35:297–300. https://doi.org/10.1111/j.1346-8138.2008.00470.
44. Futei Y, Konohana I. A case of erythema elevatum diutinum associated with B-cell lymphoma: a rare distribution involving palms, soles and nails. Br J Dermatol. 2000;142:116–9.
45. Yilmaz F, Artaç M, Ciftçioglu MA, Yilmaz E. A case of erythema elevatum diutinum associated with breast carcinoma. Int J Dermatol. 2005;44:948–50.
46. Kohler IK, Lorincz AL. Erythema elevatum diutinum treated with niacinamide and tetracycline. Arch Dermatol. 1980;116:693–5.
47. Kanitakis J, Cozzani E, Lyonnet S, Thivolet J. Ultrastructural study of chronic lesions of erythema elevatum diutinum: "extracellular cholesterosis" is a misnomer. J Am Acad Dermatol. 1993;29:363–7.
48. Takahashi H, Fukami Y, Honma M, Ishida-Yamamoto A, Iizuka H. Successful combination therapy with dapsone and cyclosporine for erythema elevatum diutinum with unusual appearance. J Dermatol. 2012;39:486–7. https://doi.org/10.1111/j.1346-8138.2011.01331.
49. Yoshii N, Kanekura T, Higashi Y, Oyama K, Azagami K, Kanzaki T. Erythema elevatum diutinum manifesting as a penile ulcer. Clin Exp Dermatol. 2007;32:211–3.
50. Lekhanont K, Patarakittam T, Mantachote K, Waiyawatjamai P, Vongthongsri A. Progressive keratolysis with pseudopterygium associated with erythema elevatum diutinum. Ophthalmology. 2011;118:927–33. https://doi.org/10.1016/j.ophtha.2010.09.013.
51. Momen SE, Jorizzo J, Al-Niaimi FJ. Erythema elevatum diutinum: a review of presentation and treatment. J Eur Acad Dermatol Venereol. 2014;28:1594–602. https://doi.org/10.1111/jdv.12566.
52. Booth SA, Moody CE, Dahl MV, Herron MJ, Nelson RD. Dapsone suppresses integrin-mediated neutrophil adherence function. J Invest Dermatol. 1992;98:135–40.
53. Zacaron LH, Gonçalves JC, Curty VM, D'Acri AM, Lima RB, Martins CJ. Clinical and surgical therapeutic approach in erithema elevatum diutinum—case report. An Bras Dermatol. 2013;88:15–8. https://doi.org/10.1590/abd1806-4841.20132150.
54. Mahoney MG, Wood MG, Wilson F. Erythema elevatum diutinum. Arch Dermatol. 1968;97:590–1.
55. Henriksson R, Hofer PA, Hörnqvist R. Erythema elevatum diutinum—a case successfully treated with colchicine. Clin Exp Dermatol. 1989;14:451–3.

Neutrophilic Urticarial Dermatosis

5

Laurence Gusdorf and Dan Lipsker

Definition

Neutrophilic urticarial dermatosis (NUD) was first described in 2009 by one of us [1] as an eruption consisting of rose or red macules or slightly elevated plaques vanishing within 24 h. The histopathologic findings are a dense perivascular and interstitial infiltrate of neutrophils with leucocytoclasia but without vasculitis.

Clinical Description (Fig. 5.1)

The individual lesion is a rose or red macule or slightly raised papule or plaque that occurs mostly on the trunk. Lower and upper limbs can also be affected. Facial swelling and palmo-plantar lesions are very rare. Exceptionally Köbner phenomenon (dermographism), annular configuration or peripheral halo of vasoconstriction can be observed. Purpura is not present and lesions are usually not edematous. There might be a slight pruritus and pain or burning sensation is unusual. Individual lesions resolve within 24–48 h without scarring, nor residual pigmentation. The eruption can either be chronic or recurrent.

Associated signs depend on the clinical context in which NUD occurs. However, fever and joint pain are commonly associated, even in the absence of associated disorders. Other clinical signs can be present such as abdominal pain and chest pain.

L. Gusdorf • D. Lipsker (✉)
Service de Dermatologie, Hôpitaux Universitaires de Strasbourg, Strasbourg, France
e-mail: dan.lipsker@chru-strasbourg.fr

D. Wallach et al. (eds.), *Neutrophilic Dermatoses*,
https://doi.org/10.1007/978-3-319-72649-6_5

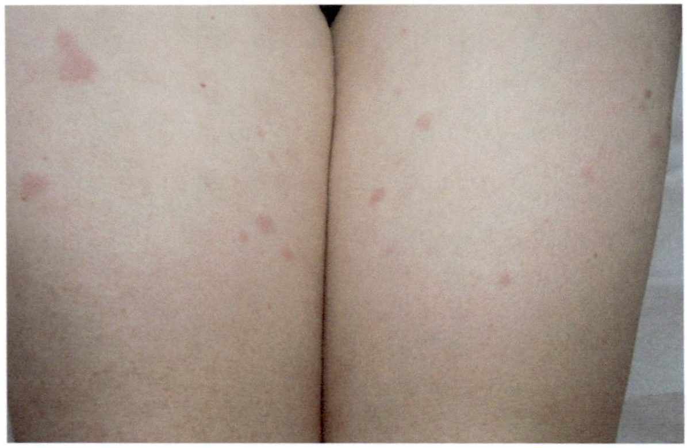

Fig. 5.1 Clinical aspect of neutrophilic urticarial dermatosis

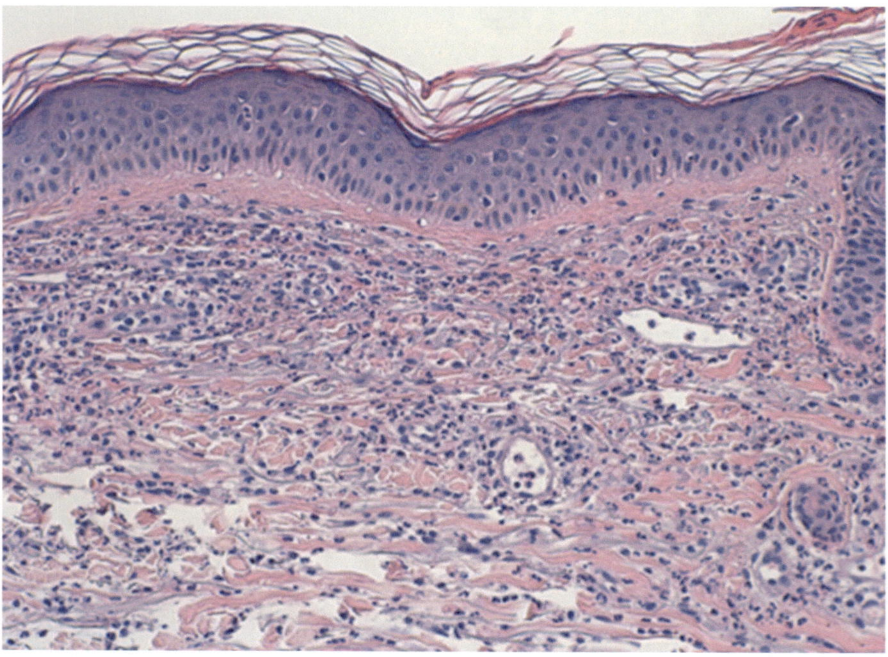

Fig. 5.2 Histological aspect of neutrophilic urticarial dermatosis

Histological Description (Fig. 5.2)

The histopathologic findings are characterized by a dense dermal neutrophilic infiltrate with interstitial involvement. In particular, neutrophils can be arranged in a single file along dermal collagen bundles. Neutrophils can also be located within ductal and secretory epithelia of sweat glands [2]. Diapedesis and leucocytoclasia are frequently seen but blood vessel walls are never damaged, fibrinoid vessel wall necrosis is always absent, which is an important clue to distinguish NUD from urticatial vasculitis. There is no dermal edema, allowing therefore, from a histopathological point of view, a distinction from Sweet syndrome. The epidermis is uninvolved. A few eosinophils and lymphocytes can also be seen within the dermal infiltrate.

Other Findings

Blood makers of inflammation such as elevated leukocyte count or increase in CRP or erythrocyte sedimentation rate may be present.

When performed, x-rays of painful joints do not show any signs of arthritis if NUD occurs without any associated disease.

Associated Diseases

The recognition of NUD is important and relevant in clinical practice. Systemic diseases are frequently associated to NUD and the practitioner should always screen them (Table 5.1). In particular, NUD is frequently seen in adult-onset Still's disease, Schnitzler syndrome, lupus erythematosus or cryopyrin-associated periodic syndrome [1, 3, 4].

Schnitzler Syndrome

Schnitzler syndrome is a rare disease with approximately 300 cases described. The mean age of disease onset is 50 years with a slight male predominance. It is characterized by the association of an urticarial rash, recurrent fever, joint and/or bone pain, elevated markers of inflammation such as CRP and leukocyte count and a monoclonal gammopathy. The monoclonal component is typically an IgM but it can sometimes be an IgG. It is not yet known if the monoclonal gammopathy precedes or succeeds the first clinical manifestations. The rash is usually the first clinical sign and is frequently accompanied by fever or bone pain. Cutaneous findings match the NUD description. Angioedema has exceptionally been described, as well as the involvement of face and extremities and dermographism. Patients also report

Table 5.1 First-line investigations

Complete blood count
CRP
Erythrocyte sedimentation rate
Serum protein electrophoresis with immunofixation
Ferritinaemia
Antinuclear antibodies, anti-dsDNA, anti-Ro/SSA, anti-La/SSB

Table 5.2 Strasbourg diagnostic criteria of Schnitzler syndrome [5]

Obligate criteria	
	Chronic urticarial rash and
	Monoclonal IgM or IgG
Minor Criteria	
	Recurrent fever[a]
	Objective findings of abnormal bone remodeling with or without bone pain[b]
	A neutrophilic dermal infiltrate on skin biopsy[c]
	Leukocytosis and/or elevated CRP[d]
Definite diagnosis if	
	Two obligate criteria AND at least two minor criteria if IgM and three minor criteria if IgG
Probable diagnosis if	
	Two obligate criteria AND at least one minor criteria if IgM and two minor criteria if IgG

[a]Must be >38 °C, and otherwise unexplained. Occurs usually—but not obligatory—together with the skin rash
[b]As assessed by bone scintigraphy, MRI or elevation of bone alkaline phosphatase
[c]Corresponds usually to the entity described as 'neutrophilic urticarial dermatosis' (Medicine 2009;88:23–31); absence of fibrinoid necrosis and significant dermal edema
[d]Neutrophils >10,000/mm^3 and/or CRP > 30 mg/L

exacerbating factors such as heat or cold exposure, alcohol consumption or physical exercise. The frequency of flares is variable, some patients experience daily flares while others describe monthly flares. The histopathological findings are important, as the presence of a neutrophilic dermal infiltrate on skin biopsy is now part of the new diagnostic criteria (also known as the Strasbourg criteria, see Table 5.2) [5]. When the skin biopsy is made on an early typical lesion, the findings may be typical of NUD. The density of the infiltrate is variable. However, other features can rarely be found such as vasculitis or urticaria [6], particularly if a late-onset lesion is biopsied. When immunofluorescence studies are performed, deposition of immunoreactants can be found around the superficial dermal vessels. The main complication of Schnitzler syndrome is the evolution into a lymphoproliferative disorder, mainly Waldenström disease, which occurs in about 20% of cases, a percentage close to IgM MGUS in general.

Lupus Erythematosus

Several types of neutrophilic dermatoses have already been reported in patients with lupus erythematosus (LE) such as pyoderma gangrenosum or Sweet's syndrome. The presence of a neutrophilic infiltrate in early and evolving lesions of cutaneous LE is a well-known phenomenon and the inclusion of neutrophilic lesions in the classification of cutaneous lesions in systemic LE has already been suggested [7].

When occurring in the setting of LE, NUD is frequently associated with joint pain, fever, abdominal pain, episcleritis, pharyngeal pain or paresthesia of fingers. Cutaneous lesions rarely occur on the face and extremities and Köbner phenomenon is exceptional. Lesions are never photodistributed. NUD can either precede the diagnosis or occur during the course of LE.

Biological findings are those typically found in LE such as polyclonal hypergammaglobulinemia, elevated sedimentation rate, antinuclear antibodies as well as anti-dsDNA, anti-Ro/SSA and anti-La/SSB antibodies. Interestingly, CRP is often elevated which is rather rare in SLE flares except when serositis or infection are present.

The association of cutaneous lesions, fever and joint pain is often mistaken for a systemic lupus flare and leads to unnecessary immunosuppressive treatment. In this case, dermatological advice and skin biopsy are essential. Histological aspect is typical of NUD, although mild vacuolar change of the basal layer can also be found. Direct immunofluorescence can show a lupus band and should not be misleading.

Cryopyrin-Associated Periodic Syndrome

Cryopyrin-associated periodic syndrome (CAPS) is a rare autoinflammatory disorder. It includes three phenotypes that increase in severity from familial cold autoinflammatory syndrome and Muckle-Wells syndrome to chronic infantile neurological, cutaneous and articular syndrome/neonatal onset multisystem inflammatory disease (CINCA/NOMID). All three phenotypes are related to heterozygous mutations of a single gene, *NLRP3* (NOD-like receptor family, pyrin domain containing 3). *NLRP3* encodes a protein called cryopyrin that plays a role in the induction of innate immune response: mutations of *NLRP3* lead to uncontrolled overproduction of IL-1β. The mode of inheritance is autosomal dominant with variable penetrance.

The diagnosis is discussed in patients with childhood onset chronic recurrent episodes of fever, urticarial rash, arthralgia and elevated markers of inflammation such as CRP and serum amyloid A (SAA) with or without neurological symptoms. NUD can also lead to the diagnosis of CAPS [8], especially in patients with late-onset disease and without family history. Typically, the urticarial rash is non-itchy, without angio-oedema and occurs on the trunk and limbs during the day as fever develop. The flare lasts up to 24 h. Skin histopathological findings correspond to the definition of NUD. In our opinion, substantial intravascular accumulation of neutrophils is the characteristic hallmark of CAPS-associated NUD.

Adult Onset Still's Disease

Adult Onset Still's disease (AOSD) is an inflammatory disorder characterized by recurrent fever, arthritis and an evanescent skin rash.

The classical skin rash of AOSD is an evanescent, salmon-colored maculopapular cutaneous eruption, which occurs during the fever spike. The skin lesions occur more frequently on the trunk and limbs and Köbner phenomenon can be present. This typical rash of Still's disease is one of the major diagnostic criteria of Yamaguchi et al. [9]. Skin biopsy is usually not indicated. When performed, it often shows non specific features, but reveals only dermal edema and mild perivascular inflammation in the superficial dermis consisting of lymphocytes and histiocytes. However, there are an increasing number of reports of other cutaneous findings including the possibility of persistent plaques and NUD [1]. The main differential diagnosis of persistent pruritic red papules and plaques occurring in the set of AOSD is a lichenoid eruption [10] with lesions arising on the trunk, the neck, face and extensor sides of the extremities. They can sometimes take a linear pattern. Histological analysis of these lesions is radically different and is characterized by multiple individual necrotic keratinocytes mainly located in the upper epidermis and infiltration of lymphocytes and neutrophils in the papillary and middermis. Basal vacuolar alteration, nuclear dust and subcorneal or intracorneal pustules may also be seen. These atypical skin rashes can appear together with the classical signs of AOSD, including the classical skin rash, or a few months after. These AOSD-like presentations could be linked to a higher risk of developing malignancies [11]. On the other hand, the classic rash of AOSD can display the typical findings of NUD. It depends possibly on the moment when the biopsy has been performed.

Serum Sickness-Like Drug Reaction

More recently, two cases of serum sickness-like drug reaction (SSLR) have been reported [12]. SSLR is related to serum sickness, a type III hypersensitivity reaction occurring after injection of heterologous serum. Clinically, it is characterized by arciform, generally fixed plaques that will persist for a few days, associated with joint pain and fever. Complement consumption, kidney and liver involvement can be observed. SSLR occurs 7–21 days following the drug exposure. Unlike serum sickness reaction, no immune complex is found in SSLR and no internal organ is affected. Skin eruption consists on edematous and annular urticarial plaques of the limbs and trunk. Facial edema and eyelid swelling can be present as well. Joint pain and fever are also found. Skin biopsy shows superficial to deep perivascular and interstitial infiltrate with prominent interstitial neutrophils and occasional eosinophils. Perieccrine involvement and scant perivascular leucocytoclasia are also observed. Patients improve when the culprit drug is stopped.

Link to Autoinflammation

The association of NUD and CAPS, a paradigm of monogenic autoinflammatory diseases, led us to consider that NUD could be a cutaneous marker of innate immunity dysfunction, thus of autoinflammation. Furthermore, Schnitzler syndrome and AOSD are polygenic acquired diseases that probably primarily involve autoinflammatory pathways. Concerning Schnitzler syndrome, no germline mutations has been reported so far, but somatic mosaicism of *NLRP3* involving the myeloid lineage has been reported in two patients with variant Schnitzler syndrome [13].

Differential Diagnosis

Urticarial Vasculitis

Urticarial vasculitis is the main differential diagnosis of NUD. Clinically, urticarial vasculitis can be indistinguishable from chronic urticaria. Other cutaneous signs can be present such as livedo reticularis, Raynaud's phenomenon and bullous lesions. Urticarial plaques and papules can be found anywhere on the body and angio-oedema is frequent. The lesions classically resolve leaving a purpuric patch, which is never the case in NUD. Skin biopsy is crucial to distinguish urticarial vasculitis from NUD. The presence of a leucocytoclastic vasculitis, swelling of endothelial cells, extravasation of erythrocytes and parietal fibrinoid necrosis are present in urticarial vasculitis and not in NUD.

Sweet Syndrome

Sweet syndrome can also be mistaken for NUD. Clinically it is characterized by erythematous to violaceous tender papules or nodules that often coalesce to form well defined plaques. The lesions are much more edematous and raised than those seen in NUD. Other clinical signs can be associated such as fever, general malaise, joint pain or episcleritis, exactly as in NUD, illustrating the overlapping nature of the neutrophilic dermatoses and their nosologic community. From a pathological point of view, the dermal neutrophilic infiltrate is much more dense and substantial dermal edema is present.

Palisaded Neutrophilic Granulomatous Dermatitis

Clinical presentation of palisaded neutrophilic granulomatous dermatitis is wide, and it can occur as erythematous urticarial plaques or papules. Histological findings are interstitial granuloma annulare-like or necrotizing extravascular granulomatous process with basophilic degenerate collage. Intense tissue neutrophilia is present as well as leucocytoclasis and particularly small vessel leukocytoclastic vasculitis.

Management

The management of NUD depends on the clinical setting (Table 5.3). Usually, anti-histamines are not efficient but can be prescribed at first.

Table 5.3 NUD management (see also text as strategy is different if an associated disease is present)

First line therapy: Antihistamines (up to 4 times the common dose; we use four different molecules)
Second line therapy: Colchicine 0.5–2 mg/day Dapsone 50–200 mg/day
Third line therapy: Anakinra 50–400 mg/day Tocilizumab 4 mg/kg every 4 weeks[a]

[a]Almost no data so far

When NUD occurs within systemic lupus erythematosus, immunosuppressive drugs are usually not effective. Classic neutrophil migration inhibitors, namely dapsone and colchicine are generally effective and should be the first-line treatment. Therapeutic dosage of dapsone ranges from 50 to 200 mg/day. Patients need to be monitored to detect adverse effects such as methemoglobinemia, hemolytic anemia (constant), hepatitis, or hypersensitivity syndrome. Therapeutic doses of colchicine range from 0.5 mg to 1 mg/day. Most of the time, this treatment is well tolerated but it may cause abdominal pain and diarrhea. The interaction with macrolides can be fatal, a notion of which the patient and his general practitioner should be informed.

When occurring in the setting of Schnitzler syndrome or CAPS, the most effective treatment are anti-IL-1 drugs such as anakinra (mainly for Schnitzler syndrome), rilonacept and canakinumab.

Therapeutic dosage of anakinra ranges from 50 to 100 mg/day in Schnitzler syndrome and from 100 to 400 mg/day (0.5 up to 12 mg/kg/day in two or three doses in children) in CAPS. It is administered subcutaneously. Patients should be free of all symptoms within hours after the first injection but this efficacy is only temporary and all the symptoms reappear if the patient omits an injection. Tapering to the lowest possible dose should be tried once the remission of symptoms is effective. Monitoring should include neutrophil count, liver enzymes, cholesterol and triglycerides. Tolerance is usually good; the most common adverse effects are injection site reactions and neutropenia. Neutropenia imposes treatment dose reduction or suspension until blood count normalization.

When NUD occurs in the set of AOSD, it resolves with the use of the conventional treatment of AOSD. Anakinra and tocilizumab are usually effective.

References

1. Kieffer C, Cribier B, Lipsker D. Neutrophilic urticarial dermatosis: a variant of neutrophilic urticaria strongly associated with systemic disease. Report of 9 new cases and review of the literature. Medicine (Baltimore). 2009;88:23–31.
2. Broekaert SMC, Boer-Auer A, Kerl K, Herrgott I, Schulz X, Bonsmann G, et al. Neutrophilic epitheliotropism is a histopathological clue to neutrophilic urticarial dermatosis. Am J Dermatopathol. 2016;38:39–49.

3. Gusdorf L, Bessis D, Lipsker D. Lupus erythematosus and neutrophilic urticarial dermatosis: a retrospective study of 7 patients. Medicine (Baltimore). 2014;93:e351.
4. Kolivras A, Theunis A, Ferster A, Lipsker D, Sass U, Dussart A, et al. Cryopyrin-associated periodic syndrome: an autoinflammatory disease manifested as neutrophilic urticarial dermatosis with additional perieccrine involvement. J Cutan Pathol. 2011;38:202–8.
5. Simon A, Asli B, Braun-Falco M, De Koning H, Fermand J-P, Grattan C, et al. Schnitzler's syndrome: diagnosis, treatment, and follow-up. Allergy. 2013;68:562–8.
6. Gusdorf L, Asli B, Barbarot S, Neel A, Masseau A, Puechal X, et al. Schnitzler syndrome: validation and applicability of diagnostic criteria in real-life patients. Allergy. 2017;72:177–82.
7. Lipsker D. The need to revisit the nosology of cutaneous lupus erythematosus: the current terminology and morphologic classification of cutaneous LE: difficult, incomplete and not always applicable. Lupus. 2010;19:1047–9.
8. Herbert VG, Ahmadi-Simab K, Reich K, Boer-Auer A. Neutrophilic urticarial dermatosis (NUD) indicating Cryopyrin-associated periodic syndrome associated with a novel mutation of the NLRP3 gene. J Eur Acad Dermatol Venereol. 2016;30:852–3.
9. Yamaguchi M, Ohta A, Tsunematsu T, Kasukawa R, Mizushima Y, Kashiwagi H, et al. Preliminary criteria for classification of adult Still's disease. J Rheumatol. 1992;19:424–30.
10. Lee JY-Y, Yang C-C, Hsu MM-L. Histopathology of persistent papules and plaques in adult-onset Still's disease. J Am Acad Dermatol. 2005;52:1003–8.
11. Sun NZ, Brezinski EA, Berliner J, Haemel A, Connolly MK, Gensler L, et al. Updates in adult-onset Still disease: atypical cutaneous manifestations and associations with delayed malignancy. J Am Acad Dermatol. 2015;73:294–303.
12. Nguyen CV, Miller DD. Serum sickness-like drug reaction: two cases with a neutrophilic urticarial pattern. J Cutan Pathol. 2017;44:177–82.
13. De Koning HD, van Gijn ME, Stoffels M, Jongekrijg J, Zeeuwen PLJM, Elferink MG, et al. Myeloid lineage-restricted somatic mosaicism of NLRP3 mutations in patients with variant Schnitzler syndrome. J Allergy Clin Immunol. 2015;135(2):561–4.

Pyoderma Gangrenosum

6

Daniel Wallach

Pyoderma gangrenosum (PG), one of the most impressive cutaneous conditions, is an inflammatory ulceration with a distinctive clinical appearance, often associated with systemic diseases. Considerations on the significance of pyoderma gangrenosum, both in its classic ulcerative form and in its clinical variants, led to its inclusion among the spectrum of the neutrophilic dermatoses. Ongoing research aims at identifying genetic factors favoring PG, as well as deciphering the mechanisms of inflammation in PG.

PG is a rare disease. Its annual incidence has been estimated in UK to be 6/million persons [1]. It has been observed at all ages, even in small children, although rarely, but predominates in the middle-age group. Women are slightly more affected in most series. There is no known ethnic predominance.

The management of a patient with suspected PG requires dermatological skills because the diagnosis only relies on the clinical presentation; there are no histological nor laboratory diagnostic criteria. These dermatological skills also include internal medicine expertise, because the majority of PG patients suffer from a multisystemic condition.

Excellent reviews on PG have been published [2–6]. Many of them have been written by researchers associated with the Mayo Clinic, Rochester [2, 4, 5].

History

Phagedaena Geometrica (Brocq)

It is worth describing in detail the clinical appearance of the PG ulceration, because even now it is one of the most valuable diagnostic arguments. This ulceration has been very accurately described in 1908, before the individualization of PG, by Louis

D. Wallach
Physician (Hon.) of Paris Hospitals, Paris, France

D. Wallach et al. (eds.), *Neutrophilic Dermatoses*,
https://doi.org/10.1007/978-3-319-72649-6_6

Brocq, one of the most talented dermatologists of his time, and his pupil Clément Simon [7]. Their report is about phagedenism. This word, derived from the Greek words meaning "to eat, to devour" and "a lot" was used to describe extensive ulcerations, showing an unusual local malignity. Phagedenism was a complication of many ulcerations, the main cause being a venereal disease, a chancre or a tertiary syphilis. But Brocq and Simon insisted on the fact that phagedenism is not specific of venereal diseases, and can complicate other infectious ulcerations. Among the eight first patients, five, or six, however had syphilis as the primary morbid process. Clinical arguments define phagedenism. The border of the ulceration is elevated, cut vertically and undermined by pustules, abscesses or purulent cavities. The periphery is inflammatory, lymphangitis-like. The lesion extends peripherally, rapidly, forming circular arcs or ovales, resembling trichophytic infections, leading to the term "phagédénisme géométrique". Phagedenism was viewed as a superinfection, staphylococci and streptococci were suspected. Wide surgical excision was successful.

Eight years after this first presentation to the *Société médicale des Hôpitaux de Paris*, Brocq felt that dermatologists had not given enough attention to his description of geometrical phagedenism. He reports to the French Society of Dermatology and Syphiligraphy his early cases, adds five new personal cases and cites an additional case, in a 12-year old boy. This publication in the *Annales de Dermatologie* includes 12 clinical photographs [8]. Brocq's patients are ten women and three men, aged 17–68 years. The phagedenism is located on the legs (six cases), and more rarely on the thighs, the buttocks, the face, the neck, the breast. Eight patients were syphilitic, which was viewed as a possible predisposing factor.

Brocq insists on the fact that geometrical phagedenism is a specific entity, of probable infectious cause, and best treated, when possible (only one of his cases), by surgery. If many of Brocq's reflections are only of historical value, his clinical description stood the test of time and is still cited. Brocq himself considered that the clinical characteristics were so striking that the differential diagnosis was not really a problem.

This pathognomonic clinical appearance includes:

- The quickness of the extension;
- The geometrical configuration of this extension, with a round or oval circular border, similar to a trichophytic parasitism;
  - The appearance of this elevated border zone, described in three parts:
    Linear culminating ridge;
    Peripheral red areola, with a gentle slope and gradual fading towards healthy skin;
    Inner border vertically cut (80°–85°), compared to a steep cliff. The walls of this cliff are riddled by small abscesses. Gentle pressure led to a purulent oozing, compared to a sponge.

The ulcerated area, inside these borders, is irregular, with no specific feature. It may be purulent, yellowish or grayish, covered with tissue debris, or hemorrhagic, or, when healing starts, granulating.

Geometrical phagedenism may destroy all the skin layers, but rarely invades deep tissues. There is no lymphadenopathy. Pain is variable, and may be absent or very violent.

Histopathology is disappointing. One case was studied in detail. The importance of the neutrophilic infiltration is stressed, but no pathognomonic tissue alteration is found.

Inasmuch as geometrical phagedenism is considered as a local microbial infection, antiseptic dressings are the best treatment, considered as efficacious. Surgical destruction or excision, although rarely possible, is still considered as the treatment of choice.

Post-operative Gangrene (Cullen)

Surgeons are familiar with postoperative complications, but Thomas Cullen was the first, in 1924, to attract attention on a particular post-operative gangrene [9]. The patient was a 50-year old man, who underwent surgery for an appendicular abscess. A few days later, a wide cutaneous sloughing area with undermined borders developed around the surgical incision. Streptococci were isolated. Many physicians were consulted; they had never seen such an ulceration. One of them thought this was ecthyma gangraenosum. Cullen insists on the fact that this gangrene developed slowly, progressively, in contrast with well-known wound dehiscences and streptococcal and other post-surgical infections. He also stresses that the ulcerative process implies only the skin and superficial tissues, sparing the intra-abdominal initial infectious lesion. The patient was cured, with the help of pinch grafts. This paper contains no bibliographic reference. Beautiful watercolors show an ulceration typical of what will soon be called pyoderma gangrenosum, including the bluish peripheral inflammation, the undermined elevated border, and the granulating ulceration (Fig. 6.1).

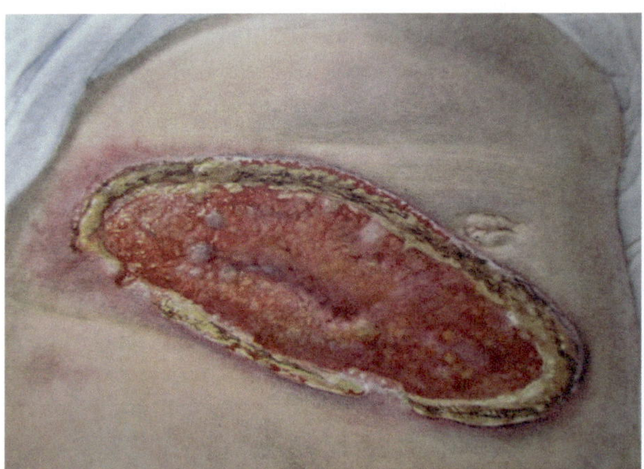

Fig. 6.1 The first accurate illustration of pyoderma gangrenosum, in form of post-operative progressive gangrene (post-operative PG). (Fig. 1 of [9], Cullen 1924, Reprinted with permission from the Journal of the American College of Surgeons, formerly Surgery Gynecology & Obstetrics)

Two years later, Brewer and Meleney published similar observations [10]. These two reports proved very helpful to guide surgeons confronted with such an unusual complication, seemingly infectious but different from well known infectious surgical complications [11].

Pyoderma (Ecthyma) Gangrenosum (Brunsting, Goeckerman, O'Leary)

The term Pyoderma gangrenosum was proposed in 1930 by Brunsting, Goeckerman and O'Leary [12], from the Rochester Mayo Clinic, to designate cases of extensive cutaneous ulcerations in which staphylococci and streptococci were found, in patients suffering from a severe, infectious, debilitating process.

In their review of the literature, Brunsting and colleagues do not cite Brocq, but a number of observations reported under various names, including post-operative gangrene. All were considered as pyodermas, or infectious skin lesions.

Their report is about five patients, four of them had severe chronic ulcerative colitis with parallel evolutions of the skin and bowel ulcerations. These four patients were three women and a man, aged 16- to 32-years old. They were suffering from very long-lasting attacks of acute diarrhea leading to cachexia and needing blood transfusions. Some had polyarthritis. The cutaneous lesions were located all over the body, mainly the lower limbs and the trunk.

The fifth patient, a 48-year old man, had chronic empyema and extensive thoracic and abdominal ulceration starting from a site of drainage. He died following another drainage attempt.

The clinical description of the lesions is very similar to Brocq's text, with a well-defined, strikingly blue, undermined border, and a serpiginous peripheral extension, at times rapid (up to 1–2 cm daily).

The patients had to stay in hospital during many months and the authors could observe elementary lesions. These were small inflammatory pustules which softened and broke down, then involuting or extending peripherally to form the typical ulceration. In some instances, pathergy is evident in the formation of ulcers. They also mention that some healed areas had a vegetative character. In one patient, the three types of lesions could be observed: inflammatory pustules, spreading ulcerations with undermined borders, and chronic, vegetative ulcerations with granulations.

Histopathology showed a chronic inflammatory process in three stages: pustules or abscess, ulceration, and a vegetative late phase.

Bacteriological studies showed in each case highly virulent staphylococci and streptococci. The authors speculate on the responsibility of these germs, isolated or in symbiosis and on the role of the state of reactivity or allergy of the host.

Whereas Brocq initially thought that geometrical phagedenism was a superinfection of an initial cutaneous lesion, Brunsting et al. considered pyoderma gangrenosum as a dissemination from an internal infection (bowel, lung) favored by a low bodily resistance.

Synthesis: The First Observations of Ulcerative Pyodermas

In 1941, Sigmund S Greenbaum [13] reviewed the literature on the reported cases of ulcerative pyodermas characterized by the special progression and the undermined borders. He notes that the term phagedena, used in France, was absent from American publications and discussions.

Greenbaum proposes a classification of these phagedenic ulcers in primary, arising on normal or traumatized (accidentally or surgically) skin, and secondary, beginning as a venereal disease or an ecthyma.

The published texts and photographs lead Greenbaum to assert the identity of pyoderma gangrenosum and geometric phagedena. He also writes that the designation gangraenosum is unsatisfactory because the tissue destruction is not a gangrene in the true sense (black, necrotic, dead tissues). The literature reviewed by Greenbaum includes reports under many terms, listed in Table 6.1.

Greenbaum reports six cases of phagedaena geometrica and performed bacteriological studies, including inoculations. He concludes that staphylococci and streptococci, alone or in symbiosis, may be "the exciting cause", but that the relationship between the organisms and the lesions remains to be determined. He adds that "non-bacterial (allergic?) factors [are] believed to be a necessary complement".

In spite of Greenbaum's plea for the term geometric phagedaena, the term Pyoderma gangrenosum will be adopted in the subsequent literature. It unifies earlier observations, including the ulcerated pyodermas, for which the bacterial cause has always appeared questionable, and postsurgical gangrenes.

Table 6.1 Denominations of ulcerated pyodermas in earlier literature (from Greenbaum, 1941, [13])

Brocq	Geometric phagedenism	1908
Cullen	Post-operative progressive gangrene (denomination by Meleney)	1924
Zurhelle, Klein	Exulcerating papillary pyoderma	1928
Bolog	Chronic ulcerative pyodermata	1928
Tischnenko, Kroiczic	Chronic serpiginous ulcerative (and erosive) pyoderma	1928
Smith	Chronic pyoderma	1929
Brunsting, Goekerman, O'Leary	Pyoderma gangraenosum	1930
Meleney	Gangrenous ecthyma or impetigo	1933
Holman	Phagedenic ulceration	1935
Fox, Maloney	Chronic serpiginous ulcerative pyoderma	1935
Meleney, Johnson	Chronic undermining burrowing ulcer	1937
Zeisler	Pyogenic lesions of the skin associated with chronic ulcerative colitis	1938
Ormsby	Dermatitis gangraenosa	1938

This list is not exhaustive. Similar cases had been reported since the end of the nineteenth century, and considered as infectious ulcerations, but only the precise clinical description initiated by Brocq allowed to group the reports under the same name, and following Brunsting et al., Pyoderma gangraenosum was rapidly adopted

Clinical Features

These pioneer observations refer to ulcerative PG, which may be called classic PG. More recent works described clinical variants, and PG is now considered as a heterogenous disease.

Classic, Ulcerative PG

There is not much to add, nor to subtract, to the initial descriptions of PG. Classic PG often starts as an inflammatory pustule, which may look like a superficial pyoderma or a carbuncle. This pustule enlarges and breaks, forming an ulceration which will gradually increase both superficially and in depth. The floor of the ulceration is covered by whitish debris, necrotic tissue, purulent material or granulating tissue. Muscles and tendons may be visible. The PG ulceration is overhanged by a well-demarcated, elevated border, slowly progressing centrifugally in forming oval or circular arcs. The characteristics of the border are important to suspect or even diagnose PG. In this typical border well described by Brocq, three parts must be described. The inner part is a clear-cut ditch with a steep slope, undermined by small purulent collections. The top of the border is indurated, of variable thickness and elevation, red-bluish or violaceous, the epidermis may be separated in sheets. The wide outer part of the border is a gentle slope, the inflammation gradually fades towards healthy skin.

About 70% of PG ulcerations occur on the legs, but the trunk and all body sites may be involved (Fig. 6.2).

PG lesions may be unique or multiple, and of variable size. Ulcerations may be enormous (30 cm or more), involving a great part of the trunk or limbs.

Lesions start in healthy skin, and may be provoked by a trauma, whether trivial or important. This pathergy is an important feature of PG and will be detailed later.

The speed of the centrifugal extension of the ulceration is variable, but may reach more than 1 cm daily.

Some patients suffer extreme pain, but in others pain is surprisingly mild. During acute extension stages, there may be moderate fever and general malaise.

In spite of the importance of the absence of skin on ulcerated areas, there is no lymphadenopathy; superinfection, lymphangitis or septicemia originating in PG lesions are extremely rare [14].

Important ulcerations may expose tendons, fascias, muscles, but do not exceed the subcutaneous tissues.

Progressive, active PG has a purulent base and an elevated, inflammatory border. When PG involutes, the border collapses, redness fades and granulation tissue appears on the ulceration.

Although clinical flares may be acute, PG is a chronic disease. Untreated PG lasts for months or years with frequent recurrences. In 2000, Bennett et al. analyzed the time to remission in treated patients [15]. Sixty-eight percent of patients cleared within 6 months and 95% within 3 years. After healing, an atrophic, cribriform scar persists.

Few cases are directly lethal, but PG patients have an increased risk of death [1, 16]. Fatal outcome may result from the associated disease or a visceral complication.

Needless to say, patients with ulcerative PG are extremely impressed by such a wound and suffer both physically and psychologically. They need to be actively supported, and reassured on the fact that their wound will heal.

PG Clinical Variants

In addition to this dramatic, ulcerative form, variants have been described, where the loss of substance is much less important [17]. These superficially ulcerated or non ulcerated PG, which may coexist with classic PG, may be viewed as PG variants or as non-PG neutrophilic dermatoses, with overlapping features with other conditions of this group. Although their incidence has not been precisely studied, the variants are less frequent than the ulcerative PG [15] (Fig. 6.3).

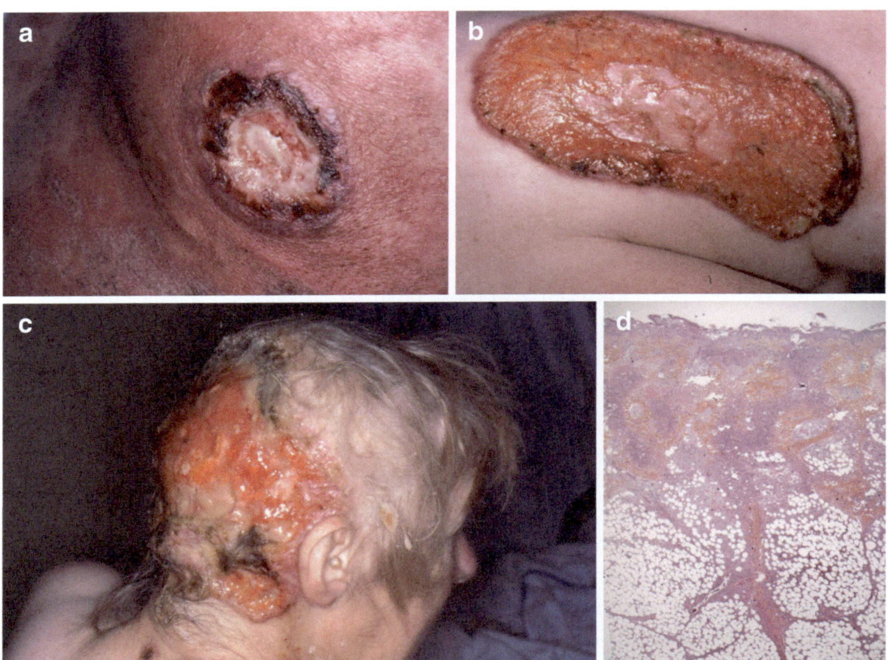

Fig. 6.2 Classical, ulcerative PG: Clinical and histological features (see the text for detailed descriptions). (**a–c**) coll. D Wallach, MD; (**d**) coll MD Vignon-Pennamen, MD

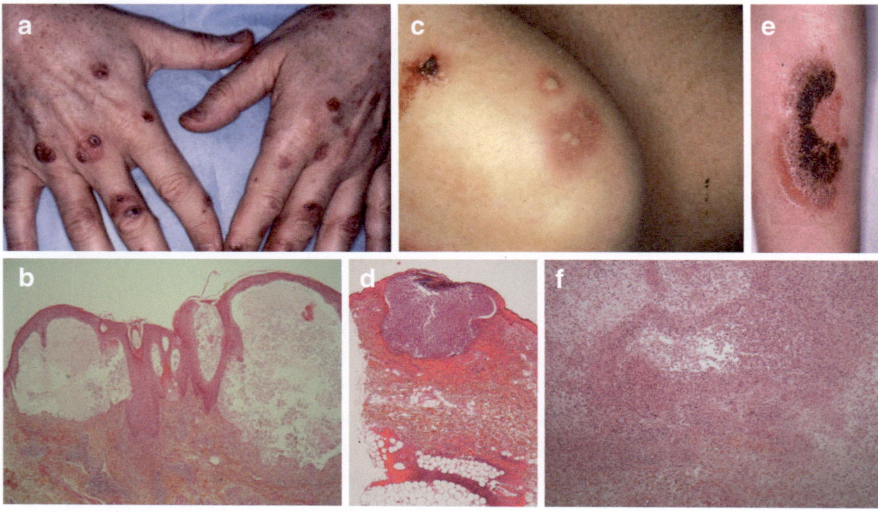

Fig. 6.3 PG variants: (**a**, **b**) Bullous PG. (**c**, **d**) Pustular PG. (**e**, **f**) Granulomatous PG (See the text for detailed descriptions). (**a**, **c**, **e**) coll. D Wallach, MD; (**b**, **d**, **f**) coll. MD Vignon-Pennamen, MD

Pustular PG

Classic PG is pustular, both at the start of the lesions and during evolution. In addition, eruptions mainly pustular, with little evolution towards ulcerations, have been described as pustular PG, mainly in patients with an inflammatory bowel disease [18] or some other gastro-intestinal condition, such as a by-pass syndrome. The number, size and distribution of the pustules are variable. They are usually surrounded by a halo of erythema. Diffuse acute pustular rashes have been observed [19]. These pustular or vesicular-pustular eruptions in patients with colitis have been described under various denominations and are clinically heterogeneous. Vesiculo-pustules, small hemorrhagic necrotic lesions, superficial ulcerations are frequently present [20]. The course of these pustular eruptions often parallels that of the digestive disorder. These eruptions represent a good illustration of the neutrophilic dermatoses spectrum, which may also be seen in other settings (blood malignancy, chronic arthritis) as well as in patients with no systemic disease.

Bullous PG

A bullous variant of PG has been described in 1972 by HO Perry and RK Winkelmann [21] in three patients who also had leukemia. These patients presented with large necrotic ulcerations diagnostic of PG, with atypical features: the ulcerations were relatively superficial, and the extension margin was bullous. The three patients soon died from myeloid leukemia; skin biopsies showed a neutrophilic infiltration, without immature hematopoietic cells. Autopsy of one of the patients showed numerous lung abscesses. This bullous PG, where the ulceration seems to result from the collapse of surrounding bullae, has been reviewed in 1992 by Ho et al. [22] who found 42 cases in the literature and also pointed out the resemblance of bullous PG with the vesiculopustular variant of Sweet's syndrome. Bullae are initially tense, their content may be clear, purulent, or hemorrhagic with a cyanotic halo. In contrast with classic PG, bullous PG is preferentially located on the upper extremities [15], including the back of the hands. Biopsy shows a neutrophilic infiltrate with various levels of splitting, and an intense dermal inflammation. Bullous PG or Sweet/PG overlap syndrome occurs often in patients with polycythemia vera, myelodysplasia [23] or leukemia, and in these patients is indicative of a poor prognosis. Many cases however are observed in the absence of a blood disorder.

Vegetative PG

The superficial, granulomatous, vegetative form of PG has been isolated by Wilson-Jones and Winkelmann [24] on the basis of the presence of a histological granuloma in 25 patients clinically diagnosed as PG at the Mayo Clinic and St John's Hospital, London. Granulomas had been mentioned by Brunsting et al. [12] in late classic PG, but vegetative PG is considered as a distinct variant [17]. The inclusion of non-ulcerated conditions in the PG group may appear questionable [3], but this remark is only of academic interest. From a practical point of view, the individualization of vegetative PG is important because the course is usually benign, associated diseases are rare, and non aggressive treatment is often effective. The preferential location is the trunk, but the legs and other areas are also affected. The lesion, often unique, appears as an infiltrated plaque with a vegetative or verrucous surface. The loss of substance is minimal and borders are only slightly elevated, nor purulent nor violaceous. The literature on vegetative PG has been reviewed in 2005 by Langan and Powell [25]. Significant associated conditions were rare. Only 39% of cases required systemic corticosteroid therapy. Dapsone, minocycline, intralesional triamcinolone, were often effective.

Pathergic PG

Pathergy is present in approximately 30% of PG cases, where lesions start at the site of skin trauma of variable importance. As a consequence, all traumas, even trivial as a seat belt pressure [26] must be avoided in PG patients. The pathergy test, which is used in Behçet's disease, is not indicated in PG.

Peristomal PG

Peristomal PG has been first described in 1984 [27] and is believed to affect as many as 5% of patients with Crohn's disease stomies. Peristomal PG is caused both by the underlying inflammatory bowel disease (ulcerative colitis or more often Crohn's disease, rarely other causes of stomies) and pathergy on the skin bearing appliances. The ulceration starts a few months after surgery at the immediate vicinity of the stoma, on the area covered by the stoma bag. It is painful and adds to the discomfort of the stoma care, but usually remains superficial. Depending on the digestive disease, stoma relocation or closure may be performed and effective, or avoided because of the risk of recurrence. Wound care, intralesional or topical corticosteroids, dapsone, may be efficient. If not, systemic treatment as indicated in other PG cases must be prescribed.

Postoperative PG

Although many modern authors do not refer to it, postoperative PG is identical to the postoperative progressive gangrene first described by Cullen in 1924 [9] and may be considered as the worst consequence of the pathergy process. Postoperative PG has been recently reviewed [28, 29]. Around 7–10 days after the operation, the surgical site becomes erythematous and painful. The wound may dehisce, or be covered and surrounded by inflammatory pustules and ulcerations. The progressive enlargement of the ulceration is that of classical PG and may affect huge surfaces.

In modern series, the majority of postoperative PG occurs after breast surgery (reduction mammoplasty, breast reconstruction, others). Postoperative PG may involve the entire breast region, often sparing the areola, which is unexplained. Thoracic, abdominal, gynecological and all other surgical interventions may be complicated by postoperative PG.

About 20–35% of patients have history of PG, or have an associated disease known to be associated with PG.

In many cases, there is no PG context, the surgical complication is the initial manifestation of the disease and the first diagnosis are wound dehiscence and/or infection. This leads to ineffective antibiotic treatment and deleterious surgical debridement. Reports of ulcerations of many months' duration, causing much distress and inadequate medical decisions, are numerous in the literature because these patients are managed by physicians unfamiliar with PG.

Consequently, all surgeons should be aware of this risk of misdiagnosing PG for surgical superinfection, because additional surgery may have disastrous consequences [30].

In rare instances, the diagnosis of cutaneous PG may lead to reevaluate the diagnosis of the disease which motivated the operation. Kitagawa and Grassi [31] published the case of a 82-year old woman who underwent surgery and chemotherapy following a diagnosis of lung cancer. The surgical wound did not heal and was diagnosed as pyoderma gangrenosum. This led to a reevaluation of the lung pathology specimens, which concluded to an inflammatory process, assimilated to primary lung PG. Field et al. reported a similar case [32] and probably these are not exceptional. As will be discussed later in this chapter, internal PG is very difficult to diagnose and postoperative PG may be one of its modes of revelation.

Drug-Induced PG

Very few PG cases have been attributed to drugs [33]. Neutrophilic dermatoses such as PG may be induced by GM-CSF and G-CSF, usually in the context of a treated blood malignancy [34]. Some cases have been observed during treatments with isotretinoin [35], interferon [36], diverse drugs or by biologic agents. It may be difficult to differentiate a true drug-induced PG from a PG progressing in spite of treatment and from PG in the setting of a treated associated disease. Some drugs may induce ulcerations described as having a "PG-like" appearance: hydroxyurea [37], hydralazine [38], oral anticoagulant therapy [39], levamisole in adulterated cocaine [40].

Iodine and broma may induce PG-like ulcerations (halogenoderma), but may also aggravate patients with authentic PG [41].

Recently, cases of PG were induced by new immunostimulants, which may provoke immune-mediated diseases [42] and by targeted anticancer drugs [43].

Special Locations

PG can affect all cutaneous and mucous surfaces, but predominates on the lower limbs (ulcerative PG), the upper limbs (bullous PG), the trunk. Some locations deserve a special mention.

Head and Face

PG of the scalp and face is impressive. It may be similar to malignant pyoderma, a facial ulceration due to Wegener's granulomatosis [44].

Hands

Bullous PG, a variant overlapping with bullous/hemorrhagic Sweet syndrome, is preferentially located on the upper extremities. Some authors have individualized a "neutrophilic dermatosis of the dorsal hands" which does not seem different from the same entity located anywhere else [45].

Genital Area

In Brocq's era, the main differential of "PG" was phagedenism from venereal lesions. To-day, PG is rarely located on the genital organs and isolated reports have been published [46, 47]. Infectious ulcerations, cutaneous Crohn's disease and Behcet's disease must be ruled out.

Oral Mucosa

Oral involvement by PG is rare and must be differentiated from malignant pyoderma, hematological malignancies and noma. Cases of PG involving the tongue, the pharynx, the larynx have been published [48]. Pyostomatitis vegetans [49] is the mucosal equivalent of pustular PG in patients with inflammatory bowel disease. Superficial flat pustules rapidly erode and form "snail-track" erosions on the gums.

Eye and Ocular Region

PG may involve the skin around the eye, including the periorbital skin and the eyelids [50]; scars may require surgical repair. Ocular involvement itself is complex. Few cases of involvement of the sclera, the cornea, have been published. The entire eye tissue may be destroyed [51]. Ulcerative keratitis is considered as an extracutaneous neutrophilic localization [52].

Histopathology

Although histological changes are not considered specific, a biopsy is always required to give essential positive information and to exclude other causes of ulceration [53, 54]. The excessive fear of a pathergy phenomenon must not be taken as a pretext to avoid a helpful biopsy.

The time and site of the biopsy must be carefully selected. It is recommended to take an elliptic specimen including the margin and the floor of the ulcer.

On a large and deep enough biopsy, the dermis and the subcutaneous fat are massively infiltrated by a suppurative inflammation that contains neutrophils, hemorraghes and necrosis. The infiltrate destroys preexisting structures, follicular units and adnexal glands. Vessels can be necrotic with thrombosis, these alterations being secondary to the neutrophilic inflammation. All these features are in favor of classic PG after exclusion of an infection.

If the biopsy is made too early in the course of the lesion and on the peripheral extension area, there is a perivascular and/or perifollicular infiltrate predominantly composed of lymphocytes and histiocytes. This aspect is non specific and does not contribute to the diagnosis.

In pustular PG and in initial pustules of ulcerative PG, the infiltrate has a tropism for the hair follicles. The infundibulum shows signs of rupture or perforation and contains and/or is surrounded by a dense neutrophilic infiltrate.

In bullous PG, lesions are characterized by subepidermal and intraepidermal collections of neutrophils. Immunofluorescence is negative or non specific.

In vegetating PG and also in some cases of classic PG, neutrophils are associated with epithelioid histiocytes and giant cells to form granulomas.

In all cases, special histochemical stains and cultures for microbiological identification are negative, this information is of paramount importance.

Diagnosis

In the absence of a specific biologic marker, the diagnosis of PG only relies on the clinical appearance in association with a neutrophilic dermal infiltration. This diagnosis may be exceedingly difficult, especially in atypical cases.

On the patient level, this difficulty is the cause of a diagnosis delay in many cases, and of many misdiagnosis. These have disastrous consequences, both when a patient mistaken for PG receives immunosuppressive therapy, and when a patient with PG is treated by aggressive surgery [55] or other inappropriate procedures.

On the academic level, the ancient literature contained only reports of isolated PG cases or small series, where the diagnostic arguments could be ascertained. The recent literature contains interesting studies of series of hundreds of patients, and there is an unavoidable doubt about the diagnostic certainty.

We are indebted to the Mayo Clinic investigators for the proposal of diagnostic criteria [5] (Table 6.2). These criteria have been widely accepted, and represent a

Table 6.2 Criteria of ulcerative PG proposed in 2004 by Su et al. [5]

Major criteria	
1.	Rapid progression of a painful, necrolytic cutaneous ulcer with an irregular, violaceous and undermined border
2.	Other causes of cutaneous ulceration have been excluded
Minor criteria	
1.	History suggestive of pathergy or clinical finding of cribriform scarring
2.	Systemic diseases associated with PG
3.	Histopathologic findings (sterile dermal neutrophilia ± mixed inflammation ± lymphocytic vasculitis)
4.	Rapid response to systemic steroid treatment

Diagnosis requires both major criteria and at least two minor criteria. Although not formally validated, these criteria are accepted by all authors. A very recent study however found that histopathological findings could be considered as the only major criterium [54]

good description of classic PG; they however have never been formally validated. Indeed, the second major criterium is of the utmost importance: all other causes of ulceration must be ruled out by appropriate investigations, which in practice necessitates a skin biopsy and some laboratory investigations. So PG is currently considered as a diagnosis of exclusion. Positive clinical and histopathological arguments must however be carefully searched for [54].

Available evidence suggests that PG criteria are underused by the authors of case reports [56] and this is probably even more true in medical practice, where exigence may be variable.

Weenig et al. [57] reviewed the charts of 240 patients seen at the Mayo Clinic for PG, as well as the relevant literature, and give a comprehensive list of differential diagnosis (Table 6.3). Ninety-five patients (49 from the Mayo Clinic) had skin ulcers resembling, or mimicking PG, and 64 of them had been inadequately treated. Even in this highly specialized referral center, 10% of PG diagnosis were found to be erroneous. A third of patients with ulcers resembling PG also had one of the diseases classically associated with PG; in half of biopsied patients, the histological findings demonstrated the alternative diagnosis.

Hafner et al. report from another reference center, specialized in leg ulcers. Among 31 patients with Martorell hypertensive ischemic leg ulcers, 16 were referred with a diagnosis of PG. The diagnosis of Martorell ulcer could only be confirmed by a wide biopsy (approximately 5.0 × 0.8 cm), including the wound border and the necrotic area, showing subcutaneous arteriosclerosis [58].

Nguyen et al. compare these PG-like ulcers with PG ulcers and similarly conclude on the difficulty of this diagnosis [59].

Adequate investigations allow to diagnose infections, malignant processes, and also vasculitis. But as well as many conditions can masquerade as PG, PG may masquerade as other conditions, such as dermatitis artefacta, with similarly hazardous consequences [60]. As long as clinical expertise remains the only way of diagnosing PG, the greatest caution is advised before claiming a diagnosis of PG, and starting a potentially toxic treatment.

Table 6.3 The differential diagnosis of pyoderma gangrenosum (Based on Weenig et al. [57])

Causes of ulcerations resembling pyoderma gangrenosum
Vascular occlusive or venous disease
Small vessel occlusive arterial disease
Hypertension/arteriosclerosis
Antiphospholipid-antibody syndrome
Livedoid vasculopathy
Cryoglobulinemia
Venous insufficiency
Vasculitis
Polyarteritis nodosa
Wegener's granulomatosis
Behçet's disease
Other vasculitis
Cutaneous malignancies
Lymphoma
Leukemia cutis
Langerhans'cell histiocytosis
Squamous cell carcinomas
Basal cell carcinomas
Primary cutaneous infection
Bacterial/mycobacterial infections
Deep fungal infections (sporotrichosis, aspergillosis, …)
Amebiasis cutis
Leishmaniasis
Drug-induced or exogenous tissue injury
Facticial disorder
Injection drug abuse
Bromoderma/iododerma
Spider bites
Other inflammatory disorders
Cutaneous Crohn's disease
Ulcerative necrobiosis lipoidica

Pyoderma Gangrenosum and the Neutrophilic Dermatoses Spectrum

The impressive ulceration typical of pyoderma gangrenosum led to consider this entity as autonomous, characterized by the frequency of associated systemic diseases, mainly digestive diseases and also blood disorders. In 1980, JL Burton attracted attention upon the vicinity of PG with acute febrile neutrophilic dermatosis, or Sweet's syndrome (SS), described in 1964 and also significantly associated with leukemia [61]. This convergence was rather unexpected, inasmuch as ulcerative PG and papular SS are distinctively different. Burton however suggested the possibility of a "nosologic continuum" linking PG and Sweet's syndrome. Caughman, Stern and Haynes reviewed the literature, and presented an additional case of the overlap between atypical bullous PG and atypical bullous SS which best illustrates this continuum [62]. They proposed the term "Neutrophilic dermatosis of myeloproliferative disorders", so expanding the term "Neutrophilic dermatosis" beyond Sweet's syndrome. In following years, it appeared that this overlapping neutrophilic dermatosis can also be found in patients with digestive disorders [63, 64], as well as in patients without any identified systemic disease [65].

In 1991, I proposed to consider a new clinical spectrum of neutrophilic dermatoses, encompassing not only PG and SS, but also other skin disorders of diverse clinical appearance, which have in common skin aseptic neutrophilia and significant association with systemic diseases [66]. These were the subcorneal pustular dermatosis described in 1956 by Ian Sneddon and Darrell Wilkinson [67], and erythema elevatum diutinum, described in 1894 and considered as a chronic neutrophilic vasculitis [68].

The criteria for inclusion in the neutrophilic dermatoses group were as follows [65]:

1. Skin disorders characterized by an infiltration of the skin by normal neutrophils;
2. No infectious cause;
3. Diverse cutaneous features (pustules, plaques, nodules, ulcerations), with associations, overlaps and transitional forms;
4. Extracutaneous symptoms;
5. Association with systemic disorders;
6. Sensitivity to steroids and other anti-inflammatory drugs.

This group of "classic" neutrophilic dermatoses evolved over time, and clinical and biological arguments led to include other entities. The classification we proposed in 2006 [69] relies on clinical-pathological relationships, and is not very different from previous classifications [70]. This classification seems to have been well accepted, and forms the basis for the present book [71].

It can thus be said that in 2017, pyoderma gangrenosum represents the most severe form, and one of the prototypical forms, of the group of the neutrophilic dermatoses [6].

The overlap between PG and Sweet's syndrome was the first indication of a clinical spectrum. In line with the above arguments, many case reports appeared in the literature to describe patients with conditions representing overlaps or transitions or associations between the typical ND. Philip Cohen reviewed these reports of multiple neutrophilic dermatoses occurring either concurrently or sequentially in the same individual in the case of oncology patients [72]. But all patients, whether they suffer or not from cancer or a systemic inflammatory condition, may present with such neutrophilic dermatoses.

In addition to Sweet's syndrome, PG has been associated with subcorneal pustular dermatosis [73, 74], erythema elevatum diutinum [75] and many authors reported on a continuum of neutrophilic dermatoses, mainly in patients with an inflammatory bowel disease [76] but also in patients with rheumatoid arthritis [52]. Dermatologists may also be consulted for such atypical patients without any associated systemic disorder.

Early reports of atypical forms of dermatitis herpetiformis in patients with PG may be tentatively interpreted as an association between PG and SPD [41, 77].

PG of Internal Organs, or Extra-cutaneous PG

The possible occurrence of extra-cutaneous aseptic neutrophilic infiltrates is one of the characteristics of the neutrophilic dermatoses and could be called the neutrophilic disease [64]. Beyond the interest of this chapter for dermatologists, it is of paramount importance to heighten the awareness of all physicians, including medical specialists and surgeons of all specialties, on these aseptic, steroid-sensitive neutrophilic infiltrates or abscesses.

These internal localizations have previously been reviewed [78] and are exposed in detail in other chapters of this book. But overlap being unavoidable when dealing with the neutrophilic dermatoses, it seems appropriate to indicate here that patients with PG are among the most prone to these localizations, which may also be called "internal PG".

Overall, all organs may be involved. The clinical presentation is highly variable. Biopsies or other samplings show neutrophils, and cultures are negative. In some patients, many organs, in addition to the skin, may be involved concurrently or sequentially.

Lungs

Pulmonary aseptic neutrophilic infiltrates are the most frequent, or the least rare, of extra-cutaneous involvement in patients with PG [79, 80]. The symptoms are non-specific: cough, fever, dyspnea, chest pain. X-ray shows patchy infiltrates, pneumonia, or abscesses. Biopies or lavages show neutrophils, all bacterial investigations are negative. Many of these patients also have an associated systemic disease [81]. Pulmonary PG may be the initial manifestation of the disease [31, 32, 78]. More often, lung and skin lesions appear simultaneously. Pulmonary neutrophilic disease may be severe and even lethal, but in the majority of cases steroids or other anti-inflammatory drugs are efficient.

Joints

Joint manifestations are frequent in PG patients. In addition to inflammatory arthralgias, spondilytis, and different patterns of polyarthritis have been described [82]. Arthritis may precede PG, and result in disabling deformities.

Colitis arthritis designates the rheumatologic manifestations of patients with IBD. Some of them also have skin manifestations, including PG [83], and the term "colitis-arthritis-dermatitis" could be proposed.

The PAPA and related syndromes, also detailed in this book, are genetic diseases with PG, arthritis, and severe acne and/or hidradenitis suppurativa (acne inversa) [84].

Bone

Two bone disorders are considered as neutrophilic manifestations: sterile osteomyelitis, which occurs mainly in children [85] (chronic recurrent multifocal osteomyelitis) but may be found in adults [86] and SAPHO syndrome [87] which is a bony, articular and cutaneous neutrophilic disease.

Intra-abdominal Viscera

Aseptic abscesses of the spleen, the liver, the pancreas, the abdominal lymph nodes, have been described in patients who usually suffer from an inflammatory bowel disease [88]. Some of them have a neutrophilic dermatosis, including PG. Intra-abdominal PG and aseptic abscesses must be considered as identical.

Other Organs

Many case reports appeared in the literature in recent years to describe patients who suffer from an internal atypical localization of the neutrophilic disease. Again, all organs may be involved in patients with PG: the eye [52, 89] the aorta [90], muscles [91], the heart [92], the pituitary gland [93], the meninges [94] the kidney [95], the fallopian tube [96], and theoretically all body organs [77]. These are informative but rare situations. The patients with extra-cutaneous PG often have a severe disease and many of them also have an associated systemic disease. The conclusion is two-fold: in patients with PG, it is important to know that any systemic symptom may result from an aseptic neutrophilic extracutaneous infiltrate. But in patients with such symptoms in isolation, as in patients with intra-abdominal aseptic abscesses, a neutrophilic disease should also be suspected.

Associated Diseases

The frequency of associated multisystemic diseases is one of the hallmarks of PG. In Brunsting et al.'s original report [12], 4 out of 5 patients suffered from a severe ulcerative colitis. In the review of 86 patients from the Mayo Clinic published in 1985 by Powell et al. [2], 67 patients (78%) suffered from an associated disease. In more recent series, the frequency of associated diseases is however lower: around 50% for Bennett et al. [15] and Al Ghazal et al. [97]. The frequency of associated diseases in published series varies according to the type of recruitment (dermatologic, gastroenterologic, hematologic, rheumatologic, wound care centers) and the type of publication (patients' reports, literature review, hospital records or administrative data bases).

Ahronowitz et al. [98] reviewed the English literature on PG associations until 2010 and could find the reports of 214 patients with an inflammatory bowel disease, 83 patients with arthritis, 35 patients with a hematologic malignancy or abnormality, 36 patients with a monoclonal gammopathy; they also cite rare or questionable associations.

In many instances, the associated disease is already known, or easily diagnosed when discovered at the time of PG diagnosis and work-up. But PG may also precede this disease, thus justifying repeated follow-up [99, 100].

Inflammatory Bowel Disease

In all published series, IBD is the most common association, present in 20–30% of PG patients. PG affects between 1 and 2% of all patients with IBD [101, 102]. The relationship between the onset, the course, the severity and the response to treatment of PG and that of colitis varies among patients and no clear pattern emerges [103].

PG in patients with IBD (Crohn's disease and ulcerative colitis) can be the classic, ulcerative type, the superficial, pustular type, the polymorphous "vesiculo-pustular eruption of colitis", peristomal PG or be part of an overlapping neutrophilic dermatosis [75, 104].

Inflammatory Arthritis

As said earlier, joint symptoms are frequent, numerous and diverse in PG patients. These "articular PG" should be differentiated from a true association of PG with rheumatoid arthritis, whether sero-positive or sero-negative [81]. Temporal relationship between the articular and cutaneous symptoms is highly variable. Both acute, rapidly enlarging PG ulcers and chronic progressive lesions can be observed. PG must be considered in the diagnosis of leg ulcers, a frequent complication of rheumatoid arthritis [105].

Leukemia, Myelodysplasia

Hematologic malignancies, mainly acute myelogenous leukemia and myelodysplastic syndromes, but also lymphoma, monoclonal gammopathies and others, may be found in association with classic PG but are significantly linked with the bullous variant, which is often acute and overlaps with bullous, hemorrhagic Sweet syndrome [21, 61]. PG and other neutrophilic dermatoses such as Sweet syndrome are classically considered as non-specific, paraneoplastic manifestations of hematologic malignancies. But recent research showed immunologic and genetic similarities between the specific infiltrate of leukemia cutis and the infiltrate of the ND [106]. This area is currently under active investigation [107, 108].

Blood diseases associated with PG are often severe and are a major cause of death of PG patients.

Monoclonal Gammopathies

Monoclonal gammopathies of undetermined significance and multiple myeloma are a classic association of PG [109] and PG, whether classic or bullous, may reveal the gammopathy. The majority of PG-associated gammopathies are of the IgA type, although IgG-type gammopathies are overall much more frequent.

The relationship between IgA immunology, its systemic and its digestive components, and neutrophils physiology and pathology warrants future investigations.

Others

A recent survey suggests that PG is not rare among patients with granulomatosis with polyangiitis (GPA, formerly Wegener's granulomatosis) [110]. Inasmuch as GPA and other ANCA-associated vasculitis are usually considered as a differential diagnosis of PG, this point deserves further research. As well, the link between ANCA (anti-neutrophil cytoplasmic antibodies) and PG and other neutrophilic dermatoses is currently not understood.

In Japan, the association of PG with Takayasu's arteritis is frequent [111].

In addition to the well-established associated diseases and of the coexistence of PG with other ND, many reviews cite other associated diseases. The significance of these associations is variable; some are currently considered as anecdotal and coincidental.

Recent surveys pointed out new possible associations, such as depression, hepatitis, diabetes mellitus, or the metabolic syndrome [16, 96]. Their significance is unclear, but they point out that all PG patients must benefit from a careful work-up, guided by clinical examination.

Pathophysiology

Pyoderma gangrenosum is characterized by a limited tissue destruction attributed to the toxic effects of enzymes and mediators contained in the neutrophil cell. It has soon become evident that infectious agents were not responsible for the neutrophil attraction, and an intrinsic neutrophilic abnormality has never been demonstrated. So current research focuses on immune disturbances and more specifically on autoinflammation [112]. Autoinflammation, recently discovered, results in an inappropriate activation of innate immunity, including an overproduction of IL-1, a master cytokine of inflammation, capable among other properties of attracting and activating PMNs [113]. Autoinflammation is the mechanism underlying many diseases, both monogenic and polygenic [114]. These diseases have very diverse clinical expressions. The precise mechanism of tissue destruction in PG has not yet been discovered. Following chapters of this book will detail the present state of knowledge on autoinflammation and its link with the pathogenesis of PG and other neutrophilic dermatoses.

Past Studies: Neutrophil Function

Studies conducted in very few cases provided inconsistent results and the role of a neutrophil dysfunction could only be suspected [115]. Drugs directly acting on the neutrophils, like dapsone or colchicine, are effective in subacute PG.

Current Studies: Genetics, Autoinflammation and Immune Regulation

In 1997, Lindor et al. [116] described the PAPA syndrome, a rare autosomal dominant disease characterized by the association of Pyogenic Arthritis, Pyoderma gangrenosum and Acne. The PAPA syndrome is due to mutations in the PSTPIP1 (proline-serine-threonine-phosphatase interactive protein) gene. PSTPIP1 is a ligand for pyrin and inhibits the activation of the inflammasome and the subsequent expression of IL-1 β. The lack of inhibition in PAPA syndrome induces the inflammatory manifestations. This discovery led to the study of the role of autoinflammation and IL-1 activation not only in PAPA and related monogenic syndromes (PASH, PAPASH) but also in non genetic PG. Nesterovitch et al. indeed evidenced genetic abnormalities of the PSTPIP1 gene in patients with non-familial, classic PG [117]. Other genetic abnormalities appear to underlie PG [118], which gives clues to the existence of genetic vartiants, which remain to be more precisely studied.

In addition to innate immune dysregulation, activation of T-cell immunity has also been investigated and researchers found evidence of T-cell clonal expansion in the blood and the skin of patients with PG [119] as well as a decrease in the ratio between regulatory T cells and effector Th17 cells [120]. These data have been confirmed by Angelo Valerio Marzano'group who showed that PG inflammation involves a TH1/TH17 activation [121].

The main cytokines implicated in PG's inflammation are IL-8 [122], IL-1 β, TNF-α and IL-17 [123]. More details will be given on the pathophysiology of PG in the second part of this book. It is important to note that targeted inhibition of the overactive cytokines may represent a valuable therapeutic approach for PG patients.

Treatment

Given the heterogeneity of the disease, the treatment of PG patients is always individualized and requires a step wise, pragmatic approach. The choice of therapy relies on the course of the disease, mild/chronic or acute/aggressive, its extent and severity, the co-morbidities, the expected tolerance of the treatment, the preferences of the patient and the experience of the physician. There are no official guidelines but the available literature provides a rather solid guide [124, 125]. Clinicians should update this guide regularly.

General Support and Pain Relief

Many patients with PG are severely affected and need hospitalization for general work-up directed at systemic PG, associated diseases and other conditions, and for the start of treatment. They also need psychological support and reassurance.

The treatment of the associated disease is always necessary, but most often fails to control PG.

Pain relief is important and relies on adequate pain medications, according to established guidelines. The rapid alleviation of pain is one of the criteria of efficacy of systemic corticosteroids. While on treatment, the side effects of the drugs used must be prevented and closely monitored. It is beyond the scope of this chapter to detail the many problems encountered by patients treated by potent anti-inflammatory/immune-suppressive agents. In this respect, PG patients do not differ from patients with other, similarly treated conditions.

Systemic Therapy

Except for mild cases and localized granulomatous PG, systemic treatment is always necessary. This treatment must alleviate acute flares, but also suppress the inflammatory process on the long term. The total duration of the treatment of PG is between 6 and 18 months.

Classic Anti-inflammatory/Immunosuppressive Agents

The two first-line agents, of proven and fast efficacy, are prednisone and cyclosporine. This has been established by a careful review of the literature [125]; these two drugs have recently been shown to be equally effective [126].

Greco and Wright were the first in 1956 to report on the efficacy of cortisone on PG [127]. This finding was important in pointing out the inflammatory nature of PG.

Prednisone is prescribed in the majority of patients, and oral doses equal or superior to 1 mg/kg daily, initially in divided doses, are necessary. The efficacy is visible in a few days: general improvement, diminution of pain, halting of the expansion, flattening of the elevated border of the ulcers, clearing of the inflammatory periphery. The subsequent tapering of prednisone is based on the clinical response and the tolerance. The total duration of the treatment is generally between 6 and 12 months. In the majority of cases, another drug is added as a steroid-sparing agent.

Mycophenolate mofetil is usually chosen [128]. Other immunosuppressive agents may be used, such as azathioprine, cyclophosphamide, or methotrexate.

Ciclosporine is also effective in the treatment of PG, the average dose being 3–5 mg/kg daily. The clinical efficacy is probably close to the one of corticosteroids. The safety may be better, and the side effects profile is different [124].

In mild, slowly progressive PG, dapsone, colchicine, thalidomide, clofazimine, minocycline, have been used with success, according to the case reports published, which have been reviewed [97, 122, 129].

In steroid-resistant, steroid-intolerant or acute refractory cases, intravenous immunoglobulins may be indicated [130].

Biologic Agents

The use of biologic agents in PG has been stimulated by its association with diseases thus treated and by recent research on the molecules implicated in autoinflammation.

A randomized clinical trial showed that infliximab is more efficient than placebo in the treatment of PG, whether it is associated with an inflammatory bowel disease or not [131]. Other anti-TNF-α agents, like adalimumab or etanercept, are probably of equal efficacy [132].

Following research on auto-inflammation, anti-IL-1 β agents have been used with success in the treatment of PG: anakinra, a recombinant IL-1 receptor antagonist [133], and canakinumab, a monoclonal antibody directed against IL-1 β [134]. Biologics directed against IL-12/IL-23, and against IL-17, will probably be tested in a near future and this field is expected to evolve rapidly.

Combination Therapy

Published clinical trials usually deal with only one agent. But the reviews on PG series and the experience of physicians managing patients with PG show that in the majority of cases, more than one agent is needed, concurrently or sequentially. These combination therapies, or multi-drug therapies, are intended to increase efficacy and decrease side effects. In practice, classic agents, biologic agents, in addition to the topical treatment which will be considered below, are all needed and their use, although common, is not standardized [16, 135].

Topical Therapy

Wound Care

PG is a chronic wound and the principles of wound care may be applied. With one caveat: pathergy is always present or threatening. So cleansing and dressing must be gentle and avoid all trauma, like aggressive debridement. Absorptive dressings are used on exudating ulcerations. Surrounding areas may be protected by petrolatum-impregnated dressings. Infection is uncommon but must be prevented and treated if present.

Topical Anti-inflammatory Agents

Topical anti-inflammatory therapy may be efficient as a monotherapy in cases of small lesions, or in the particular case of vegetating PG. In other, more common situations, it is used an as adjunct to systemic therapy and may help reducing oral steroids dosage [136]. Topical potent corticosteroids and topical tacrolimus may be used. The application of these agents to ulcerations leads to systemic absorption [137]. Intralesional corticosteroids may also be used, for example in peritsomal PG.

The Place of Surgery

In general, surgery in PG is the consequence of a misdiagnosis and has deleterious consequences. But when anti-inflammatory treatment has shown efficacy, pathergy is less likely to occur. At this time, gentle debridement can be carefully performed; various techniques of skin grafting may accelerate healing.

Conclusion

Pyoderma gangrenosum is a rare chronic cutaneous and systemic disease, considered as the most severe, and the prototype, of the neutrophilic dermatoses.

Its clinical heterogeneity is best understood in the context of its belonging to the ND spectrum.

The diagnosis of PG requires an experienced clinical evaluation, examination of a skin biopsy, and a careful exclusion of all known causes of skin ulcerations.

The possibility of extracutaneous PG must be considered in all patients.

Associated diseases are very frequent. Only about one fifth of PG have no associated disease.

The treatment of PG is a long task, requiring personalized pragmatic use of anti-inflammatory systemic therapy and wound care competences.

Ongoing research is expected to improve the diagnosis and management of PG.

Acknowledgement I am indebted to Professor Frank Powell, MD, for fruitful and friendly discussions, in addition to his outstanding writings and lectures on pyoderma gangrenosum.

References

1. Langan SM, Groves RW, Card TR, Gulliford MC. Incidence, mortality, and disease associations of pyoderma gangrenosum in the United Kingdom: a retrospective cohort study. J Invest Dermatol. 2012;132:2166–70.
2. Powell FC, Schroeter AL, Su WP, Perry HO. Pyoderma gangrenosum: a review of 86 patients. Q J Med. 1985;55:173–86.
3. Callen JP. Pyoderma gangrenosum. Lancet. 1998;351:581–5.

4. Powell FC, Collins S. Pyoderma gangrenosum. Clin Dermatol. 2000;18:283–93.
5. Su WP, Davis MD, Weenig RH, Powell FC, Perry HO. Pyoderma gangrenosum: clinicopathologic correlation and proposed diagnostic criteria. Int J Dermatol. 2004;43:790–800.
6. Wallach D, Vignon-Pennamen MD. Pyoderma gangrenosum and Sweet syndrome: the prototypic neutrophilic dermatoses. Br J Dermatol. 2015. https://doi.org/10.1111/bjd.13955.
7. Brocq L, Simon CL. Contribution à l'étude du phagédénisme. Bull. Soc Méd. Hôp. 1908;25:290–307. Paris 3eme série.
8. Brocq L. Nouvelle contribution à l'étude du phagédénisme géométrique. Ann Dermatol Syph. 1916;6:1–39. 5ème série.
9. Cullen TS. A progressively enlarging ulcer of the abdominal wall involving the skin and fat following drainage of an abdominal abscess apparently of appendiceal origin. Surg Gynecol Obstet. 1924;28:579–82.
10. Brewer GE, Meleney FL. Progressive gangrenous infection of the skin and subcutaneous tissues, following operation for acute perforative appendicitis: a study in symbiosis. Ann Surg. 1926;84:438–50.
11. Tixier, Pollosson, Arnulf. La gangrène post-opératoire progressive de la peau et son traitement. Presse médicale. 1937;64:1163–4.
12. Brunsting LA, Goeckerman WH, O'Leary PA. Pyoderma (ecthyma) gangrenosum. Arch Dermatol Syphilol. 1930;22:655–80.
13. Greenbaum SS. Phagedaena geometrica (Brocq). Arch Dermatol Syphilol. 1941;43:775–801.
14. Liu JW, Hsu NY, Huang TC. Pustules and bacteraemia. Lancet. 1997;350:860.
15. Bennett ML, Jackson JM, Jorizzo JL, Fleischer AB Jr, White WL, Callen JP. Pyoderma gangrenosum. A comparison of typical and atypical forms with an emphasis on time to remission. Case review of 86 patients from 2 institutions. Medicine (Baltimore). 2000;79:37–46.
16. Binus AM, Qureshi AA, Li VW, Winterfield LS. Pyoderma gangrenosum: a retrospective review of patient characteristics, comorbidities and therapy in 103 patients. Br J Dermatol. 2011;165:1244–50.
17. Powell FC, Su WP, Perry HO. Pyoderma gangrenosum: classification and management. J Am Acad Dermatol. 1996;34:395–409.
18. O'Loughlin S, Perry HO. A diffuse pustular eruption associated with ulcerative colitis. Arch Dermatol. 1978;114:1061–4.
19. Levitt MD, Ritchie JK, Lennard-Jones JE, Phillips RK. Pyoderma gangrenosum in inflammatory bowel disease. Br J Surg. 1991;78:676–8.
20. Fenske NA, Gern JE, Pierce D, Vasey FB. Vesiculopustular eruption of ulcerative colitis. Arch Dermatol. 1983;119:664–9.
21. Perry HO, Winkelmann RK. Bullous pyoderma gangrenosum and leukemia. Arch Dermatol. 1972;106:901–5.
22. Ho KK, Otridge BW, Vandenberg E, Powell FC. Pyoderma gangrenosum, polycythemia rubra vera, and the development of leukemia. J Am Acad Dermatol. 1992;27:804–8.
23. Jacobs P, Palmer S, Gordon-Smith EC. Pyoderma gangrenosum in myelodysplasia and acute leukaemia. Postgrad Med J. 1985;61:689–94.
24. Wilson-Jones E, Winkelmann RK. Superficial granulomatous pyoderma: a localized vegetative form of pyoderma gangrenosum. J Am Acad Dermatol. 1988;18:511–21.
25. Langan SM, Powell FC. Vegetative pyoderma gangrenosum: a report of two new cases and a review of the literature. Int J Dermatol. 2005;44:623–9.
26. Rashid RM. Seat belt pyoderma gangrenosum: minor pressure as a causative factor. J Eur Acad Dermatol Venereol. 2008;22:1273–4.
27. McGarity WC, Robertson DB, McKeown PP, Amerson JR, Darden WA. Pyoderma gangrenosum at the parastomal site in patients with Crohn's disease. Arch Surg. 1984;119:1186–8.
28. Zuo KJ, Fung E, Tredget EE, Lin AN. A systematic review of post-surgical pyoderma gangrenosum: identification of risk factors and proposed management strategy. J Plast Reconstr Aesthet Surg. 2015;68:295–303.

29. Tolkachjov SN, Fahy AS, Wetter DA, Brough KR, Bridges AG, Davis MD, et al. Postoperative pyoderma gangrenosum (PG): the Mayo Clinic experience of 20 years from 1994 through 2014. J Am Acad Dermatol. 2015;73:615–22.
30. Lê Huu S, Spertini F, Roggero P, Egloff DV, Raffoul W. Pyoderma gangrenosum: a rare pathology or an omitted diagnosis? Ann Chir Plast Esthet. 2009;54:82–7.
31. Kitagawa KH, Grassi M. Primary pyoderma gangrenosum of the lungs. J Am Acad Dermatol. 2008;59:S114–6.
32. Field S, Powell FC, Young V, Barnes L. Pyoderma gangrenosum manifesting as a cavitating lung lesion. Clin Exp Dermatol. 2008;33:418–21.
33. Roujeau JC. Neutrophilic drug eruptions. Clin Dermatol. 2000;18:331–7.
34. Lewerin C, Mobacken H, Nilsson-Ehle H, Swolin B. Bullous pyoderma gangrenosum in a patient with myelodysplastic syndrome during granulocyte colony-stimulating factor therapy. Leuk Lymphoma. 1997;26:629–32.
35. Tinoco MP, Tamler C, Maciel G, Soares D, Avelleira JC, Azulay D. Pyoderma gangrenosum following isotretinoin therapy for acne nodulocystic. Int J Dermatol. 2008;47:953–6.
36. Yurci A, Guven K, Torun E, Gursoy S, Baskol M, Akgun H, et al. Pyoderma gangrenosum and exacerbation of psoriasis resulting from pegylated interferon alpha and ribavirin treatment of chronic hepatitis C. Eur J Gastroenterol Hepatol. 2007;19:811–5.
37. Crittenden SC, Gilbert JE, Callen JP. Hydroxyurea-induced leg ulceration in a patient with a homozygous MTHFR polymorphism misdiagnosed as pyoderma gangrenosum. JAMA Dermatol. 2014;150:780–1.
38. Peterson LL. Hydralazine-induced systemic lupus erythematosus presenting as pyoderma gangrenosum-like ulcers. J Am Acad Dermatol. 1984;10:379–84.
39. Pralong P, Debarbieux S, Paret N, Balme B, Depaepe L, Nosbaum A, et al. Recurrent pyoderma gangrenosum-like ulcers induced by oral anticoagulants. Ann Dermatol Venereol. 2014;141:34–8.
40. Jiménez-Gallo D, Albarrán-Planelles C, Linares-Barrios M, Rodríguez-Hernández C, Martínez-Rodríguez A, García-Moreno E, et al. Pyoderma gangrenosum and Wegener granulomatosis-like syndrome induced by cocaine. Clin Exp Dermatol. 2013;38:878–82.
41. Perry HO, Brunsting LA. Pyoderma gangrenosum; a clinical study of nineteen cases. AMA Arch Derm. 1957;75(3):380–6.
42. Rudolph BM, Staib F, Von Stebut E, Hainz M, Grabbe S, Loquai C. Neutrophilic disease of the skin and intestines after ipilimumab treatment for malignant melanoma—simultaneous occurrence of pyoderma gangrenosum and colitis. Eur J Dermatol. 2014;24:268–9.
43. Pinato DJ, Sharma R. Imatinib induced pyoderma gangrenosum. J Postgrad Med. 2013;59:244–5.
44. Boudny C, Nievergelt H, Braathen LR, Simon D. Wegener's granulomatosis presenting as pyoderma gangrenosum. J Dtsch Dermatol Ges. 2008;6:477–9.
45. Del Pozo J, Sacristán F, Martínez W, Paradela S, Fernández-Jorge B, Fonseca E. Neutrophilic dermatosis of the hands: presentation of eight cases and review of the literature. J Dermatol. 2007;34:243–7.
46. Lebbé C, Moulonguet-Michau I, Perrin P, Blanc F, Frija J, Civatte J. Steroid-responsive pyoderma gangrenosum with vulvar and pulmonary involvement. J Am Acad Dermatol. 1992;27:623–5.
47. Farrell AM, Black MM, Bracka A, Bunker CB. Pyoderma gangrenosum of the penis. Br J Dermatol. 1998;138:337–40.
48. Kennedy KS, Prendergast ML, Sooy CD. Pyoderma gangrenosum of the oral cavity, nose, and larynx. Otolaryngol Head Neck Surg. 1987;97:487–90.
49. Storwick GS, Prihoda MB, Fulton RJ, Wood WS. Pyodermatitis-pyostomatitis vegetans: a specific marker for inflammatory bowel disease. J Am Acad Dermatol. 1994;31:336–41.
50. Rose GE, Barnes EA, Uddin JM. Pyoderma gangrenosum of the ocular adnexa: a rare condition with characteristic clinical appearances. Ophthalmology. 2003;110:801–5.
51. Newman WD, Frank HJ. Pyoderma gangrenosum of the orbit. Eye (Lond). 1993;7:89–94.

52. Wilson DM, John GR, Callen JP. Peripheral ulcerative keratitis—an extracutaneous neutrophilic disorder: report of a patient with rheumatoid arthritis, pustular vasculitis, pyoderma gangrenosum, and Sweet's syndrome with an excellent response to cyclosporine therapy. J Am Acad Dermatol. 1999;40:331–4.
53. Su WP, Schroeter AL, Perry HO, Powell FC. Histopathologic and immunopathologic study of pyoderma gangrenosum. J Cutan Pathol. 1986;13:323–30.
54. Maverakis E, Ma C, Shinkai K, Fiorentino D, Callen J, Wollina U, et al. Diagnostic criteria of ulcerative pyoderma gangrenosum: a Delphi consensus of international experts. JAMA Dermatol. 2018. https://doi.org/10.1001/jamadermatol.2017.5980.
55. Wong WW, Machado GR, Hill ME. Pyoderma gangrenosum: the great pretender and a challenging diagnosis. J Cutan Med Surg. 2011;15:322–8.
56. Hadi A, Lebwohl M. Clinical features of pyoderma gangrenosum and current diagnostic trends. J Am Acad Dermatol. 2011;64:950–4.
57. Weenig RH, Davis MD, Dahl PR, Su WP. Skin ulcers misdiagnosed as pyoderma gangrenosum. N Engl J Med. 2002;347:1412–8.
58. Hafner J, Nobbe S, Partsch H, Läuchli S, Mayer D, Amann-Vesti B, et al. Martorell hypertensive ischemic leg ulcer: a model of ischemic subcutaneous arteriolosclerosis. Arch Dermatol. 2010;146:961–8.
59. Nguyen KH, Miller JJ, Helm KF. Case reports and a review of the literature on ulcers mimicking pyoderma gangrenosum. Int J Dermatol. 2003;42:84–94.
60. Harries MJ, McMullen E, Griffiths CE. Pyoderma gangrenosum masquerading as dermatitis artefacta. Arch Dermatol. 2006;142:1509–10.
61. Burton JL. Sweet's syndrome, pyoderma gangrenosum and acute leukaemia. Br J Dermatol. 1980;102:239.
62. Caughman W, Stern R, Haynes H. Neutrophilic dermatosis of myeloproliferative disorders. Atypical forms of pyoderma gangrenosum and Sweet's syndrome associated with myeloproliferative disorders. J Am Acad Dermatol. 1983;9:751–8.
63. Benton EC, Rutherford D, Hunter JA. Sweet's syndrome and pyoderma gangrenosum associated with ulcerative colitis. Acta Derm Venereol. 1985;65:77–80.
64. Davies MG, Hastings A. Sweet's syndrome progressing to pyoderma gangrenosum—a spectrum of neutrophilic skin disease in association with cryptogenic cirrhosis. Clin Exp Dermatol. 1991;16:279–82.
65. Vignon-Pennamen MD, Wallach D. Cutaneous manifestations of neutrophilic disease. A study of seven cases. Dermatologica. 1991;183:255–64.
66. Wallach D. Les dermatoses neutrophiliques. Presse Med. 1991;20:105–7.
67. Sneddon IB, Wilkinson DS. Subcorneal pustular dermatosis. Br J Dermatol. 1956;68:385–94.
68. Radcliffe-Crocker H, Williams C. Erythema elevatum diutinum. Br J Dermatol. 1894;6:33–8.
69. Wallach D, Vignon-Pennamen MD. From acute febrile neutrophilic dermatosis to neutrophilic disease: forty years of clinical research. J Am Acad Dermatol. 2006;55:1066–71.
70. Moschella SL. Review of so-called aseptic neutrophilic dermatoses. Australas J Dermatol. 1983;24:55–62.
71. Wallach D. The neutrophilic dermatoses. Overview. In this volume.
72. Cohen PR. Neutrophilic dermatoses occurring in oncology patients. Int J Dermatol. 2007;46:106–11.
73. Scerri L, Zaki I, Allen BR. Pyoderma gangrenosum and subcorneal pustular dermatosis, without monoclonal gammopathy. Br J Dermatol. 1994;130:398–9.
74. Cartier H, Plantin P, Leroy JP, Larzul JJ. Pyoderma gangrenosum, subcorneal IgA pustulosis and recurrent neutrophilic pleural and pulmonary diseases in a patient with IgA gammopathy. Ann Dermatol Venereol. 1995;122:97–101.
75. Caucanas M, Heylen A, Rolland F, Müller G, Olemans C, Sass U, et al. Associated pyoderma gangrenosum, erythema elevatum diutinum, and Sweet's syndrome: the concept of neutrophilic disease. Int J Dermatol. 2013;52:1185–8.

76. Mendoza JL, García-Paredes J, Peña AS, Cruz-Santamaría DM, Iglesias C, Díaz Rubio M. A continuous spectrum of neutrophilic dermatoses in Crohn's disease. Rev Esp Enferm Dig. 2003;95:233–6, 229–32.
77. Ayres S Jr, Ayres S 3rd. Pyoderma gangrenosum with an unusual syndrome of ulcers, vesicles, and arthritis. AMA Arch Derm. 1958;77:269–78.
78. Vignon-Pennamen MD. The extracutaneous involvement in the neutrophilic dermatoses. Clin Dermatol. 2000;18:339–47.
79. McCulloch AJ, McEvoy A, Jackson JD, Jarvis EH. Severe steroid responsive pneumonitis associated with pyoderma gangrenosum and ulcerative colitis. Thorax. 1985;40: 314–5.
80. Vignon-Pennamen MD, Zelinsky-Gurung A, Janssen F, Frija J, Wallach D. Pyoderma gangrenosum with pulmonary involvement. Arch Dermatol. 1989;125:1239–42.
81. Fukuhara K, Urano Y, Kimura S, Hori K, Arase S. Pyoderma gangrenosum with rheumatoid arthritis and pulmonary aseptic abscess responding to treatment with dapsone. Br J Dermatol. 1998;139:556–8.
82. Holt PJ, Davies MG, Saunders KC, Nuki G. Pyoderma gangrenosum: clinical and laboratory findings in 15 patients with special reference to polyarthritis. Medicine (Baltimore). 1980;59:114–33.
83. Wright V, Watkinson G. The arthritis of ulcerative colitis. Br Med J. 1965;2(5463):670–5.
84. Marzano AV, Borghi A, Meroni PL, Cugno M. Pyoderma gangrenosum and its syndromic forms: evidence for a link with autoinflammation. Br J Dermatol. 2016;175(5):882–91. https://doi.org/10.1111/bjd.14691.
85. Schaen L, Sheth AP. Skin ulcers associated with a tender and swollen arm. Pyoderma gangrenosum (PG) in association with chronic recurrent multifocal osteomyelitis (CRMO). Arch Dermatol. 1998;134(9):1146–7, 1149–50.
86. Yoshida C, Kojima H, Ishigaki T, Katsura Y, Kaneko S, Suzukawa K, et al. Association of pyoderma gangrenosum and sterile osteomyelitis in a patient having myelodysplastic syndrome with der(1;7)(q10;q10). Eur J Haematol. 2004;72:149–53.
87. Claudepierre P, Clerc D, Cariou D, Lavabre C, Venencie PY, Bisson M. SAPHO syndrome and pyoderma gangrenosum: is it fortuitous? J Rheumatol. 1996;23:400–2.
88. André MF, Piette JC, Kémény JL, Ninet J, Jego P, Delèvaux I, et al. French Study Group on Aseptic Abscesses. Aseptic abscesses: a study of 30 patients with or without inflammatory bowel disease and review of the literature. Medicine (Baltimore). 2007;86:145–61.
89. Maringe E, Gueudry J, Joly P, Muraine M. Nodular scleritis associated with pyoderma gangrenosum. J Fr Ophtalmol. 2015;38:171–3.
90. Linck V, Sanchez B, Baubion E, Molinie V, Deligny C, Quist D, et al. Pyoderma gangrenosum and neutrophilic aortitis preceding the development of rheumatoid arthritis. Ann Dermatol Venereol. 2015;142:425–9.
91. Marie I, Levesque H, Joly P, Reumont G, Courville P, Baudrimont M, et al. Neutrophilic myositis as an extracutaneous manifestation of neutrophilic dermatosis. J Am Acad Dermatol. 2001;44:137–9.
92. Koester G, Tarnower A, Levisohn D, Burgdorf W. Bullous pyoderma gangrenosum. J Am Acad Dermatol. 1993;29:875–8.
93. Chanson P, Timsit J, Kujas M, Violante A, Guillausseau PJ, Derome PJ, et al. Pituitary granuloma and pyoderma gangrenosum. J Endocrinol Invest. 1990;13:677–81.
94. Urano S, Kodama H, Kato K, Nogura K. Pyoderma gangrenosum with systemic involvement. J Dermatol. 1995;22:515–9.
95. Carvalho LR, Zanuncio VV, Gontijo B. Pyoderma gangrenosum with renal and splenic impairment—case report. An Bras Dermatol. 2013;88:150–3.
96. Dinulescu M, Vigy P, Droitcourt C, Adamski H, Rioux N, Bretagne JF, et al. Pyoderma gangrenosum and aseptic pyosalpinx in a pregnant patient. Ann Dermatol Venereol. 2007;134:179–80.

97. Al Ghazal P, Herberger K, Schaller J, Strölin A, Hoff NP, Goerge T, et al. Associated factors and comorbidities in patients with pyoderma gangrenosum in Germany: a retrospective multicentric analysis in 259 patients. Orphanet J Rare Dis. 2013;8:136.
98. Ahronowitz I, Harp J, Shinkai K. Etiology and management of pyoderma gangrenosum: a comprehensive review. Am J Clin Dermatol. 2012;13:191–211.
99. Decherd JW, Leyden JJ, Holtzapple PG. Facial pyoderma gangrenosum preceding ulcerative colitis. Cutis. 1974;14:208–10.
100. Schlick K, Regauer S, Beham-Schmid C, Cerroni L, Rohn A, Deutsch AJ, et al. Pyoderma gangrenosum heralding acute leukemia for months: diagnostic hint written on the skin. J Clin Oncol. 2011;29:e506–8.
101. Mir-Madjlessi SH, Taylor JS, Farmer RG. Clinical course and evolution of erythema nodosum and pyoderma gangrenosum in chronic ulcerative colitis: a study of 42 patients. Am J Gastroenterol. 1985;80:615–20.
102. Farhi D, Cosnes J, Zizi N, Chosidow O, Seksik P, Beaugerie L, et al. Significance of erythema nodosum and pyoderma gangrenosum in inflammatory bowel diseases: a cohort study of 2402 patients. Medicine (Baltimore). 2008;87:281–93.
103. Marzano AV, Ishak RS, Saibeni S, Crosti C, Meroni PL, Cugno M. Autoinflammatory skin disorders in inflammatory bowel diseases, pyoderma gangrenosum and Sweet's syndrome: a comprehensive review and disease classification criteria. Clin Rev Allergy Immunol. 2013;45:202–10.
104. Salmon P, Rademaker M, Edwards L. A continuum of neutrophilic disease occurring in a patient with ulcerative colitis. Australas J Dermatol. 1998;39:116–8.
105. Seitz CS, Berens N, Bröcker EB, Trautmann A. Leg ulceration in rheumatoid arthritis--an underreported multicausal complication with considerable morbidity: analysis of thirty-six patients and review of the literature. Dermatology. 2010;220:268–73.
106. Vignon-Pennamen MD, Aractingi S. Sweet's syndrome and leukemia cutis: a common skin homing mechanism? Dermatology. 2003;206:81–4.
107. Sujobert P, Cuccuini W, Vignon-Pennamen MD, Martin-Garcia N, Albertini AF, Uzunov M, et al. Evidence of differentiation in myeloid malignancies associated neutrophilic dermatosis: a fluorescent in situ hybridization study of 14 patients. J Invest Dermatol. 2013;133:1111–4.
108. Haga N, Iwata H, Yamaguchi Y, Shirato T, Nishimura K, Yamane N, et al. Mucocutaneous pyoderma gangrenosum due to trisomy 8 neutrophilic infiltrates in a patient with myelodysplastic syndrome. Br J Dermatol. 2016;174:239–41.
109. Powell FC, Schroeter AL, Su WP, Perry HO. Pyoderma gangrenosum and monoclonal gammopathy. Arch Dermatol. 1983;119:468–72.
110. de Boysson H, Martin Silva N, de Moreuil C, Néel A, de Menthon M, Meyer O, et al. French Vasculitis Study Group, French Internal Medicine Society. Neutrophilic dermatoses in antineutrophil cytoplasmic antibody-associated vasculitis: a French multicenter study of 17 cases and literature review. Medicine (Baltimore). 2016;95:e2957.
111. Ujiie H, Sawamura D, Yokota K, Nishie W, Shichinohe R, Shimizu H. Pyoderma gangrenosum associated with Takayasu's arteritis. Clin Exp Dermatol. 2004;29:357–9.
112. Farasat S, Aksentijevich I, Toro JR. Autoinflammatory diseases: clinical and genetic advances. Arch Dermatol. 2008;144:392–402.
113. Lachmann HJ, Quartier P, So A, Hawkins PN. The emerging role of interleukin-1β in autoinflammatory diseases. Arthritis Rheum. 2011;63:314–24.
114. Butler D, Shinkai K. What do autoinflammatory syndromes teach about common cutaneous diseases such as pyoderma gangrenosum? A commentary. Dermatol Clin. 2013;31:427–35.
115. Braswell SF, Kostopoulos TC, Ortega-Loayza AG. Pathophysiology of pyoderma gangrenosum (PG): an updated review. J Am Acad Dermatol. 2015;73:691–8.
116. Lindor NM, Arsenault TM, Solomon H, Seidman CE, McEvoy MT. A new autosomal dominant disorder of pyogenic sterile arthritis, pyoderma gangrenosum, and acne: PAPA syndrome. Mayo Clin Proc. 1997;72:611–5.

117. Nesterovitch AB, Hoffman MD, Simon M, Petukhov PA, Tharp MD, Glant TT. Mutations in the PSTPIP1 gene and aberrant splicing variants in patients with pyoderma gangrenosum. Clin Exp Dermatol. 2011;36:889–95.
118. DeFilippis EM, Feldman SR, Huang WW. The genetics of pyoderma gangrenosum and implications for treatment: a systematic review. Br J Dermatol. 2015;172:1487–97.
119. Brooklyn TN, Williams AM, Dunnill MG, Probert CS. T-cell receptor repertoire in pyoderma gangrenosum: evidence for clonal expansions and trafficking. Br J Dermatol. 2007;157:960–6.
120. Caproni M, Antiga E, Volpi W, Verdelli A, Venegoni L, Quaglino P, et al. The Treg/Th17 cell ratio is reduced in the skin lesions of patients with pyoderma gangrenosum. Br J Dermatol. 2015;173:275–8.
121. Quaglino P, Fava P, Caproni M, Antiga E, De Simone C, Papini M, et al. Phenotypical characterization of circulating cell subsets in pyoderma gangrenosum patients: the experience of the Italian immuno-pathology group. J Eur Acad Dermatol Venereol. 2016;30:655–8.
122. Oka M. Pyoderma gangrenosum and interleukin 8. Br J Dermatol. 2007;157:1279–81.
123. Marzano AV, Fanoni D, Antiga E, Quaglino P, Caproni M, Crosti C, et al. Expression of cytokines, chemokines and other effector molecules in two prototypic autoinflammatory skin diseases, pyoderma gangrenosum and Sweet's syndrome. Clin Exp Immunol. 2014;178:48–56.
124. Chow RK, Ho VC. Treatment of pyoderma gangrenosum. J Am Acad Dermatol. 1996;34:1047–60.
125. Miller J, Yentzer BA, Clark A, Jorizzo JL, Feldman SR. Pyoderma gangrenosum: a review and update on new therapies. J Am Acad Dermatol. 2010;62:646–54.
126. Ormerod AD, Thomas KS, Craig FE, Mitchell E, Greenlaw N, Norrie J, et al. Dermatology Clinical Trials Network's STOP GAP Team. Comparison of the two most commonly used treatments for pyoderma gangrenosum: results of the STOP GAP randomised controlled trial. BMJ. 2015;350:h2958.
127. Greco DJ, Wright ET. Pyoderma gangrenosum; report of a case controlled by cortisone. AMA Arch Derm. 1956;74:543–6.
128. Li J, Kelly R. Treatment of pyoderma gangrenosum with mycophenolate mofetil as a steroid-sparing agent. J Am Acad Dermatol. 2013;69:565–9.
129. Reichrath J, Bens G, Bonowitz A, Tilgen W. Treatment recommendations for pyoderma gangrenosum: an evidence-based review of the literature based on more than 350 patients. J Am Acad Dermatol. 2005;53:273–83.
130. Cummins DL, Anhalt GJ, Monahan T, Meyerle JH. Treatment of pyoderma gangrenosum with intravenous immunoglobulin. Br J Dermatol. 2007;157:1235–9.
131. Brooklyn TN, Dunnill MG, Shetty A, Bowden JJ, Williams JD, Griffiths CE, et al. Infliximab for the treatment of pyoderma gangrenosum: a randomised, double blind, placebo controlled trial. Gut. 2006;55:505–9.
132. Jacob SE, Weisman RS, Kerdel FA. Pyoderma gangrenosum—rebel without a cure? Int J Dermatol. 2008;47:192–4.
133. Brenner M, Ruzicka T, Plewig G, Thomas P, Herzer P. Targeted treatment of pyoderma gangrenosum in PAPA (pyogenic arthritis, pyoderma gangrenosum and acne) syndrome with the recombinant human interleukin-1 receptor antagonist anakinra. Br J Dermatol. 2009;161:1199–201.
134. Kolios AG, Maul JT, Meier B, Kerl K, Traidl-Hoffmann C, Hertl M, et al. Canakinumab in adults with steroid-refractory pyoderma gangrenosum. Br J Dermatol. 2015;173:1216–23.
135. Patel F, Fitzmaurice S, Duong C, He Y, Fergus J, Raychaudhuri SP, et al. Effective strategies for the management of pyoderma gangrenosum: a comprehensive review. Acta Derm Venereol. 2015;95:525–31.
136. Wenzel J, Gerdsen R, Phillipp-Dormston W, Bieber T, Uerlich M. Topical treatment of pyoderma gangrenosum. Dermatology. 2002;205:221–3.
137. Ghislain PD, De Decker I, Lachapelle JM. Efficacy and systemic absorption of topical tacrolimus used in pyoderma gangrenosum. Br J Dermatol. 2004;150:1052–3.

Aseptic Abscesses Syndrome

7

Marc André

Introduction and Overview

The concept of an aseptic abscesses (AA) syndrome emerged in the late 1980s and early 1990s. Although AA share common features and are sometimes associated with neutrophilic dermatoses (ND), AA syndrome should be considered as a separate entity and not as only extra-cutaneous localizations of ND, mainly because the deep locations are in many cases the sole feature of AA syndrome. AA syndrome is rather a syndrome than a disease, first because an underlying systemic disorder is frequently encountered, second because of its definition based on (a) abscess-like collections in deep organs (b) lack of microbes, bacteria, virus and parasites after an exhaustive search (c) ineffectiveness of antibiotics (d) high sensitivity to corticosteroid therapy.

History of Aseptic Abscesses Syndrome: The Emergence of a New Entity

Evoking an inflammatory condition when deep intra-abdominal collections are discovered on a CT scan performed in a febrile patient can be surprising. When a 25-year-old male patient was admitted in June 1988 for a 2 months duration fever with abdominal pain and weight loss, a raised white blood cell count and neutrophil percentage, a high CRP level and a normal ultrasound abdominal scan a few days before, the workup followed the screening for fever of unknown origin. Blood cultures were negative. An abdominal CT scan revealed numerous abscess-like lesions

M. André
Université Clermont Auvergne, CHU Clermont-Ferrand, Service de Médecine Interne,
Hôpital Gabriel Montpied, Inserm U1071, INRA USC2018, M2iSH,
Clermont-Ferrand, France
e-mail: mandre@chu-clermontferrand.fr

D. Wallach et al. (eds.), *Neutrophilic Dermatoses*,
https://doi.org/10.1007/978-3-319-72649-6_7

of the spleen and probably of the kidney. Echocardiography was normal. Nevertheless, an infection was suspected and the patient was given broad spectrum antibiotics. Because he didn't improve, a splenectomy was decided. It demonstrated multiple round collections ranging from few mm to 4/5 cm and containing pus. Cultures remained negative and the patient improved without other treatment. Blood parameters normalized. Unfortunately, fever reappeared in March 1989 associated with episcleritis, painful erythematous nodules of the chest, the forearms and the legs. Absolute neutrophil count and CRP were increased again. Despite empiric antibiotic therapy, abdominal pain added to this situation. Abdominal CT scan showed abscesses of the liver and abdominal lymph nodes. A laparotomy was performed and biopsies demonstrated the same histological data that previously; direct examination, cultures and searches for acid-fast bacillus (AFB) were still negative. Skin biopsies showed dermo-hypodermic infiltrate of polymorphonuclear neutrophils (PMNs) so the possibility of an inflammatory illness was considered. He was given potassium iodide and his condition improved quickly. On September 1989, potassium iodide was withdrawn and he developed further abdominal lymph node abscesses and pancreatic abscesses. Transcutaneous biopsy of an abdominal lymph node yielded PMNs and remained sterile. Then, he received successfully colchicine 2 mg per day. In May 1990, he had mild diarrhea that was attributed to colchicine so, as he was clinically and biologically in remission, the treatment was stopped. One week later, he reported headaches and right chest pain. CT scan showed a brain abscess of the right frontal lobe and a lung abscess of the right lower lobe. Cerebrospinal fluid analysis demonstrated neutrophilic pleocytosis but direct examination was negative and cultures were sterile. The patient responded well to intravenous (IV) pulses of methylprednisolone followed by oral prednisone but as prednisone was decreased to 25 mg per day in June 1990, he complained of a right-sided hemiparesis and aphasia due to an abscess in the left internal capsule and in the tail of the right caudate nucleus. Pulses of methylprednisolone were renewed and he was given IV cyclophosphamide successfully.

This previously undescribed condition associating fever, pain and deep sterile collections of PMNs responsive to corticosteroids was called AA syndrome. The occurrence of a mild Crohn's disease 3 years later reinforced the suspicion of an inflammatory condition [1]. At this time, literature on this topic was almost nonexistent [2]. Given that the presentation of this case in a national meeting brought some potential other similar unclassified cases by colleagues, these patients were followed-up and gathered and it appeared that they had a new syndrome [3, 4].

Epidemiology of Aseptic Abscesses Syndrome

The incidence and prevalence of the AA syndrome are not exactly known. To better define the epidemiology of AA syndrome, a register has been created in France [5]. Nowadays, about 100 cases are identified including 60 cases directly reported to the AA syndrome register and 40 published cases. According to these data, AA syndrome has a worldwide distribution. AA syndrome affects equally men and women mainly in their third and fourth decades of life. Patients without associated inflammatory bowel disease (IBD) are on an average older. Pediatric and elderly populations may be affected too.

Pathogenesis of Aseptic Abscesses Syndrome

Histopathology

The cornerstones of AA syndrome are (a) a core of mature PMNs that are more or less altered, sometimes consisting of large necrotizing noncaseating cavities pus-filled that flow when the tissues are cut (b) a border of the lesions lined with palisading histiocytes and a few giant cells (Fig. 7.1). Lymphocytic vasculitis or mononuclear infiltration of the vascular walls next to the abscesses are rarely found and seem to be collateral damages. Different phases in the development of AA have been observed: the acute phase is the one in which neutrophils are dominant. The organization of the epithelioid border with palisading histiocytes is possibly the second stage. In the late stage, less abundant neutrophils are surrounded by fibrous tissue with few macrophages [4, 5]. Special stains for microorganisms are negative. The skin lesions encountered in the index case are probably one of the first descriptions of AA as a dermatological feature. Beside the clinical aspect, the neutrophilic involvement was deeper than in classical Sweet syndrome, localized in the deep dermis and hypodermis, with an unusual histiocytic pattern and the absence of edema in the papillary dermis. Many cases of literature are reported as necrotic/necrobiotic granulomas and are easily recognized as AA in the context in which they arise.

Genetics

Although there is no clear Mendelian pattern of inheritance for AA syndrome, family history is noteworthy in some patients with among others IBD or sarcoidosis.

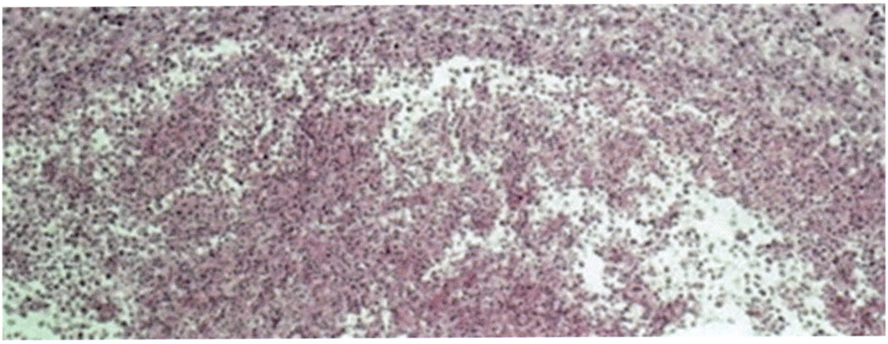

Fig. 7.1 Spleen aseptic abscess with epithelioid histiocytes (top), a multinucleated giant cell (top, right) and PMNs (bottom). (H&E, magnification ×80, courtesy of Professor Jean-Louis Kémény)

A candidate gene approach was conducted to search for predisposing polymorphisms or mutations. Given the relationship with IBDs, *NOD2* gene was screened first. The main variants associated with Crohn's disease, R702W, G908R and 1007fs, were found with an expected frequency. There was only a significant association between the severity of AA syndrome and the synonymous variant R459R [6]. The second gene of interest was *CD2BP1* or *PSTPIP1*, the gene involved in an autosomal dominant variety of Pyoderma gangrenosum called PAPA syndrome for Pyogenic Arthritis, Pyoderma gangrenosum and Acne. A long allele of a microsatellite located in the promoter of the gene was significantly associated with AA syndrome in French patients [7].

Signaling Pathways

The expression of 30 genes of interest was analyzed by RT-PCR on paraffin-embedded biopsies of AA. There was a significant over-expression of interleukin (IL)-1β and IL-6 compared with healthy tissues and microbial abscesses [8].

Diagnosis and Differential Diagnosis of Aseptic Abscesses Syndrome

Most of patients with AA syndrome have fever but some may be afebrile. There is no feature of sepsis. Weight loss is also common. Pain is often encountered depending on the location of the AA. Almost all organs may be involved. However, AA occurs mainly inside the abdomen in more than two thirds of cases. Liver and abdominal lymph nodes are frequently involved but for unknown reasons, spleen is the most often affected organ. Outside the abdomen, lung is frequently involved. Two or more organs are involved simultaneously in more than 50% of cases. Up to six sites may be involved by AA in further flares during the follow-up. Although ND may be associated, in up to 20% of patients in the first series, and at least as much in the literature since that date, they are less frequent in the register. Many of these NDs are atypical, including cutaneous abscesses. Cutaneo-mucous involvement includes also aphthous ulcers and erythema nodosum. Joint pains or arthritis are found in about 20% of cases. Uveitis or episcleritis may be present in about 10% of cases.

There is a raised neutrophil count with sometimes a leukemoid reaction, with a raised CRP, in more than 80% of cases. Liver tests are abnormal in about 40% of patients. Antineutrophil cytoplasmic autoantibodies and anti-*Saccharomyces cerevisiae* antibodies are rarely found positive. There is no frank autoimmune feature although AA syndrome has been described in rheumatoid arthritis and in one case of lupus. Procalcitonin is negative, as well as blood cultures and others searches for bacteria, virus, fungi and parasites.

CT scan is the first line diagnostic tool of choice. Unenhanced and contrast-enhanced CT scans demonstrate one or several hypodense well-defined areas, with

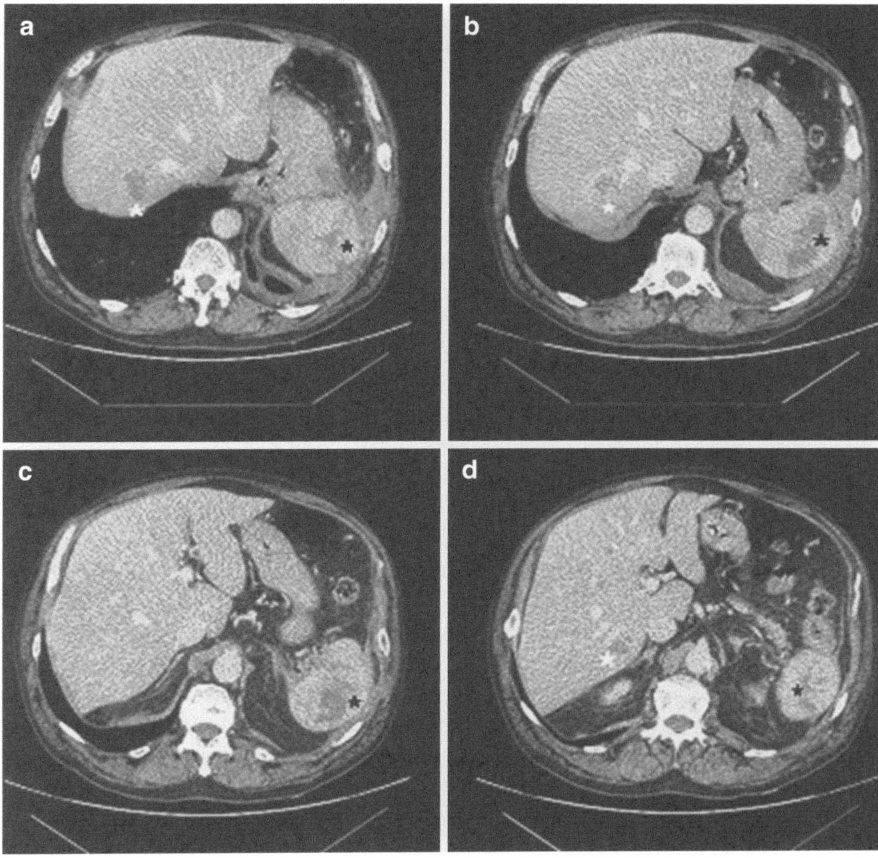

Fig. 7.2 (**a–d**) Abdominal CT scan demonstrating liver (white stars) and spleen (black stars) aseptic abscesses

diameters range from a few mm to several cm, often without significant rim enhancement in the abdominal organs (Fig. 7.2a–d). The presuppurative phase of AA is more easily detected by FDG-PET/CT scan. FDG-PET/CT scan may be performed on diagnosis or for relapses. It can demonstrate silent focus of AA and also multifocal AA, a situation often encountered [9].

Biopsy of a suspected AA is recommended for microbiological analyses including 16s and 18s rRNA polymerase chain reaction that is very sensitive to rule out an infection, and for a pathological examination. The pathologist must be aware of the possibility of AA syndrome. Many patients with AA of the spleen had undergone a splenectomy. Splenectomy may be required for diagnostic purposes. But splenectomy is preventable in some cases: bacterial abdominal abscesses are a common complication in Crohn's disease but are usually associated with a fistula. Interestingly, bacterial spleen abscesses are exceptionally encountered in Crohn's disease so the evidence of IBD and particularly Crohn's disease when spleen abscesses are discovered is highly suggestive of AA syndrome. In such a case, it seems possible to establish the diagnosis without pathological examination. So, searching for an underlying illness and particularly an IBD can give a clue to the diagnosis of AA syndrome.

A careful work-up is mandatory to rule out differential diagnoses, above all an infection. Standard blood cultures, direct examinations and cultures especially for AFB, intracellular and fastidious bacterial species, are mandatory as well as HIV and syphilis tests. Among the organisms that are involved in pyogranulomatous lesions, particular attention must be paid to *Yersinia*, *Bartonella*, *Chlamydia* and fungi. In case of spleen abscesses, an echocardiography must be performed to search for endocarditis. Responsiveness of abscesses to antibiotics requires reconsidering the diagnosis of AA syndrome. Differential diagnosis should also include vasculitis, particularly granulomatosis with polyangiitis, sarcoidosis, malignancies and chronic granulomatous disease. For this latter disease, evaluation of PMNs oxidative burst activity by nitroblue tetrazolium reduction test or dihydrorhodamine flow cytometric assay may be performed.

Clinical Spectrum of Aseptic Abscesses Syndrome

An underlying illness was present in most of early cases but in recent data from the register and the literature, up to 60% of AA syndromes are free of an associated disease. In the first series, there were only three patients without associated condition. This reflects probably a better recognition of AA syndrome even when an evocative background doesn't exist. IBDs remain the most commonly associated diseases, with often a mild form. Crohn's disease is more represented than ulcerative colitis. It may antedate AA syndrome, occur concomitantly or appear after the diagnosis. In most of cases, IBDs precede the diagnosis of AA syndrome or are simultaneous. Apart from IBDs, relapsing polychondritis and spondyloarthritis are the main associated illnesses. Behçet disease, Mouth And Genital ulcers with Inflamed Cartilage (MAGIC) syndrome, rheumatoid arthritis, lupus erythematosus, periarteritis nodosa, Synovitis Acne Pustulosis Hyperostosis Osteitis (SAPHO) syndrome, myeloma, monoclonal gammopathy of undetermined significance and amyloidosis have been also described in case reports. So, throughout the follow-up, it is mandatory to look for an underlying disease. Medical family history is also part of the clinical spectrum.

Treatment of Aseptic Abscesses Syndrome

Systemic corticosteroids are the first line treatment recommended for AA syndrome with doses ranging from 0.5 to 1 mg/kg per day of prednisone orally, sometimes with IV pulses of methylprednisolone initially. Corticosteroid treatment usually spectacularly improves symptoms of AA syndrome within a few hours or days: there is a quick relief of fever and pain. CRP levels decrease and normalize. Medical imaging demonstrates a regression of abscesses and in most of cases normalization. There are not clear recommendations for how to taper off prednisone doses gradually. According to most of the register and literature data, it seems possible to try to reach 5 mg per day of prednisone at 6 months after the first flare. Corticosteroids effectiveness is the rule but high dosages are sometimes necessary for maintenance therapy justifying immunosuppressive drugs in 50% of cases to strengthen the treatment or for corticosteroid-sparing purposes. Among them, azathioprine and anti-TNF alpha drugs such as adalimumab, infliximab or less frequently etanercept are the most commonly used agents, off-label when IBDs or spondyloarthropathies are not associated. Efficacy of anakinra, an IL-1 receptor antagonist agent whose use is in accordance to pathophysiological data has been reported [10]. The use of other drugs such as cyclophosphamide, methotrexate, thalidomide, cyclosporine and sulfasalazine has also been reported. Granulocytes apheresis was used successfully in one patient [11]. A temporary treatment with colchicine is indicated when diagnosis of AA syndrome is suspected and needs further investigations to be establish. Colchicine has been used effectively in the index case and in a few other cases as monotherapy; colchicine is also prescribed as corticosteroid sparing-treatment. Rarely, corticosteroids are not used for the induction therapy, or in cases of relapses, doses of prednisone are not increased for the induction therapy. In some of these cases, anti-TNF alpha agents have a rapid efficacy like the one we have seen with corticosteroids. Too many patients still undergo a splenectomy to cure spleen AA whereas a relapse almost constantly happens after surgery, as in the index case. Single cases reporting effectiveness of splenectomy do not demonstrate enough hindsight to validate this approach.

Prognosis of Aseptic Abscesses Syndrome

Response to systemic corticosteroids is usually dramatic but reported relapse rates are as high as 50%, generally but not only when steroids are tapered. Flares can also arise under immunosuppressive therapy or spontaneously. There is more than one relapse in 25% of cases. Relapses may involve the same organ or another site. Procalcitonin dosage may be a useful tool to distinguish a flare of AA syndrome from an infection whose risk is increased by corticosteroids and immunosuppressive drugs [5, 9]. AA syndrome doesn't seem to affect the pregnancy course: at least three women with AA syndrome became pregnant without flare during pregnancy. Many relapsing patients require long term prednisone therapy despite administration of immunosuppressive drugs. When AA syndrome runs a chronic relapsing course, morbidity is increased and this results in personal, professional or social problems. Underlying conditions are usually pushed into the background: the level of care necessary is generally higher for AA syndrome than for associated illnesses. Nevertheless, when present, diseases associated with AA syndrome must as far as possible be under control. Within almost 30 years of distance, no death was directly attributable to AA syndrome but as in many inflammatory disorders, cardiovascular risk is enhanced and two patients died prematurely of heart attack.

Conclusion

AA syndrome is now more easily recognizable provided that practitioners are aware of this condition. Beyond the individualization of a new entity, the description of the AA syndrome has brought us solutions to manage these patients that were orphans before, with neither clear diagnosis nor clear treatment plan, and has helped to define the prognosis. Patients with AA syndrome display a very specific phenotype suggesting an incomplete connection with NDs. The concept of AA syndrome and this provisional classification reflect a poor understanding of the disease and will probably evolve in the future.

References

1. André M, Aumaître O, Marcheix JC, Piette JC. Aseptic systemic abscesses preceding diagnosis of Crohn's disease by three years. Dig Dis Sci. 1995;40:525–7.
2. Dallot A, Decazes JM, Drouault Y, Rybojad M, Verola O, Morel P, Modai J, Puissant A. Subcorneal pustular dermatosis (Sneddon Wilkinson disease) with amicrobial lymph node suppuration and aseptic spleen abscesses. Br J Dermatol. 1988;119:803–7.
3. André M, Aumaître O, Marcheix JC, Piette JC. Unexplained sterile systemic abscesses in Crohn's disease: aseptic abscesses as a new entity. Am J Gastroenterol. 1995;90:1183.
4. André M, Aumaître O, Papo T, Kemeny JL, Vital-Durand D, Rousset H, Ninet J, Pointud P, Charlotte F, Godeau B, Schmidt J, Marcheix JC, Piette JC. Disseminated aseptic abscesses associated with Crohn's disease: a new entity? Dig Dis Sci. 1998;43:420–8.
5. André MF, Piette JC, Kémény JL, Ninet J, Jego P, Delèvaux I, Wechsler B, Weiller PJ, Frances C, Bletry O, Wismans PJ, Rousset H, Colombel JF, Aumaître O, The French Study Group on Aseptic Abscesses. Aseptic abscesses: a study of 30 patients with or without inflammatory bowel disease and review of the literature. Medicine. 2007;86:145–61.
6. André MF, Aumaître O, Piette JC, Grateau G, Cardoso MC, Ouchchane L, Kémény JL, Dastugue B, Delpech M, Creveaux I. Analysis of the NOD2/CARD15 gene in patients affected with the aseptic abscesses syndrome with or without inflammatory bowel disease. Dig Dis Sci. 2008;53:490–9.
7. André MFJ, Aumaître O, Grateau G, Chamaillard M, Costedoat-Chalumeau N, Cardoso MC, Henry-Berger J, Ramakrishna BS, Delpech M, Piette J-C, Creveaux I. Longest form of CCTG microsatellite repeat in the promoter of the CD2BP1/PSTPIP1 gene is associated with aseptic abscesses and with Crohn disease in French patients. Dig Dis Sci. 2010;55:1681–8.
8. Bardy A, Creveaux I, Déchelotte P, Kémény JL, Rioux-Leclercq N, Aumaître O, André M. Elévation de la transcription d'IL-1β dans les abcès aseptiques. Rev Med Interne. 2010;31:392–3s.
9. Guettrot-Imbert G, Haroche J, Grimon G, Charlotte F, Ninet J, Possenti S, Kelly A, Amoura Z, Aumaître O, André M. F-18 FDG-PET/CT in aseptic abscesses with recurrent febrile abdominal pain. Scand J Gastroenterol. 2011;46:577–82.
10. Bardy A, Guettrot-Imbert G, Aumaître O, André M. Efficacy of Il-1β blockade in refractory aseptic abscesses syndrome. Mod Rheumatol. 2014;24:217–9.
11. Kato S, Hosomi E, Amano F, Kobayashi T, Kani K, Yamamoto R, Ogawa T, Matsuda A, Sato Y, Izaki S, Mitarai T, Yakabi K. The efficacy of intensive granulocyte and monocyte adsorption apheresis in a patient with Crohn's disease complicated by extensive subcutaneous aseptic neutrophilic abscesses. J Crohns Colitis. 2012;6:787–91.

Neutrophilic Panniculitis

8

Giovanni Damiani, Daniel Wallach,
and Angelo Valerio Marzano

Introduction

Panniculitis is an inflammatory disorder of the subcutaneous fat, whose diagnosis and classification relies on histologic features, mainly the location of the subcutaneous inflammatory infiltrate (septal, lobular, mixed or vascular) [1]. In the setting of lobular panniculitis in which the inflammation predominantly involves the fat lobules, there is neutrophilic panniculitis (NP), a rare condition that belongs to the group of neutrophilic dermatoses [2]. Clinically, NP manifests as a subcutaneous nodular eruption and, histologically, shows a lobular infiltrate mainly consisting of neutrophils [3–7]. NP has been reported to be significantly associated with myelodysplasia, which is a well-known association for neutrophilic dermatoses in general [3–7]. From a therapeutic point of view, it is regarded as highly sensitive to oral corticosteroids, similarly to Sweet's syndrome [2]. In this chapter, the clinical and histological features of NP are described, with emphasis on the differential diagnosis from the main panniculitides sharing a neutrophilic histological pattern.

G. Damiani
Dipartimento di Fisiopatologia Medico-Chirurgica e dei Trapianti, Universita' degli Studi di Milano, Unita' Operativa di Dermatologia, IRCCS Fondazione Ca' Granda, Ospedale Maggiore Policlinico, Milano, Italy

Young Dermatologists Italian Network (YDIN), Study Center of the Italian Group for Epidemiologic Research in Dermatology (GISED), Bergamo, Italy

D. Wallach
Physician (Hon.) of Paris Hospitals, Paris, France

A. V. Marzano (✉)
Dipartimento di Fisiopatologia Medico-Chirurgica e dei Trapianti, Universita' degli Studi di Milano, Unita' Operativa di Dermatologia, IRCCS Fondazione Ca' Granda, Ospedale Maggiore Policlinico, Milano, Italy
e-mail: angelo.marzano@unimi.it

D. Wallach et al. (eds.), *Neutrophilic Dermatoses*,
https://doi.org/10.1007/978-3-319-72649-6_8

History

The first description of NP was made in 1982 by Leibowitz et al. [3] and described as "Sweet's disease with extension of the inflammatory infiltrate into the subcutaneous fat". In 1983, Cooper et al. assessed a case of a woman with a preleukemic state evolving to acute myeloid or myelomonocytic leukemia with a neutrophilic infiltrate in subcutaneous tissue [4]. Cullity et al. in 1991 were the first to use the term "acute febrile NP" or "Sweet' panniculitis" [6] and finally in 1997 the term "neutrophilic panniculitis" appeared in an article written by Matsumura et al. [7].

Pathogenesis

Although its pathogenesis remains still largely undefined, NP sees as central event the subcutaneous accumulation of mature neutrophils [2]. Similarly to prototypic neutrophilic dermatoses such as pyoderma gangrenosum and Sweet's syndrome, a role for autoinflammation may be *bona fide* hypothesized, with proinflammatory cytokines like interleukin (IL)-1β and IL-17 as well as chemokines, notably IL-8, being crucially involved in inducing tissue damage and neutrophil recruitment [8–12]. The role of chemokines in the pathophysiology of NP is supported by the possible occurrence of the disease after receiving granulocyte-macrophage colony-stimulating factor, a well-known stimulant of neutrophil proliferation and maturation [3–7]. The recent case report of familial Mediterranean fever, a classic autoinflammatory disease, presenting with NP as the main clinical manifestation along with periodic fever provides further evidence for the involvement of autoinflammation [13].

Histology

The sample should be taken as a deep incisional biopsy [14]. It is also cardinal to culture the sample in microbiology for all cases of NP. In NP, specimens show a neutrophilic infiltrate in the hypodermis, predominating in the fat lobules (Fig. 8.1).

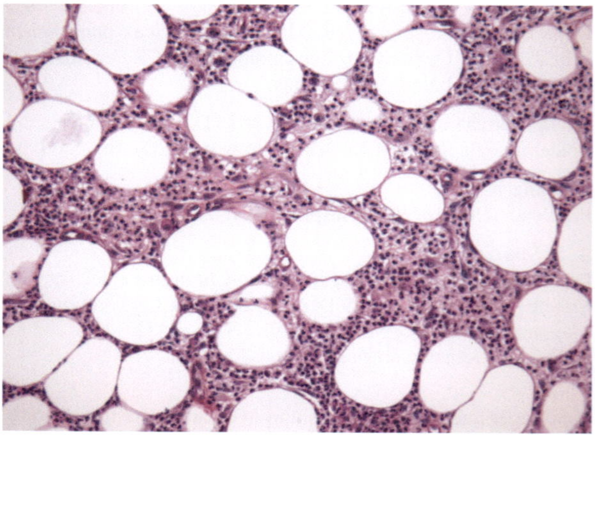

Fig. 8.1 A lobular neutrophilic infiltrate in a case of neutrophilic panniculitis (Courtesy Marie-Dominique Vignon-Pennamen, MD)

There is no vasculitis and no significant dermal involvement [2]. For the histologic differential diagnosis from other panniculitides, at the beginning, examination focuses on the location of the subcutaneous inflammatory infiltrate, in order to morphologically distinguish between septal, lobular and mixed panniculitis. The second crucial step is the characterization of the main cytotype to determine the neutrophilic, lymphocytic, histiocytic or eosinophilic nature of NP. Vascular damage assessment is the third step. The fourth step is the evaluation of the presence and pattern of fat necrosis: (1) blue grey ghost cells orients to enzymatic fat necrosis and thus to pancreatic panniculitis; (2) basophilic grungy debris in the contest of basophilic necrosis suggests infective panniculitis; (3) membranous fat necrosis, albeit non specific, is a feature frequently found in traumatic/factitial panniculitis.

Diagnostic Criteria

In 2004, Wallach et al. proposed diagnostic criteria for NP, subdividing them into positive and negative [2]. Positive criteria include five items and are useful to suspect NP: (1) nodule or plaque as the elementary lesions; (2) general symptoms as fever, arthralgia and malaise; (3) neutrophil-rich lobular infiltrate on histology; (4) concurrency with myelodysplasia; (5) high sensitivity to steroids. Negative criteria are useful for differential diagnosis: (1) neutrophils-rich infiltrate has not to be predominant in the septa; (2) no evidence of vasculitis; (3) no presence of other cause of panniculitis.

The aforementioned criteria indicate that NP is a distinctive entity, different from other panniculitides. It belongs to the group of the deep neutrophilic dermatoses, and is close to Sweet' syndrome, which may display a deep/subcutaneous presentation [2].

Clinical Aspects

NP manifests as deep-seated, erythematous, tender or painful nodules or plaques with increased skin temperature involving mainly the legs, arms, trunk and breasts (Fig. 8.2). Nodules and plaques last 15 days or more and usually heal with transient

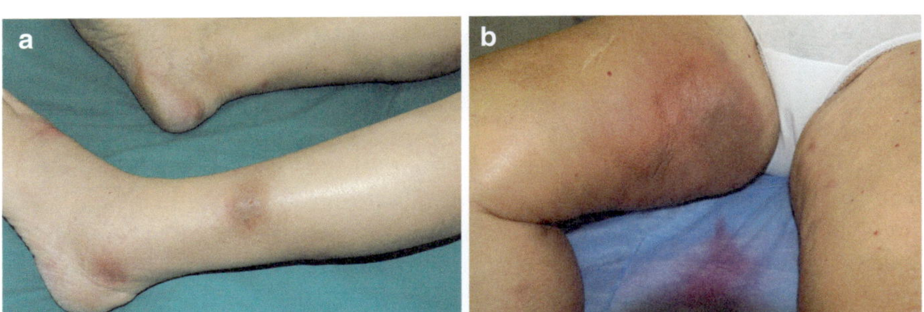

Fig. 8.2 Deep-seated erythematous-brownish nodules (panel A) and plaques (panel B) on the legs

Table 8.1 Main clinical differential diagnoses from neutrophilic panniculitis

Pancreatic panniculitis
α1-antitrypsin deficiency-associated panniculitis
Infective panniculitis
Erythema induratum
Panniculitis associated with rheumatoid arthritis
Factitial panniculitis
Subcutaneous sweet's syndrome
Early erythema nodosum
Panniculitis due to biologic therapies

post-inflammatory hyperpigmentation and atrophy [3–7, 15, 16]. Clinical differential diagnosis from other panniculitides with a neutrophilic histological pattern is mandatory (Table 8.1). Abdominal pain, acute polyarthritis and serositis orientate to pancreatic panniculitis. Mental disorder and cosmetic or therapeutic implants suggest factitial panniculitis. A history of emphysema, non-alcoholic cirrhosis, hepatitis, vasculitis and angioedema should evoke α1-antitrypsin deficiency. Likewise, acute fever, neutrophilia and elevate inflammation indexes have to remind to subcutaneous Sweet's syndrome, while concomitant rheumatoid arthritis (RA) inspires a RA-associated panniculitis. Finally, the leg calves localization, pain and scarring prompt to erythema elevatum diutinum.

Differential Diagnoses

Pancreatic Panniculitis

It is a critical diagnosis since it is a presenting sign of pancreatic disease. Pancreatic panniculitis may manifest in presence of inflammatory pancreatic diseases, both chronic and acute, pancreatic carcinomas, particularly acinar cell carcinoma [17], and congenital pancreatic abnormalities. Nodules have ulcerative behavior and exude oily brown material as result of enzymatic subcutaneous fat digestion [18]. They present mainly to distal lower extremities, but occasionally they afflict also other sites such as abdomen [19].

α1-Antitrypsin Deficiency-Associated Panniculitis

This genetic autosomic recessive disease is caused by a mutation in gene serine protease inhibitor (SERPINA) 1 (14q32.1) and has a prevalence of 1/2500 in West Europe and the most common alleles are PI Z e PI S [20]. An autoinflammatory component in the pathogenesis of this form of panniculitis has recently suggested [21]. Severe manifestations, including panniculitis, correlate with ZZ and SZ genotypes [22]. ZZ genotype usually manifests in infancy with a prolonged jaundice with conjugated hyperbilirubinemia and hypertransaminasemia in newborns [20]. Diagnosis can be established on the basis of the low levels of

α1-antitrypsin. Panniculitis may manifest in all genotypes with ulcerating subcutaneous nodules precipitated by trauma [23].

Infective Panniculitis

Direct inoculation (primary infective panniculitis) or hematogenous/lymphatic spread (secondary infective panniculitis) may result in panniculitis with a predominant neutrophilic infiltrate [24]. This entity is more common in immunosuppressed patients. Microbial culture of all lesions that histologically appear as panniculitis with a predominant neutrophilic infiltrate should be always performed [25].

Erythema Induratum

Erythema induratum is a controversial entity, regarded as an id reaction, due to an extracutaneous mycobacterial infection in a context of occult or active tuberculosis [26]. The detection of Mycobacterium tuberculosis DNA fragments in the lesional skin by means of polymerase chain reaction (with negative tissue cultures) prompts the reactive origin, namely id [26]. A rare variant of erythema induratum is panniculitic bacteroides triggered by bacteria different from Mycobacteria species [27] and presenting with painful nodules usually on the calves.

Panniculitis Associated to RA

Rarely, a pustular panniculitis occurs in patients with RA, in whom the most common form of panniculitis is erythema nodosum [28]. Typical lesions are characterized by pustules and tender erythematous nodules of lower extremities with the tendency to ulcerate and drain liquefied fat [29].

Factitial Panniculitis

Auto-referred injuries should be taken into consideration in cases of bizarre clinical presentation [30]. Foreign bodies should be searched with and without polarized light in all panniculitides, particularly those with predominant neutrophilic infiltrate. Another step is the evaluation of secondary infection that can lead to a misdiagnosis. The final step of lesion history is fibrosis that clinically has to be distinguished from scleroderma. It may be inserted into a syndromic background classically shared between Munchausen syndrome and Munchausen syndrome by proxy [31]. In Munchausen syndrome the patient purposefully injures himself, conversely in Munchausen syndrome by proxy the patient, usually a child, is injured by a child's caregiver. The cutaneous involvement is rarely described in literature suggesting either that diagnosis is not made readily or that it is an uncommon disorder.

Subcutaneous Sweet's Syndrome

The presence of subcutaneous infiltrates in Sweet syndrome is well known [4]. The rare subcutaneous variant of Sweet's syndrome may merely involve only subcutaneous fat; in this case, its distinction from neutrophilic panniculitis has been discussed [32]; the interest of this distinction is mainly academic, inasmuch as these conditions require the same work-up, focusing on the association with blood disorders. It may also deepen into fascia and skeletal muscles, assuming a necrotizing behavior [33]. Clinically, representative lesions are deep-seated tender and erythematous nodules and plaques on extremities, that in the case of the necrotizing variant may mimic fasciitis [33]. All variants respond to corticosteroids [32]. Anecdotal cases were refractory to corticosteroids and need biological therapy [34].

Early Erythema Nodosum

Although erythema nodosum is a typical example of lymphocytic or granulomatous septal panniculitis, the early presentation is characterized by a wide variety of histological features [35], among which the main one is the neutrophil-rich form. Patients typically exhibit tender erythematous nodules on shins without surface changes. Early erythema nodosum resolves spontaneously or with non-steroidal anti-inflammatory drugs [35].

NP due to Biologic Therapies

The advent of biologic therapies defined a new field of interest in the context of panniculitides. Many reports suggested a possible implication of many classes of biologics in developing an actual form of ND. Neutrophilic panniculitis is described to be a side effect of B-Rapidly Accelerated Fibrosarcoma (BRAF) inhibitors, estimated to have a prevalence of 13% in patients treated with the BRAF inhibitor vemurafenib [36]. Tyrosine kinase inhibitors (TKIs) have also been reported to be responsible for triggering NP, especially imatinib and dasatinib [37]. A solitary case of NP due to ponatinib, a new third generation tyrosine-kinase inhibitor is reported [37]. Due to the wide spectrum of cutaneous side effects of new biologic therapies, NPs should be always insert in differential diagnosis of deep seated nodules and plaques in these patients.

Treatment

The first line treatment for NP are systemic corticosteroids [38]. Immunomodulating agents like dapsone, which acts as inhibitor of neutrophil migration, may be used as steroid-sparing drug and is useful in preventing possible relapses. Steroidal approach is favorite in literature and almost always decisive [38]. Second line therapy includes biologics, which are reserved to severe cases unresponsive to corticosteroids. The main biological drugs described to be functional in NP are anakinra [38] and tumor necrosis factor (TNF) antagonists, used as off-label drugs. Only few reports describe the use of these drugs in NP. Anakinra is a IL-1 receptor antagonist reported as rapidly effective particularly in cryopyrinopathies but also in neutrophilic dermatoses [39]. Anti-TNF therapies are widely adopted in neutrophilic dermatoses [40].

References

1. Black MM, Cunliffe WJ. Subcutaneous fat. In: Champion RH, editor. Rook/Wilkinson/Ebling textbook of dermatology. 6th ed. Oxford: Blackwell.
2. Sutra-Loubet C, Carlotti A, Guillemette J, Wallach D. Neutrophilic panniculitis. J Am Acad Dermatol. 2004;50:280–5.
3. Leibowitz MR, Rippey JJ, Bezwoda WR, Carman HA. Unusual aspects of febrile neutrophilic dermatosis (Sweet's syndrome). S Afr Med J. 1982;62:375–8.
4. Cooper PH, Frierson HF, Greer KE. Subcutaneous neutrophilic infiltrates in acute febrile neutrophilic dermatosis. Arch Dermatol. 1983;119:610–1.
5. Morioka N, Otsuka F, Nogita T, et al. Neutrophilic dermatosis with myelodysplastic syndrome: nuclear segmentation anomalies of neutrophils in the skin lesion and in peripheral blood. J Am Acad Dermatol. 1990;23:247–9.
6. Cullity J, Maguim B, Gebauer K. Sweet's panniculitis. Australas J Dermatol. 1991;32:61–4.
7. Matsumura Y, Tanabe H, Wada Y, et al. Neutrophilic panniculitis associated with myelodysplastic syndromes. Br J Dermatol. 1997;136:142–3.
8. Marzano AV, Ishak RS, Saibeni S, et al. Autoinflammatory skin disorders in inflammatory bowel diseases, pyoderma gangrenosum and Sweet's syndrome: a comprehensive review and disease classification criteria. Clin Rev Allergy Immunol. 2013;45:202–10.
9. Marzano AV, Cugno M, Trevisan V, et al. Role of inflammatory cells, cytokines and matrix metalloproteinases in neutrophil-mediated skin diseases. Clin Exp Immunol. 2010;162:100–7.
10. Marzano AV, Fanoni D, Antiga E, et al. Expression of cytokines, chemokines and other effector molecules in two prototypic autoinflammatory skin diseases, pyoderma gangrenosum and Sweet's syndrome. Clin Exp Immunol. 2014;178:48–56.
11. Marzano A, Damiani G, Ceccherini I. Autoinflammation in pyoderma gangrenosum and its syndromic form PASH. Br J Dermatol. 2017;176(6):1588–98. https://doi.org/10.1111/bjd.15226.
12. Satoh TK, Mellett M, Contassot E, French LE. Are neutrophilic dermatoses autoinflammatory disorders? Br J Dermatol. 2016 Nov 30. https://doi.org/10.1111/bjd.15105. [Epub ahead of print].
13. Leiva-Salinas M, Betlloch I, Arribas MP, et al. Neutrophilic lobular panniculitis as an expression of a widened spectrum of familial mediterranean fever. JAMA Dermatol. 2014;150:213–4.
14. Chan MP. Neutrophilic panniculitis: algorithmic approach to a heterogeneous group of disorders. Arch Pathol Lab Med. 2014;138:1337–43.
15. Qian L, Shen J, Cen J, et al. Myelodysplastic syndrome with neutrophilic panniculitis: a report of two cases and a literature review. Oncol Lett. 2015;9:1954–6.
16. Jagdeo J, Campbell R, Long T, et al. Sweet's syndrome—like neutrophilic lobular panniculitis associated with all-trans-retinoic acid chemotherapy in a patient with acute promyelocytic leukemia. J Am Acad Dermatol. 2007;56:690–3.
17. Naeyaert C, de Clerck F, De Wilde V. Pancreatic panniculitis as a paraneoplastic phenomenon of a pancreatic acinar cell carcinoma. Acta Clin Belg. 2016;71:448–50.
18. Rongioletti F, Caputo V. Pancreatic panniculitis. G Ital Dermatol Venereol. 2013;148:419–25.
19. Zelger B. Panniculitides, an algorithmic approach. G Ital Dermatol Venereol. 2013;148:351–70.
20. Campos MA, Lascano J. α1 Antitrypsin deficiency: current best practice in testing and augmentation therapy. Ther Adv Respir Dis. 2014;8:150–61.

21. Marzano AV, Damiani G. Neutrophilic panniculitis and autoinflammation: what's the link? Br J Dermatol. 2016;175:646–7.
22. Stockley RA. Alpha1-antitrypsin review. Clin Chest Med. 2014;35:39–50.
23. Laureano A, Carvalho R, Chaveiro A, Cardoso J. Alpha-1-antitrypsin deficiency-associated panniculitis: a case report. Dermatol Online J. 2014;20:21245.
24. Morrison LK, Rapini R, Willison CB, Tyring S. Infection and panniculitis. Dermatol Ther. 2010;23:328–40.
25. Niebuhr M, Völker B, Kapp A, Wedi B. Recurrent neutrophilic panniculitis secondary to bacterial cystitis. Eur J Dermatol. 2007;17:89–91.
26. Gilchrist H, Patterson JW. Erythema nodosum and erythema induratum (nodular vasculitis): diagnosis and management. Dermatol Ther. 2010;23:320–7.
27. Cho KH, Lee DY, Kim CW. Erythema induratum of Bazin. Int J Dermatol. 1996;35:802–8.
28. Anstey A, Wilkinson JD, Wojnarowska F, et al. Pustular panniculitis in rheumatoid arthritis. J R Soc Med. 1991;84:307–8.
29. Kuniyuki S, Shindow K, Tanaka T. Pustular panniculitis in a patient with rheumatoid arthritis. Int J Dermatol. 1997;36:292–3.
30. Winkelmann RK, Barker SM. Factitial traumatic panniculitis. J Am Acad Dermatol. 1985;13:988–94.
31. Boyd AS, Ritchie C, Likhari S. Munchausen syndrome and Munchausen syndrome by proxy in dermatology. J Am Acad Dermatol. 2014;71:376–81.
32. Nobeyama Y, Nakagawa H. Subcutaneous Sweet's syndrome and neutrophilic panniculitis. J Dermatol. 2014;41:861–2.
33. Kroshinsky D, Alloo A, Rothschild B, et al. Necrotizing Sweet syndrome: a new variant of neutrophilic dermatosis mimicking necrotizing fasciitis. J Am Acad Dermatol. 2012;67:945–54.
34. Kluger N, Gil-Bistes D, Guillot B, Bessis D. Efficacy of anti-interleukin-1 receptor antagonist anakinra (Kineret®) in a case of refractory Sweet's syndrome. Dermatology. 2011;222:123–7.
35. Passarini B, Infusino SD. Early erythema nodosum. G Ital Dermatol Venereol. 2013;148:413–7.
36. Choy B, Chou S, Anforth R, Fernandez-Penas P. Panniculitis in patients treated with BRAF inhibitors: a case series. Am J Dermatopathol. 2014;36:492–7.
37. Zhang M, Hassan KM, Musiek A, Rosman IS. Ponatinib-induced neutrophilic panniculitis. J Cutan Pathol. 2014;41:597–601.
38. Lipsker D, Perrigouard C, Foubert A, Cribier B. Anakinra for difficult-to-treat neutrophilic panniculitis: IL-1 blockade as a promising treatment option for neutrophil-mediated inflammatory skin disease. Dermatology. 2010;220:264–7.
39. Lopalco G, Rigante D, Giannini M, et al. Safety profile of anakinra in the management of rheumatologic, metabolic and autoinflammatory disorders. Clin Exp Rheumatol. 2016;34:531–8.
40. Alexis AF, Strober BE. Off-label dermatologic uses of anti-TNF-a therapies. J Cutan Med Surg. 2005;9:296–302.

Superficial Neutrophilic Dermatoses: From Subcorneal Pustular Dermatosis (Sneddon-Wilkinson Disease) to Intercellular IgA Dermatoses

9

Laurence Feldmeyer, Takashi Hashimoto, and Luca Borradori

Introduction

Since the initial description of the subcorneal pustular dermatosis by Sneddon and Wilkinson in 1956 [1], our understanding of the pathophysiology of diseases associated with the accumulation of neutrophils in the epidermis and intraepidermal blistering has significantly evolved. Sneddon-Wilkinson disease is now regarded as condition belonging to the spectrum of neutrophilic dermatoses characterized by neutrophilic infiltration of the skin and potential extracutaneous involvement, such as Sweet syndrome and pyoderma gangrenosum [2–4]. This group of inflammatory conditions, which show considerable clinical and histological overlap, is frequently associated with systemic diseases. Recently, it has been suggested to use the term of *superficial neutrophilic dermatoses* for all neutrophilic diseases associated with intraepidermal neutrophil accumulation [5]. Intriguingly, there is a group of patients who develop a superficial neutrophilic disease very similar to Sneddon-Wilkinson disease, showing either subcorneal or intraepidermal pustule formation. However, in contrast to Sneddon-Wilkinson disease, these patients show characteristically IgA deposits on the cell surface of epidermal keratinocyte in a pemphigus-like pattern or more rarely linear deposits in the subcorneal zone.

Wallach et al. [6] first described the case of a patient with a subcorneal pustular dermatosis and intercellular IgA deposits. The presence of epidermal IgA had been mentioned earlier by Varigos [7] and by Sneddon and Wilkinson [8]. Following Wallach

L. Feldmeyer (✉) • L. Borradori
Department of Dermatology, Inselspital, Bern University Hospital, University of Bern, Bern, Switzerland
e-mail: Laurence.Feldmeyer@insel.ch; Luca.Borradori@insel.ch

T. Hashimoto
Department of Dermatology, Osaka City University Graduate School of Medicine, Osaka, Japan
e-mail: hashimot@med.kurume-u.ac.jp

D. Wallach et al. (eds.), *Neutrophilic Dermatoses*,
https://doi.org/10.1007/978-3-319-72649-6_9

et al. report, an increasing number of patients with intraepidermal IgA deposition has been reported under a variety of names: i.e., *intraepidermal IgA pustulosis* [9, 10], *atypical neutrophilic dermatosis with subcorneal IgA deposits* [11], *intercellular IgA dermatosis* [12], *intraepidermal neutrophilic IgA dermatosis* (IEN) [13], *intercellular IgA vesicopustular dermatosis* [14], *IgA pemphigus* or *IgA pemphigus foliaceus* [12, 13].

Whether these conditions with intraepidermal IgA deposits belong to a group of autoimmune diseases mediated by IgA antibodies or are integrated in the group of superficial neutrophilic dermatoses remains a matter of debate. In line with the seminal critical review of Wallach in 1992, we favor the concept that these intraepidermal IgA pustulosis should be included in the group of the neutrophilic dermatoses, in which an exaggerated innate immunity response plays a critical role. Nevertheless, it is likely that in a subset of these patients a specific IgA autoantibody response to specific target epidermal antigens contributes to the tissue damage and inflammatory reaction. We recently propose to classify this group of patients as "*intercellular IgA dermatosis*" (IAD) [15] with six distinct subtypes based on clinical, pathological and immunopathological criteria [16] (Table 9.1).

Although in a review of 20 cases Geller et al. proposed the term "*IgA pemphigus spectrum*" [17], this name is not appropriate in our view. First, pemphigus vulgaris and pemphigus foliaceus are characterized by a specific autoantibody response to desmoglein 1 (Dsg1) and Dsg3, which is only found in a subset of these patients. Second, acantholysis and vesiculobullous lesions are not always observed in affected patients, who rather present with pustular lesions. Third, these conditions are often reported in association with systemic diseases, such as lymphoid proliferations, MGUS, and chronic and inflammatory conditions that are not usually found in the classic pemphigus group.

Table 9.1 Proposed classification of intercellular IgA dermatosis and its subtypes, as well as classical subcorneal pustular dermatosis (SPD) [13]

Diagnoses	Cases	Clinical and histopathological features	Immunoreactivity
All IAD	49	Variable	Exclusively IgA antibodies
IAD subtypes			
– SPD-type IAD	17	SPD-like features	Dsc1 (weak Dsc3 in one case)
– IEN-type IAD	12	IEN-like features	None (weak Dsc3 in one case)
– IgA-PVeg	2	PVeg-like features	Unknown (Dsc2 in one case)
– IgA-PF	4	Variable	Dsg1 (Dscs)
– IgA-PV	6	Variable	Dsg3 (Dsg1 or Dscs)
Unclassified IAD	8	Variable	Dsg1, Dsg3, Dscs
Classical SPD	13	SPD-like features	None

IAD intercellular IgA dermatosis, *SPD* subcorneal pustular dermatosis, *IEN* intraepidermal neutrophilic IgA dermatosis, *PVeg* pemphigus vegetans, *PF* pemphigus foliaceus, *PV* pemphigus vulgaris, *Dsc* desmocollin, *Dsg* desmoglein

Subcorneal Pustular Dermatosis (Sneddon-Wilkinson Disease)

Subcorneal pustular dermatosis (SPD) is a rare condition with pustular eruption described by Sneddon and Wilkinson in 1956 [1, 18]. SPD is clinically characterized by the presence of symmetrically distributed annular or polycyclic lesions, which are often localized on the trunk, particularly around the axillary and inguinal folds and in the submammary region. Palmoplantar pustules may occur but the face and the mucous membranes are spared. The primary lesion consists of a pea-sized superficial pustule that may present with a gravity-induced demarcation between clear fluid in the upper part and pus in the lower part (also called hypopion pustule). New lesions spread within a day or two days in the annular, circinate or serpiginous pattern with central clearing and peripheral pustules [19]. The pustules heal, leaving superficial scaling and occasionally postinflammatory hyper or hypopigmentation. The 13 cases of classical SPD reported by Hashimoto et al. [16] presented with skin lesions on the whole body (one case), trunk (eight), extremities (six) and intertriginous areas (four), with frequent involvement of the lower extremities (five) and axillae (three). One case each had oral and nasal mucosal lesions. Clinical features were pustules (seven cases), blisters (six), erythema (seven) and erosion (three). Two cases reported itch.

In rare instances SPD is accompanied by constitutional symptoms, such as malaise, fever, and arthralgias. Affected patients may concomitantly or in the disease course present with other neutrophilic dermatoses, such as pyoderma gangrenosum [2–4]. Furthermore, extracutaneous manifestations may occur: abnormalities of hepatic enzymes, renal involvement with glomerulonephritis or aseptic neutrophilic abscesses have been described [20]. The disease is chronic and often shows a relapsing course. The disease, which predominates in women, often occur between the age of 40 and 50 years [18], whereas childhood cases have been only anecdotally reported [21–23].

Light microscopy studies show nonfollicular subcorneal pustules filled with neutrophils, and occasional eosinophils, accompanied by a mixed superficial perivascular inflammatory infiltrate. Neutrophils migrate into the epidermis, forming typically unilocular subcorneal pustules rather than spongiotic pustules [1]. In contrast to what observed in pustular psoriasis, mitotic figures are usually absent in the epidermis [24]. Acantholysis may be present in older lesions [1]. All 11 cases examined histopathologically in our laboratory [16] presented with subcorneal pustules with infiltrations of neutrophils and eosinophils in nine and three cases, respectively. One case showed acantholysis.

Direct immunofluorescence (DIF) is negative [18]. In the past, some cases of SPD have been associated with the presence of intercellular deposits of IgA. These cases would now be classified within the heterogeneous group of IAD (see below).

SPD has been reported in association with a monoclonal gammopathy, most frequently of the IgA type [4, 25–27], as well as with IgA myeloma [28–31]. They can develop before and after the diagnosis of SPD. Other, more anecdotally described associations include rheumatoid arthritis [32–35], SAPHO (synovitis, acne, pustulosis, hyperostosis, osteitis) syndrome [36], systemic lupus erythematodes [37], Sjögren's syndrome [38], Crohn's disease [39], hyperthyroidism [40], multiple sclerosis [41], aplastic anemia [42], and infections (mycoplasma pneumoniae, and HIV) [43–46]. In addition to IgA myeloma, other associated malignancies encompass chronic lymphocytic leukemia [47], thymoma [48], apudoma [49] and lung carcinoma [50].

Clinically, SPD has to be primarily differentiated from a group of IAD (see below), the pemphigus group, including pemphigus herpetiformis and pemphigus vegetans, as well as dermatitis herpetiformis. IAD are characteristically distinguished from SPD based on the positive DIF microscopic findings with detection of cell surface IgA deposits. It is unclear how to regard the isolated cases of SPD, in which immunofluorescence studies have become positive years after the first signs of the disease [18]. These observations may be due to either technical factors, a variable interpretation of the immunofluorescence findings or the possible existence of transitional forms. Finally, halogenodermas, pustular psoriasis and acute generalized exanthematous pustulosis may also be discussed and distinguished based on patient's history, disease course and clinical findings [1] (Table 9.2).

Table 9.2 Differential diagnosis [17, 69]

Diagnosis	Clinical features	Histology and immunopathology	Immunoserology Other tests
Subcorneal pustular dermatosis/ Sneddon-Wilkinson disease	Pustular lesions, annular or polycyclic pattern Hypopion pustules Axillary, inguinal folds	Nonfollicular subcorneal pustules DIF negative	No circulating Ab
Intercellular IgA dermatosis: SPD type	Flaccid vesicles and pustules, annular circinate pattern, central crusting	Subcorneal pustules with mild or no acanthosis DIF: cell surface IgA deposits in the upper epidermis	IgA anti-Dsc1 Ab
Intercellular IgA dermatosis: IEN type	Lesions with central crusts and peripheral vesiculation (sunflower lesions)	Intraepidermal pustules DIF: cell surface IgA deposits in the whole epidermis	Unknown target antigen
Pemphigus foliaceus	Flaccid bullae, localized or generalized exfoliation	Acantholysis in granular layer DIF[a]: cell surface IgG deposits mostly in superficial layers	IgG anti-Dsg1 Ab
Pemphigus vulgaris	Mucosal erosions, flaccid bullae, mouth, groin, scalp, face, neck, extremities	Suprabasilar acantholysis with intraepidermal blisters DIF: cell surface deposits of IgG, mostly in the lower epidermis	IgG anti-Dsg3 Ab ± anti-Dsg1 Ab
Dermatitis herpetiformis	Grouped papules and vesicles, prurigo-like lesions, excoriations, extensor surfaces, buttocks, scalp or back	Subepidermal blister, neutrophilic microabscesses in dermal papillae DIF: granular IgA deposits in upper dermal papillae	IgA and IgG anti-epidermal TG and anti-tissue TG Ab IgG and IgA anti-deamidated gliadin Ab

Table 9.2 (continued)

Diagnosis	Clinical features	Histology and immunopathology	Immunoserology Other tests
Pustular psoriasis	Varied distribution with pustules and erythema History of psoriasis	Intraepidermal pustules with different stages of involvement	
Acute generalized exanthematous pustulosis	Widespread tiny pustules on, erythematous basis on face , trunk, intertriginous areas; fever, leukocytosis; drug-related	Subcorneal pustules, usually subcorneal; dyskeratosis, necrotic keratinocytes, mixed interstitial and mid-dermal infiltrates	
Amicrobial pustulosis of the folds	Pustules on erythematous skin; in cutaneous folds, scalp, extensor surfaces, periorificial areas, females	Spongiform pustules with acanthosis and parakeratosis, dermal polymorphonuclear infiltrates	
Candidal intertrigo	Intertriginous areas; satellite lesions	PAS stain: budding yeast cells and pseudo-hyphae	
Bullous impetigo	Mostly face and extremities	Subcorneal bullae, few acantholytic cells, some neutrophils and Gram-positive cocci, mixed dermal inflammatory infiltrate	
Necrolytic migratory erythema (glucagonoma syndrome)	Erythematous patches, vesicles, crusting; arcuate pattern; predominant intertriginous and periorificial involvement	Parakeratosis and vacuolization within the cytoplasm of the upper epidermal keratinocytes; subcorneal pustule formation; necrotic keratinocytes	Increased blood glucagon levels
Halogenoderma	Papulopustular vegetating lesions, acneiform appearance	Papillomatosis, intraepidermal abscesses with neutrophils, neutrophilic infiltrate, some leukocytoclasia	Increased serum or urine bromide and iodide levels

[a]*DIF* direct immunofluorescence microscopy, *IIF* indirect immunofluorescence microscopy, *Ab* autoantibodies, *Dsg* desmoglein, *Dsc* desmocollin, *TG* transglutaminase, *PAS* Periodic acid–Schiff

The accumulation of neutrophils in the epidermis implies the presence of chemotactic factors, such as tumor necrosis factor alpha (TNF-α), interleukin-8, and complement fragment C5a [20, 51]. Increased expression of TNF-α has been found both in the blisters and in the serum of affected patients [51, 52]. The observation that SPD is associated with other TNF-α-related diseases, such as inflammatory bowel disease, rheumatoid arthritis and psoriasis as well as the response of SPD to anti-TNF-α inhibitors suggest a contribution of this cytokine in tissue damage.

Intercellular IgA Dermatosis (IAD)

IAD encompass a heterogeneous group of pustular dermatoses associated with tissue-bound IgA in the epidermis showing overlapping clinical and pathological features [10]. These conditions have in common the presence of IgA immunoreactants on the cytoplasmic cell membrane of keratinocytes of either the entire epidermis or within the subcorneal region. These IgA deposits are detectable either alone or in combination with C3, while circulating anti-keratinocyte cell surface IgA antibodies are detectable by different technical approaches in some but not all patients [10, 15, 17]. Affected patients have been described under a variety of sometimes confusing denominations (*see* "Introduction"), including intercellular IgA dermatosis, intraepidermal neutrophilic IgA dermatosis, and intercellular IgA vesiculopustular dermatosis.

Based on a critical review of more than >50 case reports and 30 years of research interest in this field, in our view, IAD most likely consists of different entities associated with distinctive and peculiar immunological findings.

We have proposed a working classification of IAD comprising six subtypes [16]: subcorneal pustular dermatosis (SPD)-type IAD, intraepidermal neutrophilic dermatosis (IEN)-type IAD, IgA-pemphigus vulgaris, IgA-pemphigus foliaceus, IgA pemphigus vegetans and as yet unclassified subset of IAD.

Clinical Features

The two most frequent forms of IAD are the SPD-type and the IEN-type [16].

The SPD-type is clinically characterized by recurring crops of pruritic papules and vesicles, showing sometimes an annular distribution. These lesions evolve into eroded and crusted plaques on the trunk and proximal extremities, evocating dermatitis herpetiformis [10, 15, 17]. In our recent review involving 49 IAD cases [16], there were 17 SPD-type cases (35%). There was a characteristic involvement of intertriginous areas (six cases) including the axillae (five cases) and inguinal areas (three cases). The entire body (five cases), trunk (six cases) and extremities (six cases) were involved in five, six and six cases, respectively. There was no oral mucosal involvement. The cutaneous lesions in the SPD-type consisted specifically of blisters (17 cases), pustules (16 cases) and erythema (5 cases). Annular erythema, vesicles and superficial flaccid blisters/vesicles were observed in two cases each. Itch was reported in three cases. Histopathologically subcorneal neutrophilic pustules are typically observed, while IgA deposits are confined to the upper epidermis.

The IEN-type often presents with central crusts and peripheral vesiculation, giving rise to so-called sunflower lesions [53] (Fig. 9.1). In contrast to the SPD type,

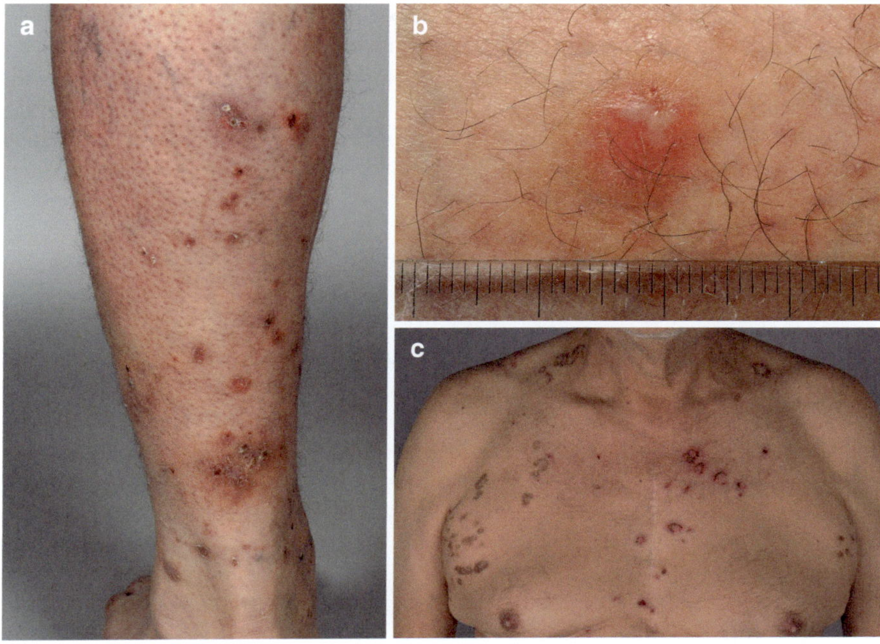

Fig. 9.1 Patient 1: 55-y.o. male patient with intercellular IgA dermatosis (**a** lower left leg, **b** detail of a pustule). Patient 2: 60-y.o. male patient with intercellular IgA dermatosis (**c** thorax)

mucosal involvement has been described with an associated colitis [54]. In our series [16] encompassing 12 IEN-type cases (24%) there was frequent involvement of the trunk (9 cases), extremities (10 cases), as well as of the back and buttock (6 cases). One case showed oral mucosal lesions. Specifically, cutaneous lesions in IEN-type comprised blisters (11 cases), pustules (8 cases) and erythema (7 cases). Annular erythema (three cases) and vesicles (four cases) were also observed. Itch was reported in only one case.

Clinical features of IgA-PV-type and PF-type are more variable and their diagnosis primarily depends on immunological findings. In contrast to the IgG-mediated pemphigus forms, pustules formation is more frequently observed. IgA-PF may show the same clinical presentation as the classic IgG-mediated counterpart [55]. In our four cases of IgA-PF, there was in once case each generalized or trunk involvement. Blisters, pustules and erythema were variably observed. There were no oral lesions. In IgA-PV oral involvement is not constant. In our series, only two out of six patients had oral lesions. Blistering was observed in three cases, whereas pustules also occurred in one case.

Diagnosis of IgA-PVeg critically relies on the clinical presence of typical vegetating lesions with PVeg-like histopathological changes. Our two IgA PVeg cases showed involvement of intertriginous areas with pustules and vegetating lesions.

In one case, lesions affected also the trunk. Erythema and erosions were variably observed. Itch may be present. IgA pemphigus cases have also been reported in children [17]. In these cases, circulating autoantibodies were found to react with either Dsg1 or Dsg3 [56].

Finally, all IAD cases that cannot be categorized into one of these five previous subtypes are referred as unclassified IAD subtype. In our series, there were eight such patients with unclassified IAD subtype.

Histopathological Features

Light microscopy studies in IAD are helpful and provide some diagnostic clues, at least for the SPD-type and IEN-type. In our series there were 37 cases , for which detailed histopathological findings were available [16]. Overall, we found intraepidermal lesions (26 cases) located in either the upper epidermis (18 cases) or the entire/middle epidermis (8 cases). Formation of pustules or blisters was found in 17 and 3 cases, respectively. Intraepidermal infiltrations of neutrophils, eosinophils and lymphocytes were found in 23, 11 and 4 cases, respectively, while acantholysis was present in 17 cases.

Specifically, the 16 studied SPD-type cases showed intraepidermal lesions at the upper epidermis or subcorneal areas (so called SPD-features), while 5 of 9 IEN-type cases showed intraepidermal lesions with pustule formation (IEN-like features) (Fig. 9.2). Acantholysis was present in two out of nine IEN-type cases. In the three IgA-pemphigus-types (IgA-PV, IgA-PF and IgAPVeg) as well as in the unclassified-IAD-type histopathological findings were more variable. Noteworthy, acantholysis was observed in only two out of the four cases of IgA pemphigus, but in six out of the seven unclassified IAD cases, which showed often intraepidermal pustules [16].

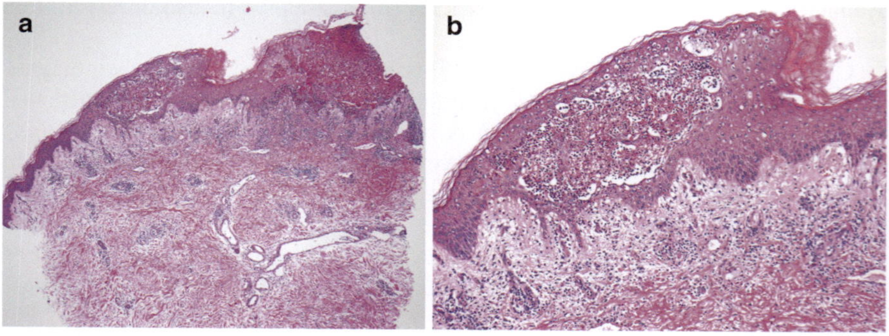

Fig. 9.2 Histology of a skin biopsy (inguinal right) showing an intraepidermal pustule with neutrophils and eosinophils, with isolated acantholytic keratinocytes. Dermal infiltrates with perivascular and interstitial neutrophilic and eosinophilic granulocytes (magnification 40× (**a**) and 100× (**b**))

Characterization of Target Antigens

The autoantigen of the SPD-type was identified as desmocollin 1 (Dsc1) [57], whereas the autoantigen of the IEN-type is still unknown. In single cases of SPD-type and IEN-type, weak IgA reactivity with Dsc3 may also be observed, the significance of which is unclear [56, 58–61]. In IgA-PVeg, IgA immunoreactivity remains unknown.

In unclassified IAD, the immunological profile is more heterogeneous and complex. Reactivities with Dsg1, Dsg3 and/or Dscs are occasionally detectable. In this unclassified IAD group, one could include cases which we previously reported under the term of IgA/IgG vesiculopustular dermatosis associated with both IgA and IgG deposits [62]. In fact we identified five patients with both IgG and IgA tissue-bound antibodies showing atypical clinical features. There was no specific reactivity of IgA antibodies with either Dsg1 or Dsg3 by immunoblot analysis. In one case each, IgG antibodies recognized Dsg1 or Dsg3. By immunoblotting of desmosome enriched fraction obtained from bovine snout epidermis, IgA antibodies in three cases and IgG antibodies in four cases showed reactivity with either Dsg1 or Dsc [62]. Noteworthy, presence of both IgG and IgA anti-Dsg3 antibodies is relatively common in sera from PV patients [63]. Nevertheless, the vast majority of these patients do not show intercellular IgA deposits.

We acknowledge that the proposed classification with six different IAD-subtypes has limitations and may appear arbitrary because of the existing clinicopathological and immunopathological overlap. For example, some cases classified as IgA-PV type due to the detection of IgA antibodies to Dsg3 present clinical features of IEN-type with sunflower-like lesions [54]. Furthermore, we have described patients with PVeg with both IgG and IgA anti-Dsg3 antibodies [64] as well as SPD-type pemphigus with anti-Dsg1 IgA and IgG antibodies, but no anti-Dsc antibodies [65]. These observations highlight the existing overlap between certain IAD types and the pemphigus group. However, this tentative classification provides the basis for future studies aimed at better delineating the immunopathological characteristics of the various IAD types and will be surely subject of further adjustments.

Associated Diseases

IgA pemphigus or IAD in general may be associated with an IgA monoclonal gammopathy. The latter has thus to be searched and excluded systematically [17], and may develop years after the onset of the dermatosis [10]. IgA monoclonal gammopathy may evolve to multiple myeloma [66]. Associations with other hematologic disorders [67], such as large B cell lymphoma [67], peripheral T-cell lymphomas [68], as well as with lung cancer [69, 70] have been described in cases of IgA pemphigus. A case with features of both IgA pemphigus and paraneoplastic pemphigus related to chronic lymphocytic leukemia has been reported [71].

Gastrointestinal diseases may also be associated with IAD: One case each of Crohn's disease and gluten-sensitive enteropathy have been reported [10].

Therapy of SPD and IAD

SPD. Subcorneal pustular dermatosis responds well to oral dapsone at doses of 50–150 mg daily [18]. The therapeutic response is less spectacular than in dermatitis herpetiformis. There is often a partial remission characterized by attenuated flares. Suspending dapsone between two flares is possible without causing immediate recurrence. Oral steroids, even high dosed, do not seem superior to dapsone [72]. In the series of Hashimoto et al. [16], dapsone was effective in one case, but not in another case. Systemic steroids were ineffective in two cases.

Alternative therapies include acitretin [21, 73–75], and etretinate [76, 77], as well as psoralen ultraviolet (UV)A [77–79] and narrowband UVB [80, 81], alone or in combination with dapsone and/or retinoids. Topical and systemic corticosteroids have also been used [82]. Furthermore, tacalcitol [83], sulfapyridine and sulfamethoxypyridazine, ketoconazole, tetracycline, cyclins, vitamin E, ciclosporin, colchicine, mizoribine and mebhydroline have also been tried with variable success [18]. Infliximab [84, 85] or etanercept [52, 86] have been anecdotally effective. Treatment of the associated myeloma may also lead to improvement of the SPD [25, 87].

IAD. Dapsone (50–200 mg/day) is the first choice therapy, used alone or in combination with topical steroids and colchicine [17]. Retinoids (acitretin, etretinate) may be used in cases where dapsone is not tolerated or inefficient [88]. Therapeutic alternatives are methotrexate [89], oral corticosteroids, retinoids [90], cyclins, and adalimumab with mycophenolate mofetil [91], as well as an anecdotic report of a therapeutic success with the macrolide azithromycin [92].

Pathogenicity of IgA Anti-cell Surface Antibodies in IAD

In over 50% of the cases the serum of IAD patients contains circulating IgA (and sometimes IgG) autoantibodies directed against epidermal components, like desmocollins (Dscs) (mostly Dsc1, but also Dsc2 and Dsc3), Dsg1, Dsg3 or other still uncharacterized antigens [15, 57].

Compared to the ample data demonstrating the pathogenicity of anti-Dsg IgG antibodies in classic pemphigus [93], the significance of IgA auto-antibodies against Dsgs, Dscs and other as-yet uncharacterized antigens is still incompletely understood.

Despite the fact that IgA reactivity is found in a substantial number of patients with classic forms of pemphigus, there is somehow surprisingly little functional data about the effect of IgA anti-Dsg antibodies on cell-cell adhesion, signaling and inflammation. There is some *in vitro* evidence suggesting that IgG anti-Dsc3 antibodies can cause cell-cell dissociation with loss of keratinocyte adhesion [94], but it is unknown if IgA anti-Dsc antibodies can also induce acantholysis [54]. IgA autoantibodies may induce the accumulation of neutrophils in the epidermis by binding to Fc alpha receptors [95].

In addition to the characterization of the various antigens bound by IgA antibodies, the antigenic sites on Dsgs and Dscs recognized by circulating IgA antibodies should be defined. These studies will disclose whether these IgA auto-antibodies bind to the same EC1 and EC2 domains of desmogleins as the pathogenic IgG antibodies in PV. These antibodies were found to disrupt trans- and potentially cisadhesion between Dsg3 molecules [96].

To gain better insight into the mechanisms causing tissue damage and accumulation of neutrophils, it will be very useful to generate human monoclonal IgA antibodies directed against Dscs, Dsgs and other targeted antigens for both in vitro and in vivo studies. The clinical phenotype of IAD characterized by a benign evolution is most likely related to the predominant IgA response, the pathogenic effects of which are inferior to the IgG4-mediated immune response to Dsg1 and Dsg3 found in patients with PV or PF.

Diagnostic Approach

In case of suspicion, diagnosis of IAD relies on the finding of direct immunofluorescence microscopic studies showing epidermal cell surface tissue-bound IgA.

In the SPD-type of IAD, IgA is predominantly confined to the upper epidermal layers, whereas in the IEN-subtype IgA deposits have a broader distribution and may be found in the entire epidermis [16] (Fig. 9.3). In case of IgA-PF and Ig-PV, the distribution of IgA deposits varies according to the targeted antigens, either Dsg1 or Dsg3 with predominant superficial staining or basal epidermal staining, respectively.

If IgA deposits are found in the epidermis, it is necessary to perform immunoserological tests to search for circulating IgA antibodies. Routinely used approaches include indirect immunofluorescence microscopic studies using normal human skin and monkey esophagus as substrate. In our series of 49 patients with IAD cases, 60% and 25% of the tested serum samples had IgA anti-keratinocyte cell surface antibodies using these two substrates, respectively. IgG reactivity is almost never observed and if present, it is weak [16].

To further characterize the specificity of the circulating IgA antibodies, there are actually few routinely available approaches. The standard ELISAs for IgG anti-Dsg1 and anti-Dsg3 antibodies are almost invariably negative. In contrast, in modified ELISA in which Dsg1 and Dsg3 are reacted by second step anti-IgA antibodies, IgA reactivities with Dsg1 and Dsg3 were found in 15.8% of 38 tested IAD sera. Such findings allow classifying the IAD cases as IgA-PF and Ig-PV, respectively.

To demonstrate the presence of IgA anti-Dsc autoantibodies, it is necessary to take advantage of more sophisticated approaches, such as COS-7 cell cDNA transfection methods with immunofluorescence studies of cells expressing human Dsc1, Dsc2, or Dsc3. Alternatively, we also developed novel ELISAs using eukaryotic recombinant forms of human Dsc1, Dsc2 and Dsc3. In SPD-type of IAD patients' sera characteristically bind to Dsc1 and, in rare instances, also to Dsc3. Patients

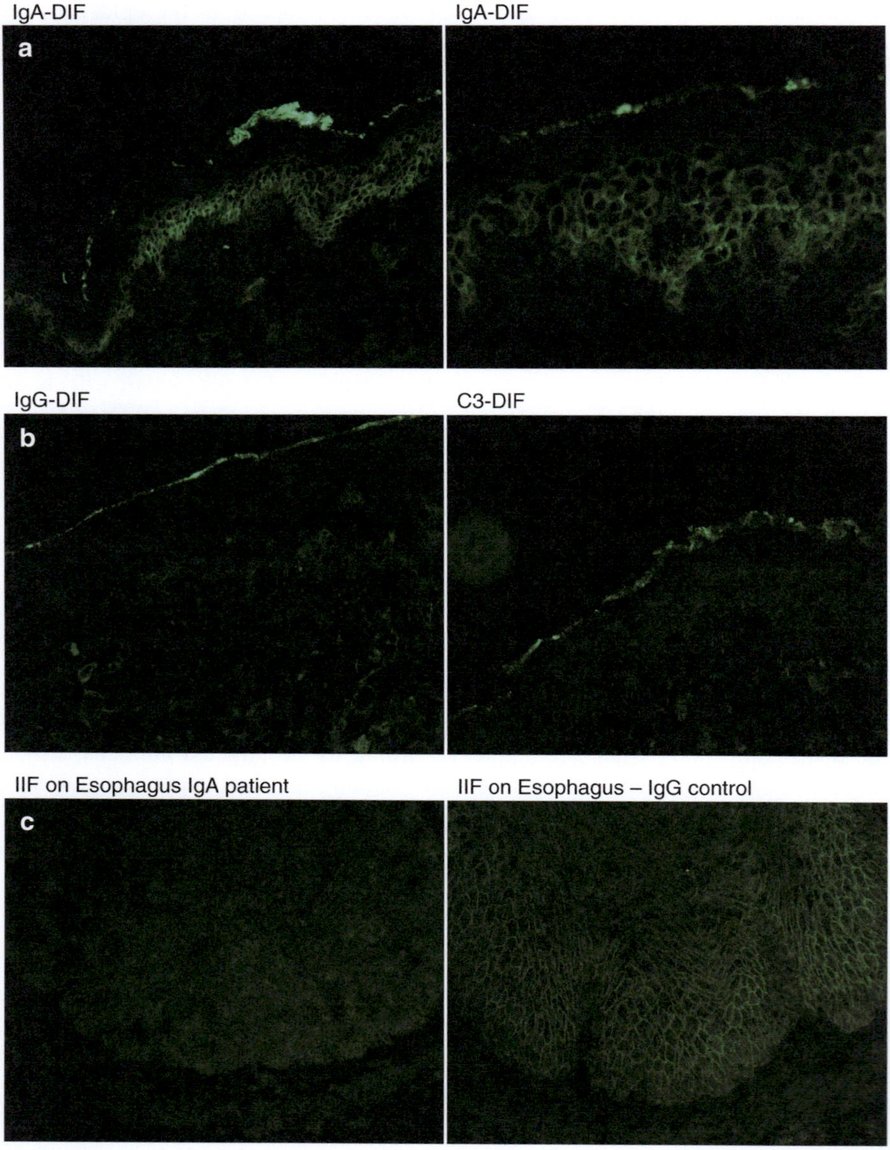

Fig. 9.3 (**a**) Direct immunofluorescence shows intercellular deposition of IgA in the epidermis and IIF (magnification 40× and 100×). (**b**) With no deposits of IgG. (**c**) Indirect immunofluorescence on rabbit esophagus shows intercellular deposition of IgA in the epithelium

with IEN-type of IAD show almost invariably no reactivity with the various Dsc isoforms. In our series, only 1 of 11 IEN-type cases reacted with Dsc3.

Finally, immunoblotting techniques using normal human epidermal keratinocytes have low sensitivities. We found IgA reactivities with Dsg3 and Dsc only in single cases of IAD.

For detection of IgA antibodies to Dsgs, immunoblotting is less sensitive than ELISAs. Therefore, when the results obtained by ELISA and immunoblotting are discordant, it is recommended to give priority to the ELISA findings. Regardless of the clinical and histopathological diagnoses of the four IAD sub-types, cases with positive IgA ELISA results for Dsg1 and Dsg3 are diagnosed as IgA-PF and IgA-PV, respectively. Cases with typical clinical and histopathological features of SPD but without tissue-bound and circulating IgA antibodies are diagnoses as classical SPD. By using normal human skin and recombinant forms of BP180, it is occasionally possible to detect anti-BP180 and anti-BP230 IgG and IgA antibodies, the significance of which is unclear. These reactivities may account for the IgA deposits found along the epidermal basement membrane zone in 10% of IAD cases [72].

By modifying the commercially available ELISA-Dsg1- and Dsg3 for IgA reactivity, it is however possible to at least distinguish patients with IgA-PF and IgA-PV with IgA anti-Dsg antibodies from other IAD patients, including cases with the SPD-type and IEN-type subtypes.

Since the techniques described here above are currently available in only a few laboratories and because of the clinicopathological and immunological overlap, many IAD cases cannot be precisely classified.

Acknowledgments We thank Dr. Michael Horn, Head Autoimmunediagnostics, University Institute of clinical chemistry, Inselspital, Bern University Hospital, University of Bern, Switzerland, for the immunofluorescence pictures.

References

1. Sneddon IB, Wilkinson DS. Subcorneal pustular dermatosis. Br J Dermatol. 1956;68(12):385–94.
2. Scerri L, Zaki I, Allen BR. Pyoderma gangrenosum and subcorneal pustular dermatosis, without monoclonal gammopathy. Br J Dermatol. 1994;130(3):398–9.
3. Powell FC, Su WP, Perry HO. Pyoderma gangrenosum: classification and management. J Am Acad Dermatol. 1996;34(3):395–409. 412
4. Marsden JR, Millard LG. Pyoderma gangrenosum, subcorneal pustular dermatosis and IgA paraproteinaemia. Br J Dermatol. 1986;114(1):125–9.
5. Wallach D, Vignon-Pennamen M-D. From acute febrile neutrophilic dermatosis to neutrophilic disease: forty years of clinical research. J Am Acad Dermatol. 2006;55(6):1066–71.
6. Wallach D, Foldès C, Cottenot F. [Subcorneal pustulosis, superficial acantholysis and monoclonal IgA]. Ann Dermatol Venereol. 1982;109(11):959–63.
7. Varigos GA. Subcorneal pustulosis with IgA abnormalities in serum and small bowel mucosa: case report. Australas J Dermatol. 1979;20(2):75–7.
8. Sneddon IB, Wilkinson DS. Subcorneal pustular dermatosis. Br J Dermatol. 1979;100(1):61–8.
9. Borradori L, Saada V, Rybojad M, Flageul B, Kuffer R, Lémann M, et al. Oral intraepidermal IgA pustulosis and Crohn's disease. Br J Dermatol. 1992;126(4):383–6.
10. Wallach D. Intraepidermal IgA pustulosis. J Am Acad Dermatol. 1992;27(6 Pt 1):993–1000.
11. Wallach D, Janssen F, Vignon-Pennamen MD, Lemarchand-Venencie F, Cottenot F. Atypical neutrophilic dermatosis with subcorneal IgA deposits. Arch Dermatol. 1987;123(6):790–5.
12. Hashimoto T, Inamoto N, Nakamura K, Nishikawa T. Intercellular IgA dermatosis with clinical features of subcorneal pustular dermatosis. Arch Dermatol. 1987;123(8):1062–5.
13. Huff JC, Golitz LE, Kunke KS. Intraepidermal neutrophilic IgA dermatosis. N Engl J Med. 1985;313(26):1643–5.

14. Ebihara T, Hashimoto T, Iwatsuki K, Takigawa M, Ando M, Ohkawara A, et al. Autoantigens for IgA anti-intercellular antibodies of intercellular IgA vesiculopustular dermatosis. J Invest Dermatol. 1991;97(4):742–5.
15. Hashimoto T, Nishikawa T. Nomenclature for diseases with IgA antikeratinocyte cell surface autoantibodies. Br J Dermatol. 2015;173(3):868–9.
16. Hashimoto T, Teye K, Ishii N. Clinical and immunological studies of 49 cases of various types of intercellular IgA dermatosis and 13 cases of classical subcorneal pustular dermatosis examined at Kurume University. Br J Dermatol. 2017;176(1):168–75.
17. Geller S, Gat A, Zeeli T, Hafner A, Eming R, Hertl M, et al. The expanding spectrum of IgA pemphigus: a case report and review of the literature. Br J Dermatol. 2014;171(3):650–6.
18. Cheng S, Edmonds E, Ben-Gashir M, Yu RC. Subcorneal pustular dermatosis: 50 years on. Clin Exp Dermatol. 2008;33(3):229–33.
19. Naik HB, Cowen EW. Autoinflammatory pustular neutrophilic diseases. Dermatol Clin. 2013;31(3):405–25.
20. Watts PJ, Khachemoune A. Subcorneal pustular dermatosis: a review of 30 years of progress. Am J Clin Dermatol. 2016;17(6):653–71.
21. Yayli S, Bahadir S, Alpay K, Cimşit G, Reis A. A case of juvenile subcorneal pustular dermatosis successfully treated with acitretin. Int J Dermatol. 2006;45(9):1131–3.
22. Garg BR, Sait MA, Baruah MC. Subcorneal pustular dermatosis in a young boy. Indian J Dermatol. 1985;30(4):21–3.
23. Johnson SA, Cripps DJ. Subcorneal pustular dermatosis in children. Arch Dermatol. 1974;109(1):73–7.
24. Ryan TJ. Sneddon and Wilkinson's pustular dermatosis does exist. Am J Dermatopathol. 1981;3(4):383–4.
25. Kasha EE, Epinette WW. Subcorneal pustular dermatosis (Sneddon-Wilkinson disease) in association with a monoclonal IgA gammopathy: a report and review of the literature. J Am Acad Dermatol. 1988;19(5 Pt 1):854–8.
26. Lautenschlager S, Itin PH, Hirsbrunner P, Büchner SA. Subcorneal pustular dermatosis at the injection site of recombinant human granulocyte-macrophage colony-stimulating factor in a patient with IgA myeloma. J Am Acad Dermatol. 1994;30(5 Pt 1):787–9.
27. Aste N, Fumo G, Pinna AL, Biggio P. IgA pemphigus of the subcorneal pustular dermatosis type associated with monoclonal IgA gammopathy. J Eur Acad Dermatol Venereol JEADV. 2003;17(6):725–7.
28. Vaccaro M, Cannavò SP, Guarneri B. Subcorneal pustular dermatosis and IgA lambda myeloma: a uncommon association but probably not coincidental. Eur J Dermatol EJD. 1999;9(8):644–6.
29. Atukorala DN, Joshi RK, Abanmi A, Jeha MT. Subcorneal pustular dermatosis and IgA myeloma. Dermatol Basel Switz. 1993;187(2):124–6.
30. Bölcskei L, Husz S, Hunyadi J, Varga G, Dobozy A. Subcorneal pustular dermatosis and IgA multiple myeloma. J Dermatol. 1992;19(10):626–8.
31. Dal Tio R, Di Vito F, Salvi F. Subcorneal pustular dermatosis and IgA myeloma. Dermatologica. 1985;170(5):240–3.
32. Weiner S. Subcorneal pustular dermatosis and rheumatoid arthritis. Arthritis Rheum. 1981;24(9):1213–4.
33. Brantley EI, Sheth P. Subcorneal pustular dermatosis in a patient with rheumatoid arthritis and diffuse scleroderma. Dermatol Online J. 2009;15(3):5.
34. Scheinfeld NS, Worth R, Mallea J, Shookster L, Weinberg JM. Subcorneal pustular dermatosis developing in a patient with rheumatoid arthritis; rheumatoid, antimicrosomal, and antimitochondrial autoantibodies; and a goiter. Skinmed. 2003;2(4):258–9.
35. Roger H, Thevenet JP, Souteyrand P, Sauvezie B. Subcorneal pustular dermatosis associated with rheumatoid arthritis and raised IgA: simultaneous remission of skin and joint involvements with dapsone treatment. Ann Rheum Dis. 1990;49(3):190–1.
36. Scarpa R, Lubrano E, Cozzi R, Ames PR, Oriente CB, Oriente P. Subcorneal pustular dermatosis (Sneddon-Wilkinson syndrome): another cutaneous manifestation of SAPHO syndrome? Br J Rheumatol. 1997;36(5):602–3.

37. Saulsbury FT, Kesler RW. Subcorneal pustular dermatosis and systemic lupus erythematosus. Int J Dermatol. 1984;23(1):63–4.
38. Tsuruta D, Matsumura-Oura A, Ishii M. Subcorneal pustular dermatosis and Sjögren's syndrome. Int J Dermatol. 2005;44(11):955–7.
39. Delaporte E, Colombel JF, Nguyen-Mailfer C, Piette F, Cortot A, Bergoend H. Subcorneal pustular dermatosis in a patient with Crohn's disease. Acta Derm Venereol. 1992;72(4): 301–2.
40. Taniguchi S, Tsuruta D, Kutsuna H, Hamada T. Subcorneal pustular dermatosis in a patient with hyperthyroidism. Dermatol Basel Switz. 1995;190(1):64–6.
41. Köhler LD, Möhrenschlager M, Worret WI, Ring J. Subcorneal pustular dermatosis (Sneddon-Wilkinson disease) in a patient with multiple sclerosis. Dermatol Basel Switz. 1999;199(1):69–70.
42. Park BS, Cho KH, Eun HC, Youn JI. Subcorneal pustular dermatosis in a patient with aplastic anemia. J Am Acad Dermatol. 1998;39(2 Pt 1):287–9.
43. Papini M, Cicoletti M, Landucci P. Subcorneal pustular dermatosis and mycoplasma pneumoniae respiratory infection. Acta Derm Venereol. 2003;83(5):387–8.
44. Bohelay G, Duong TA, Ortonne N, Chosidow O, Valeyrie-Allanore L. Subcorneal pustular dermatosis triggered by Mycoplasma pneumoniae infection: a rare clinical association. J Eur Acad Dermatol Venereol JEADV. 2015;29(5):1022–5.
45. Lombart F, Dhaille F, Lok C, Dadban A. Subcorneal pustular dermatosis associated with Mycoplasma pneumoniae infection. J Am Acad Dermatol. 2014;71(3):e85–6.
46. Calista D. Subcorneal pustular dermatosis in a patient with AIDS. J Eur Acad Dermatol Venereol JEADV. 2003;17(4):478–9.
47. Brown SJ, Barrett PD, Hendrick A, Langtry JA. Subcorneal pustular dermatosis in association with chronic lymphocytic leukaemia. Acta Derm Venereol. 2003;83(4):306–7.
48. Agarwal A, Shivaswamy KN, Raja B, Thappa DM, Verma SK. Subcorneal pustular dermatosis and thymoma: an association or a coincidence? Indian J Dermatol. 2006;51(4):272.
49. Villey MC, Ehrsam E, Marrakchi S, Colombel JF, Thomas P. Apudoma and subcorneal pustular dermatosis (Sneddon-Wilkinson disease). Dermatol Basel Switz. 1992;185(4):269–71.
50. Buchet S, Humbert P, Blanc D, Derancourt C, Beckerich D, Ranfaing E, et al. [Subcorneal pustular dermatosis associated with epidermoid carcinoma of the lung]. Ann Dermatol Venereol. 1991;118(2):125–8.
51. Grob JJ, Mege JL, Capo C, Jancovicci E, Fournerie JR, Bongrand P, et al. Role of tumor necrosis factor-alpha in Sneddon-Wilkinson subcorneal pustular dermatosis. A model of neutrophil priming in vivo. J Am Acad Dermatol. 1991;25(5 Pt 2):944–7.
52. Berk DR, Hurt MA, Mann C, Sheinbein D. Sneddon-Wilkinson disease treated with etanercept: report of two cases. Clin Exp Dermatol. 2009;34(3):347–51.
53. Heng A, Nwaneshiudu A, Hashimoto T, Amagai M, Stanley JR. Intraepidermal neutrophilic IgA/IgG antidesmocollin 1 pemphigus. Br J Dermatol. 2006;154(5):1018–20.
54. Tajima M, Mitsuhashi Y, Irisawa R, Amagai M, Hashimoto T, Tsuboi R. IgA pemphigus reacting exclusively to desmoglein 3. Eur J Dermatol EJD. 2010;20(5):626–9.
55. Beutner EH, Chorzelski TP, Wilson RM, Kumar V, Michel B, Helm F, et al. IgA pemphigus foliaceus. Report of two cases and a review of the literature. J Am Acad Dermatol. 1989;20(1):89–97.
56. Hashimoto T, Komai A, Futei Y, Nishikawa T, Amagai M. Detection of IgA autoantibodies to desmogleins by an enzyme-linked immunosorbent assay: the presence of new minor subtypes of IgA pemphigus. Arch Dermatol. 2001;137(6):735–8.
57. Hashimoto T, Kiyokawa C, Mori O, Miyasato M, Chidgey MA, Garrod DR, et al. Human desmocollin 1 (Dsc1) is an autoantigen for the subcorneal pustular dermatosis type of IgA pemphigus. J Invest Dermatol. 1997;109(2):127–31.
58. Hegazy S, Bouchouicha S, Khaled A, Laadher L, Sellami MK, Zeglaoui F. IgA pemphigus showing IgA antibodies to desmoglein 1 and 3. Dermatol Pract Concept. 2016;6(4):31–3.
59. Prost C, Intrator L, Wechsler J, Lebbe C, Bagot M, Roujeau JC, et al. IgA autoantibodies bind to pemphigus vulgaris antigen in a case of intraepidermal neutrophilic IgA dermatosis. J Am Acad Dermatol. 1991;25(5 Pt 1):846–8.

60. Wang J, Kwon J, Ding X, Fairley JA, Woodley DT, Chan LS. Nonsecretory IgA1 autoantibodies targeting desmosomal component desmoglein 3 in intraepidermal neutrophilic IgA dermatosis. Am J Pathol. 1997;150(6):1901–7.
61. Kárpáti S, Amagai M, Liu WL, Dmochowski M, Hashimoto T, Horváth A. Identification of desmoglein 1 as autoantigen in a patient with intraepidermal neutrophilic IgA dermatosis type of IgA pemphigus. Exp Dermatol. 2000;9(3):224–8.
62. Hashimoto T, Ebihara T, Nishikawa T. Studies of autoantigens recognized by IgA anti-keratinocyte cell surface antibodies. J Dermatol Sci. 1996;12(1):10–7.
63. Spaeth S, Riechers R, Borradori L, Zillikens D, Büdinger L, Hertl M. IgG, IgA and IgE autoantibodies against the ectodomain of desmoglein 3 in active pemphigus vulgaris. Br J Dermatol. 2001;144(6):1183–8.
64. Morizane S, Yamamoto T, Hisamatsu Y, Tsuji K, Oono T, Hashimoto T, et al. Pemphigus vegetans with IgG and IgA antidesmoglein 3 antibodies. Br J Dermatol. 2005;153(6):1236–7.
65. Maruyama H, Kawachi Y, Fujisawa Y, Itoh S, Furuta J, Ishii Y, et al. IgA/IgG pemphigus positive for anti-desmoglein 1 autoantibody. Eur J Dermatol EJD. 2007;17(1):94–5.
66. Szturz P, Adam Z, Klincová M, Feit J, Krejčí M, Pour L, et al. Multiple myeloma associated IgA pemphigus: treatment with bortezomib- and lenalidomide-based regimen. Clin Lymphoma Myeloma Leuk. 2011;11(6):517–20.
67. Asahina A, Koga H, Suzuki Y, Hashimoto T. IgA pemphigus associated with diffuse large B-cell lymphoma showing unique reactivity with desmocollins: unusual clinical and histopathological features. Br J Dermatol. 2013;168(1):224–6.
68. Chen L, Yang B, Fan J, Yang K, Liu H, Wu G. Peripheral T-cell lymphoma complicated by immunoglobulin A pemphigus: a case report and literature review. Oncol Lett. 2014;8(1):62–6.
69. Cetkovská P, Komorousová M, Lomicová I. Management of a pemphigus with IgA and IgG antibodies and coexistent lung cancer. Dermatol Ther. 2014;27(4):236–9.
70. Petropoulou H, Politis G, Panagakis P, Hatziolou E, Aroni K, Kontochristopoulos G. Immunoglobulin A pemphigus associated with immunoglobulin A gammopathy and lung cancer. J Dermatol. 2008;35(6):341–5.
71. Taintor AR, Leiferman KM, Hashimoto T, Ishii N, Zone JJ, Hull CM. A novel case of IgA paraneoplastic pemphigus associated with chronic lymphocytic leukemia. J Am Acad Dermatol. 2007;56(5 Suppl):S73–6.
72. Navarini AA, Borradori L, Saurat J-H. Pustuloses amicrobiennes. In: Dermatologie et infections sexuellement transmissibles. 6th ed. Elsevier Masson; 2017.
73. Marlière V, Beylot-Barry M, Beylot C, Doutre M. Successful treatment of subcorneal pustular dermatosis (Sneddon-wilkinson disease) by acitretin: report of a case. Dermatol Basel Switz. 1999;199(2):153–5.
74. Teixeira M, Lves RA, Seloresi M. Subcorneal pustular dermatosis in association with a monoclonal IgA/k gammopathy: successful treatment with acitretin. Eur J Dermatol EJD. 2006;16(5):588–90.
75. Canpolat F, Akpinar H, Cemil BC, Eskioğlu F, Oztürk E. A case of subcorneal pustular dermatosis in association with monoclonal IgA gammopathy successfully treated with acitretin. J Dermatol Treat. 2010;21(2):114–6.
76. Iandoli R, Monfrecola G. Treatment of subcorneal pustulosis by etretinate. Dermatologica. 1987;175(5):235–8.
77. Todd DJ, Bingham EA, Walsh M, Burrows D. Subcorneal pustular dermatosis and IgA paraproteinaemia: response to both etretinate and PUVA. Br J Dermatol. 1991;125(4):387–9.
78. Bauwens M, De Coninck A, Roseeuw D. Subcorneal pustular dermatosis treated with PUVA therapy. A case report and review of the literature. Dermatol Basel Switz. 1999;198(2):203–5.
79. Khachemoune A, Blyumin ML. Sneddon-Wilkinson disease resistant to dapsone and colchicine successfully controlled with PUVA. Dermatol Online J. 2003;9(5):24.
80. Orton DI, George SA. Subcorneal pustular dermatosis responsive to narrowband (TL-01) UVB phototherapy. Br J Dermatol. 1997;137(1):149–61.

81. Cameron H, Dawe RS. Subcorneal pustular dermatosis (Sneddon-Wilkinson disease) treated with narrowband (TL-01) UVB phototherapy. Br J Dermatol. 1997;137(1):150–1.
82. Laifaoui J, Guillen E, Worret W, Ring J. A case of subcorneal pustular dermatosis (Sneddon-Wilkinson disease) not responding to dapsone: therapeutic alternatives. Acta Dermatoven APA. 2003;12:109.
83. Mühlhoff C, Megahed M. Therapy of subcorneal pustulosis (Sneddon-Wilkinson disease) with tacalcitol. Hautarzt Z Dermatol Venerol Verwandte Geb. 2009;60(5):369–70.
84. Voigtländer C, Lüftl M, Schuler G, Hertl M. Infliximab (anti-tumor necrosis factor alpha antibody): a novel, highly effective treatment of recalcitrant subcorneal pustular dermatosis (Sneddon-Wilkinson disease). Arch Dermatol. 2001;137(12):1571–4.
85. Bonifati C, Trento E, Cordiali Fei P, Muscardin L, Amantea A, Carducci M. Early but not lasting improvement of recalcitrant subcorneal pustular dermatosis (Sneddon-Wilkinson disease) after infliximab therapy: relationships with variations in cytokine levels in suction blister fluids. Clin Exp Dermatol. 2005;30(6):662–5.
86. Bedi MK. Successful treatment of long-standing, recalcitrant subcorneal pustular dermatosis with etanercept. Skinmed. 2007;6(5):245–7.
87. von dem Borne PA, Jonkman MF, van Doorn R. Complete remission of skin lesions in a patient with subcorneal pustular dermatosis (Sneddon-Wilkinson disease) treated with anti-myeloma therapy: association with disappearance of M-protein. Br J Dermatol. 2017;176(5):1341–4.
88. Ruiz-Genao DP, Hernández-Núñez A, Hashimoto T, Amagai M, Fernández-Herrera J, García-Díez A. A case of IgA pemphigus successfully treated with acitretin. Br J Dermatol. 2002;147(5):1040–2.
89. Gniadecki R, Bygum A, Clemmensen O, Svejgaard E, Ullman S. IgA pemphigus: the first two Scandinavian cases. Acta Derm Venereol. 2002;82(6):441–5.
90. Yasuda H, Kobayashi H, Hashimoto T, Itoh K, Yamane M, Nakamura J. Subcorneal pustular dermatosis type of IgA pemphigus: demonstration of autoantibodies to desmocollin-1 and clinical review. Br J Dermatol. 2000;143(1):144–8.
91. Howell SM, Bessinger GT, Altman CE, Belnap CM. Rapid response of IgA pemphigus of the subcorneal pustular dermatosis subtype to treatment with adalimumab and mycophenolate mofetil. J Am Acad Dermatol. 2005;53(3):541–3.
92. Bliziotis I, Rafailidis P, Vergidis P, Falagas ME. Regression of subcorneal pustular dermatosis type of IgA pemphigus lesions with azithromycin. J Infect. 2005;51(2):E31–4.
93. Di Zenzo G, Amber KT, Sayar BS, Müller EJ, Borradori L. Immune response in pemphigus and beyond: progresses and emerging concepts. Semin Immunopathol. 2016;38(1):57–74.
94. Rafei D, Müller R, Ishii N, Llamazares M, Hashimoto T, Hertl M, et al. IgG autoantibodies against desmocollin 3 in pemphigus sera induce loss of keratinocyte adhesion. Am J Pathol. 2011;178(2):718–23.
95. Smith AD, Streilein RD, Hall RP. Neutrophil CD11b, L-selectin and Fc IgA receptors in patients with dermatitis herpetiformis. Br J Dermatol. 2002;147(6):1109–17.
96. Di Zenzo G, Di Lullo G, Corti D, Calabresi V, Sinistro A, Vanzetta F, et al. Pemphigus autoantibodies generated through somatic mutations target the desmoglein-3 cis-interface. J Clin Invest. 2012;122(10):3781–90.

Aseptic Pustulosis of the Folds

10

Angelo Valerio Marzano, Riccardo Lazzari, and Alessandro Borghi

Introduction

Aseptic (or amicrobial) pustulosis of the skin folds (APF) is a rare neutrophilic dermatosis, occurring mostly in young females affected with autoimmune or dysimmune disorders, characterized by relapsing sterile pustular eruptions mainly involving the skin folds. The disease was first reported in 1991 by Crickx and colleagues [1], who described two young women with systemic lupus erythematosus (SLE) and outbreaks of amicrobial pustules involving the scalp, major folds, and external ear canals. Subsequently, two other similar cases have been described in association with SLE and incomplete SLE, respectively [2, 3]. On reporting three additional cases in young women with subacute cutaneous lupus erythematosus (SCLE), celiac disease and various serum autoantibodies, respectively, Marzano et al. speculated that APF may represent a new entity within the spectrum of neutrophilic dermatoses [4]. Moreover, the same authors emphasized the concept that this form may be associated not only with lupus, but also with a broad spectrum of underlying autoimmune diseases or immunological abnormalities [4]. Since then, similar clinical features have been described in association with a number of other autoimmune disorders [5–13]. More recently, the inclusion of APF within the spectrum of autoinflammatory diseases has opened a new prospective in the pathophysiology of this condition [14], paving the way to

A. V. Marzano (✉) • R. Lazzari
Dipartimento di Fisiopatologia Medico-Chirurgica e dei Trapianti,
Università degli Studi di Milano, Unità Operativa di Dermatologia, IRCCS Fondazione Ca' Granda, Ospedale Maggiore Policlinico, Milano, Italy
e-mail: angelo.marzano@unimi.it

A. Borghi
Dipartimento di Scienze Mediche, Sezione di Dermatologia e Malattie Infettive,
Università degli Studi di Ferrara, Ferrara, Italy
e-mail: alessandro.borghi@unife.it

D. Wallach et al. (eds.), *Neutrophilic Dermatoses*,
https://doi.org/10.1007/978-3-319-72649-6_10

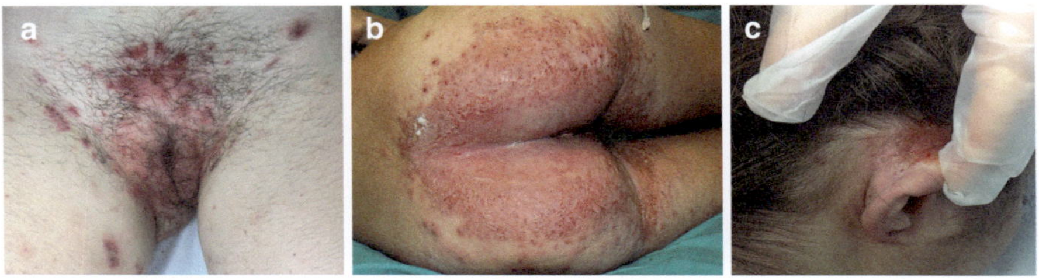

Fig. 10.1 Amicrobial pustulosis of the folds presenting with pustular lesions, erosions and crusts on the anogenital area (panels **a** and **b**) and retroauricolar region (panel **c**)

the use of biologic agents targeting the main pro-inflammatory cytokines for the management of refractory or highly relapsing APF cases.

Clinical and Histopathological Features

APF is a rare chronic relapsing dermatosis that affects almost exclusively young women with varying underlying autoimmune or dysimmune diseases. It is characterized by sudden onset of follicular and nonfollicular sterile pustular lesions involving the main cutaneous folds, usually with symmetrical distribution, anogenital area and scalp as well as the minor skin folds, particularly the area around the nostrils, retroauricular regions, and external auditory canals (Fig. 10.1). Generalised forms of pustulosis may be rarely observed [10]. The pustules overly erythematous, eczematous, or macerated skin surfaces, may tend to coalesce forming oozing, crusted or erosive areas and are usually accompanied by burning or frank pain. Onychodystrophy with suppurative vegetating paronychia is a common finding [10]. Although APF is typically amicrobial in origin, various bacterial species may secondarily colonize older pustular lesions and macerated erosive areas. Long term remissions of APF have been only rarely reported [9] and relapses of the disease following tapering or discontinuation of treatment are common.

Laboratory Findings

An increase in the acute phase reactants, namely erythrocyte sedimentation rate (usually ranging from 60 mm/1st h to 100 mm/1st h) and serum levels of C reactive protein (usually ranging from 1 to 6 mg/dL; normal values <0.5 mg/dL) is a common finding in APF patients. Various serum autoantibodies are frequently detected (Table 10.1). However, it is noteworthy that autoantibodies can be found in patients' serum regardless of the presence of an underlying autoimmune/dysimmune disease [14], suggesting that these autoantibodies do not necessarily have a clinical relevance.

Table 10.1 Major and minor criteria for the diagnosis of amicrobial pustulosis of the folds

Major criteria	Minor criteria
Pustulosis involving one or more major folds, one or more minor folds, and the anogenital area	Association with one or more autoimmune or autoinflammatory disorders
Histologic pattern consisting of intraepidermal spongiform pustules and a mainly neutrophilic dermal infiltrate	Positive ANA at a titer of 1/160 or higher
Negative culture from unopened pustule	One or more serum autoantibodies (anti-ENA, anti-dsDNA, antiphospholipid, antihistone, antismooth muscle, antimitochondrial ,antigastric parietal cell, and antiendomysial)

The diagnosis of amicrobial pustulosis of the folds can be ascertained if major criteria and at least one minor criterion are fulfilled. *ANA* antinuclear antibodies, *dsDNA* double-stranded DNA, *ENA* extractable nuclear antigens

Histopathological Aspects and Direct/Indirect Immunofluorescence Findings

The histopathological findings include subcorneal or intraepidermal spongiform pustules and a dermal inflammatory infiltrate predominantly consisting of neutrophils, without vasculitis [4, 10, 15]. Older plaques show psoriasiform hyperplasia with parakeratosis, neutrophil exocytosis and a dermal lymphocytic infiltrate. Direct and indirect immunofluorescence are typically negative. Due to its histological features, APF has been included in the spectrum of neutrophilic dermatoses (NDs) [4], which represent a clinically heterogeneous group of disorders hallmarked by an accumulation of neutrophils in the skin and rarely internal organs [16, 17]. In 2006, Wallach and Vignon-Pennamen proposed a clinicopathological classification for NDs based on the localization of the neutrophilic infiltrate and subdividing the NDs into three groups: (1) superficial ND, characterized by an epidermal neutrophilic infiltrate, and including subcorneal pustular dermatosis as the most representative form; (2) ND "en plaques" characterized by a dermal neutrophilic infiltrate, and whose prototype is Sweet's syndrome (SS); (3) deep ND, characterized by a dermal and hypodermal infiltrate, and whose paradigm is pyoderma gangrenosum (PG) [16]. Like subcorneal pustular dermatosis, APF may be regarded as another prototypic superficial ND.

Diagnostic Criteria and Differential Diagnosis

The diagnosis of APF remains challenging, as it shares clinical and histological features with other pustular conditions. Firstly, it is necessary to exclude possible primary infectious causes of subcorneal pustules, such as candidosis, folliculitis and impetigo, which are by far the most frequent forms of pustulosis. The clinical picture of APF is similar to that of pustular psoriasis, mainly its inverse type, which, however, usually spares the minor folds and often presents with psoriasis lesions in other sites of the body. APF must also be differentiated from a number of other conditions, including subcorneal pustular dermatosis or Sneddon-Wilkinson disease, acute generalized exanthematous pustulosis (AGEP), pemphigus foliaceus, and autoimmune bullous diseases with pustular or erythematous presentation such as pemphigus foliaceous and IgA pemphigus, respectively. A set of criteria to assist with differential diagnosis of APF has been proposed by Marzano et al. [10], mainly both major and minor diagnostic criteria on the basis of involved sites, histopathological features and immunological findings (Table 10.1). In particular, obligate features include the occurrence of pustules along either one major or minor flexure and the anogenital area, intraepidermal pustules with a dermal mainly neutrophilic infiltrate on histology and negative microbial cultures from unopened pustule. Minor criteria include autoimmune comorbidities and antinuclear antibody titers of at least 1/160 or positivity in a number of circulating autoantibodies, particularly anti-extractable nuclear antigen (ENA), anti-dsDNA, anti-smooth muscle, anti-mitochondrial, anti-parietal cell or anti-endomysium. The authors suggested that diagnosis of APF can be ascertained if all the obligate criteria and at least one minor criterion are fulfilled. It is well known that APF often occurs in patients affected with autoimmune/dysimmune or autoinflammatory diseases, mostly systemic lupus erythematosus. Numerous other underlying diseases have been also reported, including subacute cutaneous lupus erythematosus, systemic lupus erythematosus/scleroderma overlap syndrome [14], mixed connective tissue disease [7, 18], myasthenia gravis [5], Sjögren syndrome [8, 19], celiac disease [4], rheumatoid arthritis [20], idiopathic thrombocytopenic purpura (ITP) [5], immunoglobulin A nephropathy [19], Hashimoto's thyroiditis [21], and autoimmune hepatitis [13]. It is noteworthy that the course of APF not always parallels that of the associated condition and isolated cases can uncommonly be seen [14]. Skin reactions manifesting as APF developed after treatment with anti-tumour necrosis factor (TNF) agents, namely infliximab and adalimumab given for inflammatory bowel diseases (IBD), have been reported in the literature [22, 23]. APF resolution upon TNF blocker withdrawal combined with a corticosteroid cycle strongly suggested a triggering role of these drugs. The observation of these paradoxical reactions following anti-TNF therapy for IBD expanded both the clinical context in which APF may occur and the spectrum of cutaneous adverse effects of anti-TNF biologics.

Etiopathogenesis

The etiology of APF remains still unclear. However, since the first observations, the association of APF with autoimmune diseases suggested a possible etiological relationship between immunological imbalance and this disease [4]. In particular, as neutrophils clearly appeared to play an important role in triggering APF, as suggested by the histology, their functions had been evaluated *in vitro*. After the first conflicting results on neutrophil chemotaxis and bactericidal activity [18], Marzano et al. found that a true defect in neutrophil function would be unlikely in APF, while

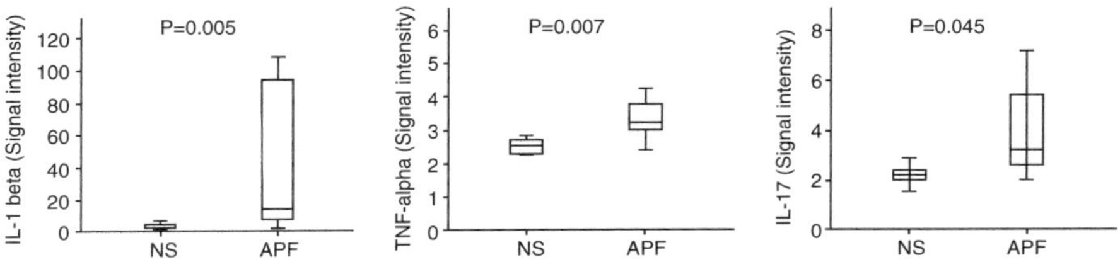

Fig. 10.2 Expression of interleukin (IL)-1β, tumor necrosis factor (TNF)-α, IL-17 in homogenate samples of lesional skin from nine patients with amicrobial pustulosis of the folds (APF). Six normal subjects (NS) served as controls. Numerical values represent signal intensity in a cytokine array assay. Median values, interquartile ranges (boxes), and 5th and 95th percentiles (whiskers)

it was conceivable that defective neutrophil chemotaxis was only a secondary phenomenon playing an autoregulatory role in neutrophil-mediated inflammation [4, 10, 24]. Thus, although the relationship between APF and the underlying autoimmune disease as well as its pathophysiology in itself remained unclarified, the authors concluded that APF should be classified within the spectrum of NDs [4].

Lipsker and Saurat, who suggestively called APF a 'neutrophilic cutaneous lupus', considered this disorder as a paradigm for a neutrophilic pattern of inflammation, potentially involving predominantly autoinflammatory pathways [25]. In line with this intriguing hypothesis, the overexpression of cytokines/chemokines and molecules amplifying the inflammatory network recently observed in skin samples from APF patients, by means of both immunohistochemistry and a cytokine array method, supported the view that APF has an important autoinflammatory component in analogy with PG, SS and, theoretically, the whole spectrum of NDs [14]. Indeed, two prototypic NDs like PG and SS have recently been included among the autoinflammatory diseases [26], which are characterized by recurrent episodes of sterile inflammation in the affected organs, including the skin, without circulating autoantibodies and autoreactive T cells [27–29]. In this concern, Marzano et al. found an overexpression of interleukin (IL)-1β and its receptors in all the APF patients evaluated [14] (Fig. 10.2). This finding may be linked to a dysregulation of the inflammasome, a molecular platform which induces the activation of caspase 1, an enzyme that proteolytically cleaves the inactive pro-IL-1β to its functionally active isoform, IL-1β. IL-1β is recognized to induce the formation and release of other proinflammatory cytokines, notably TNF-α and IFN-γ, and numerous chemokines [30]. Consistently, TNF-α, another key cytokine in the inflammatory scenario, and chemokines, such as IL-8, CXCL 1/2/3, CXCL16, and regulated on activation, normal T cell expressed and secreted (RANTES), which are responsible for neutrophil recruitment and activation, were overexpressed in the patients affected with APF investigated by the same authors [14]. Moreover, in all these patients an overexpression of both IL-17 and its receptor was found. IL-17 is known to contribute to neutrophil and monocyte chemotaxis by stimulating the tissue production of chemokines and acting in combination with other proinflammatory cytokines, thus being likely that this cytokine plays a role in the pathogenesis of NDs [31, 32]. In addition, IL-17, synergizing with IL-1 and TNFα, increases the production by neutrophils of metalloproteinase (MMP)-2 and MMP-9 [33]. The excessive production of MMPs contributes to tissue damage by destroying the extracellular matrix and inducing the release of chemokines.

As a whole, the most recent investigations showed high values of proinflammatory cytokines, chemokines, and tissue damage effector molecules in the lesional skin of APF patients, often in association with various circulating autoantibodies regardless of a frank underlying autoimmune/dysimmune disease, supporting the autoinflammatory origin of APF [14]. This is in line with an increasing evidence that indicates clinical and immunological similarities between autoinflammatory and autoimmune diseases, giving rise to the view on them as a single spectrum of diseases having at one end pure autoinflammatory diseases and at the other end pure autoimmune diseases [14, 25, 34]. According to this view, APF may be regarded as a condition at the border between innate and acquired immunity [25]. Whether genetic alterations predispose for the neutrophil-mediated autoinflammation in APF patients remains so far unknown.

Treatment

Systemic corticosteroids (prednisone or methylprednisolone) administered at mean doses of 0.5–1 mg/kg/day are effective in most cases and represent the first-choice treatment for APF [12–14]. Although corticosteroid therapy is currently regarded as the most effective treatment, the lesions can reappear once dosage is reduced or treatment is stopped. High strength topical corticosteroids can be coadministered. Systemic antibiotics are only useful in treating secondary impetiginization. Oral cimetidine (800 mg twice daily) combined with ascorbic acid (3 g/daily) has been found effective in some patients [10]. Several other treatments have been anecdotally reported, such as dapsone, colchicine, hydroxychloroquine, ciclosporin, cyclophosphamide, methotrexate, oral retinoids and zinc supplementation [6–9, 15, 35]. In a chronic-relapsing disease like APF, immunomodulating agents, particularly dapsone, or immunosuppresants, notably ciclosporin, can be used also as steroid-sparing drugs. Biologics, particularly the TNF-α blocker infliximab has successfully been used [14]. Interestingly, in a recent report the increased expression of IL-1α found in skin samples from an APF female patient prompted the authors to use the IL-1 receptor antagonist anakinra, which led to complete and stable remission of the clinical picture [36]. As for the other NDs, the near future for treating refractory cases of APF is a combined therapy targeting different pathways implicated in the pathogenesis of the disease, such as for example an IL-1 antagonist in combination with a TNF-α blocker [37].

Conclusions

APF is an uncommon entity characterized by peculiar clinical and histopathological features as well as by autoimmune or dysimmune comorbidities. It is included within the spectrum of NDs, which encompass a heterogeneous group of conditions that are hallmarked by an accumulation of neutrophils in the skin and rarely internal organs, in the absence of infection or true vasculitis. The definition of ND is closely similar to that of autoinflammatory diseases, which are characterized, from a physiopathological point of view, by an overactivation of innate immune signaling pathways. Recently, an upregulation of cytokines crucially involved in autoinflammation has been demonstrated in the lesional skin of patients with APF, suggesting an important autoinflammatory component in the pathogenesis of this disease. Together with an increasingly detailed definition of the inflammatory profile of APF, it could be expected that the identification of the disease pathomechanisms could further improve as well. This, in turn, could lead to advance the therapeutic approach of this distressing condition.

References

1. Crickx B, Diego ML, Guillevin L, Picard C, Grossin M, Belaïch S. Pustulose amicrobienne et lupus érythémateux systémique. Communication no. 11. Journées Dermatologiques de Paris. París; 1991.
2. Oberlin P, Bagot M, Perrussel M, Leteinturier F, Wechsler J, Revuz J. Pustulose amicrobienne et lupus érythémateux systémique. Ann Dermatol Vénéréol. 1991;118:824–5.
3. Saiag PH, Blanc F, Marinho E, De La Blanchardière A, Leconte I, Cocheton JJ, Tulliez M. Pustulose amicrobienne et lupus érythémateux systémique: un cas. Ann Dermatol Vénéréol. 1993;120:779–81.
4. Marzano AV, Capsoni F, Berti E, Gasparini G, Bottelli S, Caputo R. Amicrobial pustular dermatosis of cutaneous folds associated with autoimmune disorders: a new entity? Dermatology. 1996;193:88–93.
5. Lagrange S, Chosidow O, Flette JC, Wechsler B, Godeau P, Frances C. A peculiar form of amicrobial pustulosis of the folds associated with systemic lupus erythematosus and other autoimmune diseases. Lupus. 1997;6:514–20.
6. Stefanidou MP, Kanavaros PE, Stefanaki KS, Tosca AD. Amicrobial pustulosis of the folds: a cutaneous manifestation associated with connective tissue disease. Dermatology. 1998;197:394–6.
7. Bénéton N, Wolkenstein P, Bagot M, Cosnes A, Wechsler J, Roujeau JC, Revuz J. Amicrobial pustulosis associated with autoimmune diseases: healing with zinc supplementation. Br J Dermatol. 2000;143:1306–10.
8. Kuyama M, Fujimoto W, Kambara H, Egusa M, Saitoh M, Yamasaki O, Maehara K, Ohara A, Arata J, Iwatsuki K. Amicrobial pustular dermatosis in two patients with immunological abnormalities. Clin Exp Dermatol. 2002;27:286–9.
9. Kerl K, Masouyé I, Lesavre P, Saurat JH, Borradori L. A case of amicrobial pustulosis of the folds associated with neutrophilic gastrointestinal involvement in systemic lupus erythematosus. Dermatology. 2005;211:356–9.
10. Marzano AV, Ramoni S, Caputo R. Amicrobial pustulosis of the folds. Report of 6 cases and a literature review. Dermatology. 2008;216:305–11.
11. Claeys A, Bessis D, Cheikhrouhou H, Pouaha J, Cuny JF, Truchetet F. Amicrobial pustulosis of the folds revealing asymptomatic autoimmune thyroiditis. Eur J Dermatol. 2011;21:641–2.
12. Lim YL, Ng SK, Lian TY. Amicrobial pustulosis associated with autoimmune disease in a patient with Sjögren syndrome and IgA nephropathy. Clin Exp Dermatol. 2012;37:374–8.
13. Méndez-Flores S, Charli-Joseph Y, Saeb-Lima M, Orozco-Topete R, Fernández Sánchez M. Amicrobial pustulosis of the folds associated with autoimmune disorders: systemic lupus erythematosus case series and first report on the association with autoimmune hepatitis. Dermatology. 2013;226:1–4.

14. Marzano AV, Tavecchio S, Berti E, Gelmetti C, Cugno M. Cytokine and chemokine profile in amicrobial pustulosis of the folds: evidence for autoinflammation. Medicine (Baltimore). 2015;94:e2301.
15. Boms S, Gambichler T. Review of literature on amicrobial pustulosis of the folds associated with autoimmune disorders. Am J Clin Dermatol. 2006;7:369–74.
16. Wallach D, Vignon-Pennamen MD. From acute febrile neutrophilic dermatosis to neutrophilic disease: forty years of clinical research. J Am Acad Dermatol. 2006;55:1066–71.
17. Prat L, Bouaziz JD, Wallach D, Vignon-Pennamen MD, Bagot M. Neutrophilic dermatoses as systemic diseases. Clin Dermatol. 2014;32:376–88.
18. Vignon-Pennamen MD, Wallach D. Cutaneous manifestations of neutrophilic disease. Dermatologica. 1991;183:255–64.
19. Natsuga K, Sawamura D, Homma E, Nomura T, Abe M, Muramatsu R, Mochizuki T, Koike T, Shimizu H. Amicrobial pustulosis associated with IgA nephropathy and Sjögren's syndrome. J Am Acad Dermatol. 2007;57:523–6.
20. Hoch O, Herbst RA, Gutzmer R, Kiehl P, Kapp A, Weiss J. Amicrobial intertriginous pustulosis in autoimmune disease: a new entity? Hautarzt. 1998;49:634–40.
21. López-Navarro N, Alcaide A, Gallego E, Herrera-Acosta E, Gallardo M, Bosch RJ, Herrera E. Amicrobial pustulosis of the folds associated with Hashimoto's thyroiditis. Clin Exp Dermatol. 2009;34:e561–3.
22. Marzano AV, Tavecchio S, Berti E, Gelmetti C, Cugno M. Paradoxical autoinflammatory skin reaction to tumor necrosis factor alpha blockers manifesting as amicrobial pustulosis of the folds in patients with inflammatory bowel diseases. Medicine (Baltimore). 2015;94:e1818.
23. Lee HY, Pelivani N, Beltraminelli H, Hegyi I, Yawalkar N, Borradori L. Amicrobial pustulosis-like rash in a patient with Crohn's disease under anti-TNF-alpha blocker. Dermatology. 2011; 222:304–10.
24. Schroder JM, Szperalski B, Koch CJ, Christophers E. IgA-associated inhibition of polymorphonuclear leukocyte chemotaxis in neutrophilic dermatoses. J Invest Dermatol. 1981;77:464–8.
25. Lipsker D, Saurat JH. Neutrophilic cutaneous lupus erythematosus. At the edge between innate and acquired immunity? Dermatology. 2008;216:283–6.
26. Marzano AV, Ishak RS, Saibeni S, Crosti C, Meroni PL, Cugno M. Autoinflammatory skin disorders in inflammatory bowel diseases, pyoderma gangrenosum and Sweet's syndrome: a comprehensive review and disease classification criteria. Clinic Rev Allerg Immunol. 2013; 45:202–10.
27. de Jesus AA, Canna SW, Liu Y, Goldbach-Mansky R. Molecular mechanisms in genetically defined autoinflammatory diseases: disorders of amplified danger signaling. Annu Rev Immunol. 2015;33:823–74.
28. Marzano AV, Cugno M, Trevisan V, Fanoni D, Venegoni L, Berti E, Crosti C. Role of inflammatory cells, cytokines and matrix metalloproteinases in neutrophil-mediated skin diseases. Clin Exp Immunol. 2010;162:100–7.
29. Marzano AV, Cugno M, Trevisan V, Lazzari R, Fanoni D, Berti E, Crosti C. Inflammatory cells, cytokines and matrix metalloproteinases in amicrobial pustulosis of the folds and other neutrophilic dermatoses. Int J Immunopathol Pharmacol. 2011;24:451–60.
30. Dinarello CA. A clinical perspective of IL-1ß as the gatekeeper of inflammation. Eur J Immunol. 2011;41:1203–17.
31. Isailovic N, Daigo K, Mantovani A, Selmi C. Interleukin-17 and innate immunity in infections and chronic inflammation. J Autoimmun. 2015;60:1–11.
32. Donetti E, Cornaghi L, Gualerzi A, Baruffaldi Preis FW, Prignano F. An innovative three-dimensional model of normal human skin to study the proinflammatory psoriatic effects of tumor necrosis factor-alpha and interleukin-17. Cytokine. 2014;68:1–8.
33. Agarwal S, Misra R, Aggarwal A. Interleukin 17 levels are increased in juvenile idiopathic arthritis synovial fluid and induce synovial fibroblasts to produce proinflammatory cytokines and matrix metalloproteinases. J Rheumatol. 2008;35:515–9.

34. Navarini AA, Satoh TK, French LE. Neutrophilic dermatoses and autoinflammatory diseases with skin involvement—innate immune disorders. Semin Immunopathol. 2016;38:45–56.
35. Antille C, Frei M, Sorg O, Tran C, Kaya G, Masouyé I, Fontao L, Prins C, Saurat JH. Amicrobial pustulosis of the folds associated with autoimmune disorders. Dermatology. 2008;216:324–9.
36. Amazan E, Ezzedine K, Mossalayi MD, Taieb A, Boniface K, Seneschal J. Expression of interleukin-1 alpha in amicrobial pustulosis of the skin folds with complete response to anakinra. J Am Acad Dermatol. 2014;71:e53–6.
37. Chokoeva AA, Cardoso JC, Wollina U, Tchernev G. Pyoderma gangrenosum—a novel approach? Wien Med Wochenschr. 2017;167:58–65.

Pustular Psoriasis

11

Andrew Johnston

Pustular Psoriasis

Psoriasis is one of the most common and well-studied inflammatory skin diseases, affecting about 2% of the population [1]. The pathogenesis of plaque psoriasis (*psoriasis vulgaris*), involves the interplay of keratinocytes, T cells, antigen-presenting cells and to a limited extent, neutrophils as the central cellular components of the disease [2]. A number of pustular variants of psoriasis have been described, their pustular nature betraying the prominent role of neutrophils in the disease process. Although often categorized as subtypes or variants of psoriasis, as detailed below, these diseases have conspicuous genetic, environmental, temporal, mechanistic, and histological characteristics which set them apart from common plaque psoriasis (Table 11.1). These differences are heightened by the recent discovery of a number of pustular disease-associated genetic loci which have driven great strides in our understanding of the pathogenic mechanisms behind pustular psoriasis.

Generalized Pustular Psoriasis

Several variants of pustular psoriasis have been described, occurring as either localized or systemic (generalized) diseases. Generalized pustular psoriasis (GPP), also known as acute pustular psoriasis of von Zumbusch, after the disease's first description in 1910 [3], is a rare (prevalence of 1 in 10,000), debilitating and life-threatening disease, characterized by episodic infiltration of neutrophils into the skin, pustule development, generalized erythema and desquamation (Fig. 11.1, left). The disease manifests as clearly defined, raised bumps on the skin that are filled with pus (pustules). In contrast to plaque psoriasis, the onset of GPP is acute and frequently

A. Johnston
Department of Dermatology, University of Michigan, Ann Arbor, MI, USA
e-mail: andjoh@med.umich.edu

D. Wallach et al. (eds.), *Neutrophilic Dermatoses*,
https://doi.org/10.1007/978-3-319-72649-6_11

Table 11.1 Contrasting characteristics of plaque and pustular psoriasis

	Plaque psoriasis	Pustular psoriasis
Genetics	Complex genetics: 80+ risk loci identified *HLA-Cw*0602*	3 loci identified: *IL36RN, CARD14, AP1S3*
Onset	Gradual (plaque), although guttate psoriasis onset is acute (often following streptococcal pharyngitis)	Onset is acute, often with high-grade fever and chills
Systemic signs	Elevated skin and serum cytokines	Markers of systemic inflammation elevated
Effector cells	T cell driven; neutrophils present	Neutrophils predominate
Histology	Acanthosis (uniform elongation of the rete ridges), parakeratosis and orthokeratosis, loss of granular layer, pustules can be present in spinous layer (Munro's microabscess), upper part of epidermis (spongiform pustules of Kogoj), beneath the normal cornified layer or within the parakeratotic layer (intracorneal pustule)	Widespread intraepidermal or subcorneal pustules in erythrodermic and edematous skin, spongiosis, massive epidermal neutrophil infiltrate eosinophils, apoptotic keratinocytes

Pustular psoriasis is often classified as a variant of plaque psoriasis yet striking clinical, histological and genetic differences suggest that the two diseases have distinct pathogenic mechanisms

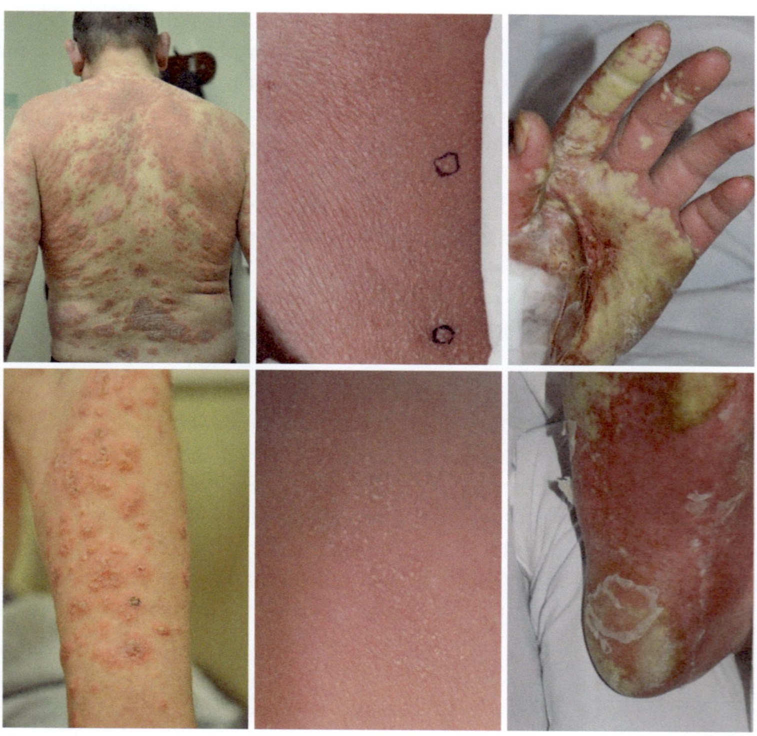

Fig. 11.1 Generalized pustular psoriasis (left images), acute generalized exanthematous pustulosis (AGEP, middle), and palmo-plantar pustulosis (PPP, right images). Images courtesy of Dr. Johann E. Gudjonsson (Department of Dermatology, University of Michigan, Ann Arbor, MI, USA)

accompanied by chills, high-grade fever, fatigue and neutrophilia which can be potentially life-threatening and require hospitalization [4, 5]. Cases of GPP can occur either as a distinct entity or are preceded by, concurrent with, or followed by chronic plaque psoriasis, a phenomenon that has confounded the study of the disease [5]. GPP can be difficult to treat, and until recently, therapeutic options have been limited to those that have proven efficacy for plaque psoriasis such as retinoids (acitretin), methotrexate, cyclosporine A, 6-thioguanine, hydroxyurea; however, these drugs typically do not completely control the disease, with resistance to existing treatments and disease recurrence commonly associated with GPP [6]. This shortfall in the efficacy of these treatments likely comes from an incomplete overlap of the pathobiology of plaque psoriasis and pustular forms of psoriasis [7] and there are ongoing efforts to improve our understanding of these disease mechanisms to aid the development of new therapies [7, 8]. Critical to these efforts are recent genetic findings which, as detailed below, have reshaped our understanding and management of these diseases.

A second pustular form of psoriasis is a severe cutaneous inflammatory drug reaction, acute generalized exanthematous pustulosis (AGEP). This is characterized by widespread sterile, non-follicular, fine, pinhead-sized pustules arising on edematous and erythemic skin (Fig. 11.1, middle). AGEP has a predilection for the major flexures, and is often accompanied with systemic inflammatory symptoms. AGEP is rare, occurring in one to five individuals per million per year [9], and the vast majority of cases are adverse reactions to medications; However, in rare instances AGEP has also been reported to be induced by triggers as diverse as spider bites, bacterial or viral infections, foods, and herbal remedies [9–11]. Offending medications include a variety of antibiotics, antimycotics and anticonvulsants. Several of the drugs reported to trigger AGEP are also known triggers of Stevens-Johnson syndrome [11, 12] a cutaneous drug reaction in which cytotoxic $CD8^+$ T cell responses predominate; However, unlike Stevens-Johnson syndrome, no confirmed associations with HLA alleles exist for AGEP patients [13] and cutaneous responses in AGEP are typically much more rapid (24–48 h versus 1–3 weeks) [13]. Notwithstanding, the activation of drug-specific $CD4^+$ and $CD8^+$ T cells is proposed to be involved in the initial triggering of neutrophil activation and infiltration of the skin in AGEP [14]. As with other severe cutaneous inflammatory drug reactions, the identification and withdrawal of the offending drug are the essential first therapeutic steps, with subsequent glucocorticosteroids to induce disease remission. Despite their seemingly divergent initial triggers, to date no clear histological or immunohistochemical differences have been demonstrated between GPP and AGEP, and the recent identification of shared genetic mutations between these diseases strengthens the idea that they share pathological mechanisms and therapeutic targets [15–17]. Carriage of certain genetic mutations may also influence the disease phenotype [15], suggesting that as the disease allele influences the disease process, further subphenotyping based on genetics and clinical features will be necessary to better understand this disease and to optimize effective treatments. Other systemic forms of pustular psoriasis have been described, including impetigo herpetiformis (a form of pustular psoriasis occurring in pregnancy) [18], and annular pustular psoriasis where lesions develop in ring-like, circular forms.

Localized Forms of Pustular Psoriasis

Localized forms of pustular psoriasis include palmo-plantar pustulosis (PPP) and acrodermatitis continua of Hallopeau (ACH), where the disease has a predilection for the palms and soles, or the tips of the fingers and toes, respectively. PPP manifests as cyclic and erupting sterile pustules on the palms and soles, often under a thick cornified layer (Fig. 11.1, right). The pustules may be present on clear skin or erythematous and hyperkeratotic lesions. Despite its restricted anatomical pattern, patients with severe symptoms may have significant pain and be unable to stand, walk or do manual work, thus this disease has a profound impact on quality of life [19, 20]. PPP has a worldwide distribution and is associated with plaque psoriasis in about 20% of cases; PPP, without concomitant plaque psoriasis, has an incidence estimated between 1 and 5 in 10,000 [21, 22]. Onset of the disease occurs mostly between the ages of 20 and 60 years and, unlike plaque psoriasis, has a strong predilection for women [22, 23]. As with GPP, a number of early [24, 25] and more recent [23, 26] genetic observations, together with clinical and epidemiological features have suggested that PPP is an entity distinct from plaque psoriasis [27].

The cause of the disease predilection for the palms and soles is unknown, but these areas are differentiated by the presence of numerous eccrine sweat glands (acrosyringium) which have been implicated in the pathogenesis of PPP [28–30]. A number of studies found that the majority of their PPP cohort was either current or former tobacco smokers [22, 23, 31]. This led to the suggestion that PPP is an autoimmune reaction induced by tobacco smoking against the acrosyringium and the papillary endothelium [31]. PPP has been associated with tonsillitis, in particular infections with α-streptococci have been implicated in triggering the disease. In support of this, increased numbers of α-streptococci-reactive T cells, have been detected in the tonsils of PPP compared with recurrent tonsillitis patients [32]. Elevations in the frequency of both cutaneous lymphocyte-associated antigen positive (CLA, a molecule expressed by the majority of T cells in the skin) and CCR6 positive T cells have been detected in the tonsils of PPP patients compared with non-PPP (recurrent tonsillitis) patients [32, 33]. Moreover, the abundance of these CLA+ or CCR6+ T cells was reduced in the peripheral blood of these PPP patients in the months following tonsillectomy [32, 33]. These populations are thought to represent streptococci-specific skin-homing T cells, which on entering the skin can initiate an inflammatory reaction after misrecognition of their cognate antigens. This scenario is analogous to that posited for chronic plaque and guttate psoriasis patients, wherein β-hemolytic streptococcus is suspected of initiating the disease, particularly for patients carrying one or two copies of the *HLA-Cw*0602* allele [34–36]. This contrasts with PPP, where no strong class I HLA association is known and α-streptococcus a suspected culprit. The mechanism whereby a bout of streptococcal tonsillitis leads to the elicitation of a chronic skin pustulosis is currently unknown, however tonsillectomy has been anecdotally associated with disease remission. The efficacy of tonsillectomy for PPP has not been properly assessed, yet is regarded as a routine treatment for PPP in Japan [32, 37–39].

Genetic Clues to Disease Mechanisms in Pustular Psoriasis

Until recently, the etiology and pathogenic mechanisms of pustular psoriasis were unknown, which critically stalled the development of specific and effective treatments. During the last decade, the situation has radically changed with the identification of inherited mutations in three genes each of which, through altered function of their respective proteins, cause inflammatory mechanisms to be dysregulated, leading to the development of neutrophilic skin disease.

The first gene found to be associated with GPP is *IL36RN* [40, 41]. These seminal observations brought IL-36, a cytokine which at the time was more of a curiosity than a critical and disease-inducing cytokine, into the limelight. The GPP-associated missense mutations in *IL36RN* affect the structure and function of the IL-36 receptor antagonist (IL-36Ra). Loss of functional IL-36Ra leads to unrestricted IL-36 activity, as evidenced by induction of IL-1β, IL-6, and CXCL8 production, and neutrophil infiltration of skin [40, 41]. Since these initial observations, mutations in *IL36RN* have been identified in numerous studies of GPP with and without concomitant plaque psoriasis, as well as cases of AGEP [15–17, 42], but not PPP [17, 23, 43], suggesting different a different etiology for PPP.

The three isoforms of IL-36 exist: IL-36α, β and γ, which form a trio of pro-inflammatory IL-1-like cytokines that are overexpressed in lesions of plaque psoriasis [44–46], GPP [7], and AGEP [8], where they can drive keratinocyte inflammatory responses [44], synergize with other pro-inflammatory cytokines [44, 47], and promote dendritic cell activation [48, 49]. The effects of IL-36 on skin have been modeled in mice [44, 45], where the transgenic expression of IL-36α in murine epidermis led to epidermal thickening, hyperkeratosis, mixed inflammatory cell infiltrate, and elevated chemokine expression [45]. Backcrossing to an *IL36RN*-deficient mouse resulted in more severe skin lesions, reflecting the effect of nonsense *IL36RN* mutations in GPP. This phenotype was partly reversed by the use of a neutrophil-depleting antibody, suggesting a causative role for neutrophils in this IL-36α-induced skin hyperplasia. This is supported by our own observations that subcutaneous administration of IL-36α to mice induces acanthosis and prominent neutrophilic infiltration [48]. IL-36 expression is also elevated in the skin of psoriasiform KC-Tie2 mice [44] and during imiquimod-induced skin inflammation [44, 50]. One of the early features of imiquimod-treated mouse skin is neutrophil infiltration, and the inflammatory phenotype is ablated in IL-36 receptor deficient mice [50] adding further support for a neutrophil/IL-36 axis as a central driver in the development of skin inflammation in GPP. Like their IL-1 family counterparts IL-1β, IL-18 and IL-33, the IL-36 cytokines require post-translational N-terminal peptide cleavage for activity [51] and it was recently demonstrated that IL-36 cleavage could be carried out by the neutrophil serine proteases elastase and cathepsin G [7, 52] as well as keratinocyte-derived cathepsin S [53]. Cathepsin S is strongly upregulated in psoriasis lesions, likely by the synergistic actions of TNF and IFN-γ, and, unlike elastase and cathepsin G, cathepsin S has been demonstrated to cleave IL-36γ into its most potent form [53]. Interestingly, these processes appear to be regulated by the activities of endogenous protease inhibitors expressed by the keratinocytes of psoriasis skin lesions, indicating the presence of a potential feedback inhibitory mechanism to restrain IL-36 driven inflammation [7].

Mutations in *IL36RN* have been shown to account for between 46 and 82% of cases of GPP without associated plaque psoriasis [54, 55]. The proportion of *IL36RN* mutant carriage is much lower (10–17%) in cases of GPP with concomitant plaque psoriasis [56], supporting the idea that divergent pathogenic mechanisms may be active in the two diseases. A recent meta-analysis of 233 GPP cases revealed that carriage of one or two *IL36RN* mutant alleles conferred a more severe clinical phenotype with an earlier age of onset and increased risk of systemic inflammation than non-carriage [56]. Moreover, a gene-dosage effect was also evident as homozygous carriers had an earlier age of onset than heterozygotes.

Mutations in *AP1S3* affecting the structure and function of the AP-1 complex subunit σ1C have been identified in ACH [57], GPP and PPP [26] patients. AP-1 is a member of the adaptor protein (AP) family which is a group of cytosolic heterotetrameric complexes that direct the assembly and trafficking of small transport vesicles [58]. Each of the five known complexes (AP-1, AP-2, AP-3, AP-4, and AP-5) is active in a distinct subcellular compartment, where it mediates the delivery of transmembrane proteins to specific target organelles [59]. AP-1 is involved in the transport of cargo between the trans-Golgi network and the endosomes, a process that requires the formation of specialized clathrin-coated vesicles [58]. Similar to other AP complexes, AP-1 consists of two large (γ1 and β1), one medium (μ1), and one small (σ1) subunit. The σ1 subunit exists in three forms, σ1A, σ1B, and σ1C, encoded by AP1S1, AP1S2, and AP1S3 respectively. Of particular interest here, the σ subunit stabilizes the tetrameric complex and thus non-synonymous mutations in *AP1S* genes are predicted to destabilize the entire AP-1 complex disrupting protein transport [57]. The two pustular psoriasis-associated *AP1S3* mutations described (p.Phe4Cys and p.Arg33Trp) lead to loss of AP1S3 function by reducing the stability of AP1-σ1C and by disrupting the interaction between the AP1-σ1C and AP1-μ1A subunits, respectively [26, 57]. Loss of AP1S3 function was found to result in reduced autophagy, a process shown to modulate NF-κB signaling by degrading p62, an adaptor molecule which binds TRAF6 leading to NF-κB activation. Carriage of mutant alleles resulted in p62 accumulation, and enhanced IL-1β, IL-8 and IL-36γ cytokine production in response to Toll-like receptor or IL-1R stimulation by keratinocytes from patients carrying *AP1S3* mutations [26].

Mutations in *CARD14* leading to structural and functional changes in caspase recruitment family member 14 (CARD14, previously known as CARMA2), have been associated with plaque psoriasis [60, 61], GPP [60, 62, 63], PPP [23], and pityriasis rubra pilaris, a papulosquamous condition phenotypically related to psoriasis [64, 65]. CARD14 is a member of the CARD-containing membrane-associated guanylate kinase (MAGUK) protein (CARMA) family of scaffold proteins. The other two members, CARD11 (CARMA1) and CARD10 (CARMA3) are critical for the activation of NF-κB in response to antigen and G-protein-coupled receptor stimulation respectively. On activation, CARD14 forms a signaling complex with BCL10 and MALT1, leading to activation of NF-κB, JNK, and p38 MAP kinase pathways

[66–68]. Thirty-two *CARD14* mutations have been described for plaque and pustular psoriasis [69] with the majority of the variants affecting the CARD or coiled-coil domains of the protein. These disease-associated mutations alter the structure of an inhibitory domain which normally keeps CARD14 activity in check, thus bypassing the need for an activating stimulus [62, 66, 68]. The psoriasis-associated CARD14 mutant proteins induce spontaneous formation of CARD14-BCL10-MALT1 complexes, which triggers MALT1 to promote inflammation in two key ways: first, by initiating pro-inflammatory signal transduction via its scaffold function; second, as a paracaspase MALT1 has the ability to cleave A20, CYLD, and RelB, three negative regulators of NF-κB, thus disabling feedback inhibition and further driving the inflammatory response. Like AP1S3 [26], CARD14 appears to be preferentially expressed by epidermal keratinocytes, and also to a lesser extent endothelial cells [60, 70]. CARD14 expression is strongly upregulated in psoriasis skin lesions [60], particularly in the upper epidermis which is also the zone where many NF-κB response genes (e.g., IL-36, CCL20, CXCL1, CXCL8) are overexpressed in lesional psoriasis skin. This pattern of AP1S3 and CARD14 tissue expression likely explains why these gain of function mutations lead to inflammatory skin disease.

Common, or at least overlapping, mechanisms may underlie the pathology of these diseases. Different gene mutations (*IL36RN, AP1S3, CARD14*) leading to activation of different molecules (IL-36R, p62, MALT1) which feed into common, or at least overlapping, signaling pathways (NF-κB, MAP kinases) to drive unwarranted and dysregulated inflammatory responses (Fig. 11.2). In some cases a single dominant mutation may be sufficient to cause disease as is the case with *CARD14* where mutations may be sufficient to cause disease (at least without contributions from *IL36RN* mutations or *HLA-Cw*0602* carriage [23, 60]). Likewise, the initial study on AP1S3 focused on finding mutations in a group of ACH patients who had been typed as non-carriers of *IL36RN* and *CARD14* mutations [57]. However there are indications of epistasis between mutant loci: an individual carrying deleterious mutations in *AP1S3* and *IL36RN* was found to have a much more severe disease phenotype than her sibling carrying only the *IL36RN* mutation [26]. As the gain-of-function mutations in *CARD14*, and loss-of-function *AP1S3* and *IL36RN* mutants all result in a net increase in NF-κB activity, it is not unexpected to see additive effects resulting from the carriage of multiple disease alleles (Fig. 11.2).

Emerging Treatments for Pustular Psoriasis

Pustular psoriasis utilizes signaling pathways both overlapping and separate from plaque psoriasis, and because of their efficacy in moderate-severe plaque psoriasis, a number of therapies specifically targeting cytokines are in use for GPP. Several reports describe the use of anakinra, an IL-1 receptor antagonist [71–73] or canakinumab, a human monoclonal antibody targeted at IL-1β [74], to treat GPP. Anakinra appears to induce a rapid normalization of systemic inflammatory symptoms followed by improvement of the pustular skin eruption. The responses to IL-1 receptor inhibition in the skin tend to be incomplete however, with erythema

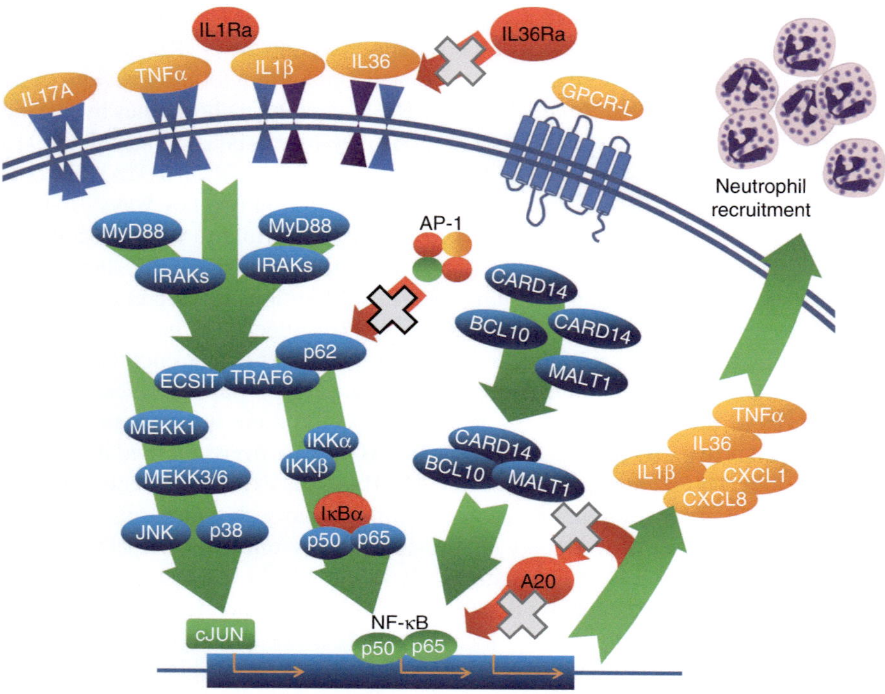

Fig. 11.2 Pustular psoriasis-associated *IL36RN, AP1S3,* and *CARD14* mutations activate overlapping pathways leading to inflammatory gene expression, chemokine production and neutrophil infiltration. *IL36RN* mutations giving rise to loss of function of the IL-36 receptor antagonist (IL-36Ra) lead to unrestrained IL-36 activity at the IL-36 receptor. This signal is transduced via NF-κB driving inflammatory cytokine (IL-1, IL-36, TNF) and chemokine (CXCL1, CXCL2, CXCL8, CCL20) production, drawing neutrophils into the skin. Mutations in *AP1S3* result in loss of AP-1 function and defective autophagy, leading to an accumulation of the adaptor protein p62, which drives cellular inflammatory responses downstream of Toll-like (e.g., TLR2/4) and cytokine receptors (including IL-17, TNF, IL-1, IL-36), again signaling via TRAF6 and the NF-κB pathway. Lastly, the disease-associated mutations in *CARD14* result in structural alterations in the protein's CARD or coiled-coil domains leading to loss of an inhibitory motif and spontaneous formation of CARD14-BCL10-MALT1 complexes that drive NF-κB activity. This is likely augmented by the paracaspase activity of MALT1 which can degrade a number of negative regulators of NF-κB signaling such as the deubiquitinases A20 and CYLD

and hyperkeratosis remaining in some cases, which suggests that IL-1 is not playing a central role in GPP but acts in a positive feedback loop inducing and being induced by IL-36 [44]. The relevance of using IL-1 receptor antagonism to tackle a disease which may be primarily driven by deviations in IL-36 signaling, particularly when *IL36RN* mutations are present, has recently been questioned [75]. However, clinical trials are ongoing in the UK (APRICOT) and USA (NIH NCT01794117) assessing the efficacy of anakinra and PPP and pustular skin diseases (including PPP) respectively. The premise for these trials is the effectiveness of anakinra for treatment of diseases caused by IL-1RA deficiency and the elevated IL-1 and IL-36 activity in observed PPP. The outcome of these trials will be interesting given the reported lack of genetic associations between PPP and *IL1RN* and *IL36RN* mutations [17, 23, 43].

TNF-α is a central mediator in chronic plaque psoriasis as evidenced by the effectiveness of therapies that block TNF-α activity. Of the three TNF biologics in use for plaque psoriasis, infliximab has most commonly been used for GPP [76, 77] and as such has become one of the recommended treatment options for severe acute GPP despite the lack of adequate clinical trials [6]. Infliximab has been reported to have a rapid effect, with systemic inflammation and skin pustules starting to recede in as little as 2 days from the first infusion. In this context, the efficacy of infliximab likely stems from the rapid availability of the drug following infusion, and its inhibition of the synergy between TNF and multiple inflammatory cytokines including IL-36, IL-17A, IL-1β [44, 47, 78, 79].

Given the plethora of recent studies highlighting the effectiveness of targeting of IL-17A in plaque psoriasis, this approach has now also been tested with success for treating GPP. The notion that IL-17 may have a prominent role in pustular psoriasis is not only supported by the efficacy of blocking IL-17, and the presence of increased tissue IL-17A [80], skin-homing Th17 T cells [81], IL-17^{+} neutrophils [82], and strong IL-17A signatures in the lesions [7, 8], but also the clinical observations of severe pustular flare after sudden discontinuation of IL-17 axis suppression by brodalumab in psoriasis patients [83]. IL-17 is a key cytokine in the induction of chemokine-mediated neutrophil infiltration of skin [84], and neutrophils are an obvious and central mechanistic component of pustular diseases. Not only do neutrophils express IL-17 [82, 85, 86] but they have also been shown to respond to IL-17A [87] as they express both prerequisite receptor subunits for IL-17A response. Secukinumab, a biologic targeting IL-17A, was recently shown to rapidly improve both systemic symptoms and the skin disease in GPP patients [88–90]. Likewise brodalumab, a biologic targeting the IL-17 receptor A chain, was also shown to induce clinical improvement in 11 out of 12 GPP patients [91]. Given the encouraging findings from biologics targeting IL-17, there are now several ongoing trials examining inhibition of IL-23, a cytokine thought to act upstream of IL-17, as a master regulator of IL-17 expression by T cells [92, 93] and neutrophils [87] . Both guselkumab (NIH NCT02343744) and risankizumab (NIH NCT03022045) are biologics targeting IL-23p19 under test for treating GPP. Given the seemingly central role of the IL-36/IL-36R system in GPP, supported by a glut of genetic and mechanistic data, this is surely an attractive target for the development of new therapies for GPP [94, 95].

PPP is a very difficult disease to treat and is commonly recalcitrant to existing therapeutic options, a situation that is confounded by the paucity of robust clinical trials of new medications. As such, therapeutic recommendations have often relied on case reports, thus less rigorous data is currently available for the efficacy of biologics in PPP. Unlike GPP, reports on the usage of anti-TNF biologics in PPP have revealed only modest to poor responses with all three of the TNF biologics used for plaque psoriasis [96–98]. Moreover there exist several reports of new onset PPP following anti-TNF treatment of other diseases [99–103]. Studies using ustekinumab, an antibody directed at IL-12p40 (a shared subunit of IL-12 and IL-23), for PPP have also generated equivocal results [104–107]. Much more promising data have emerged for two of the IL-17 biologics (secukinumab and ixekizumab), the use of which is supported by the detection of elevated levels of IL-17 [108, 109] and enrichment of IL-17 signature genes in PPP lesions [8]. A recent study of secukinumab for moderate to severe PPP demonstrated a 50% improvement in disease severity and significant improvements in quality of life scores [90]. Given that increased IL-23 has been detected in PPP lesions [109, 110], inhibition of IL-23p19 may also be an effective approach for PPP therapy.

Concluding Remarks

The discovery of mutations in *IL36RN*, *CARD14* and *AP1S3* that lead to dysregulated inflammation have increased enormously our understanding of pustular psoriasis over the last decade; However, several pieces of the puzzle remain to be revealed. It is likely that carriage of a mutant allele in itself is not enough for disease initiation: many pustular psoriasis patients have their first episode of the disease as adults, despite being lifelong mutant allele carriers, and patients can be heterozygous at disease loci, suggesting that either a yet to be identified second disease locus, or environmental trigger may be necessary to precipitate the disease. The co-occurrence of plaque psoriasis, GPP, PPP, or AGEP has confounded the genetic and mechanistic study of these diseases, which highlights the importance of clear phenotyping and sequential screening of disease-associated genes to increase the power to detect new pathogenic mutations and thus shed more light on the disease mechanisms. Thus, despite recent major advances in the study and treatment of pustular skin diseases, there remain key genetic, environmental and mechanistic pieces to be identified to solve these puzzling and difficult to treat diseases.

References

1. Parisi R, Symmons DP, Griffiths CE, Ashcroft DM. Global epidemiology of psoriasis: a systematic review of incidence and prevalence. J Invest Dermatol. 2012;133:377–85.
2. Di Meglio P, Villanova F, Nestle FO. Psoriasis. Cold Spring Harb Perspect Med. 2014;4(8).
3. von Zumbush L. Psoriasis and pustuloses exanthem. Arch Derm Syph. 1910;99:335–46.
4. Mengesha YM, Bennett ML. Pustular skin disorders: diagnosis and treatment. Am J Clin Dermatol. 2002;3:389–400.
5. Gudjonsson JE, Elder JT. Psoriasis (Chapter 18). In: Goldsmith LA, Katz SI, Gilchrest BA, Paller AS, Leffell DJ, Wolff K, editors. Fitzpatrick's dermatology in general medicine, vol. 1. 8th ed. New York: McGraw-Hill Medical; 2012.
6. Robinson A, Van Voorhees AS, Hsu S, et al. Treatment of pustular psoriasis: from the Medical Board of the National Psoriasis Foundation. J Am Acad Dermatol. 2012;67:279–88.
7. Johnston A, Xing X, Wolterink L, et al. IL-1 and IL-36 are dominant cytokines in generalized pustular psoriasis. J Allergy Clin Immunol. 2016;140(1):109–20.
8. Liang Y, Xing X, Beamer MA, et al. Six-transmembrane epithelial antigens of the prostate comprise a novel inflammatory nexus in patients with pustular skin disorders. J Allergy Clin Immunol. 2017;139(4):1217–27.
9. Sidoroff A, Halevy S, Bavinck JN, Vaillant L, Roujeau JC. Acute generalized exanthematous pustulosis (AGEP)—a clinical reaction pattern. J Cutan Pathol. 2001;28:113–9.

10. Szatkowski J, Schwartz RA. Acute generalized exanthematous pustulosis (AGEP): a review and update. J Am Acad Dermatol. 2015;73:843–8.
11. Sidoroff A, Dunant A, Viboud C, et al. Risk factors for acute generalized exanthematous pustulosis (AGEP)-results of a multinational case-control study (EuroSCAR). Br J Dermatol. 2007;157:989–96.
12. Mockenhaupt M, Viboud C, Dunant A, et al. Stevens-Johnson syndrome and toxic epidermal necrolysis: assessment of medication risks with emphasis on recently marketed drugs. The EuroSCAR-study. J Invest Dermatol. 2008;128:35–44.
13. Paulmann M, Mockenhaupt M. Severe drug hypersensitivity reactions: clinical pattern, diagnosis, etiology and therapeutic options. Curr Pharm Des. 2016;22:6852–61.
14. Schmid S, Kuechler PC, Britschgi M, et al. Acute generalized exanthematous pustulosis: role of cytotoxic T cells in pustule formation. Am J Pathol. 2002;161:2079–86.
15. Navarini AA, Valeyrie-Allanore L, Setta-Kaffetzi N, et al. Rare variations in IL36RN in severe adverse drug reactions manifesting as acute generalized exanthematous pustulosis. J Invest Dermatol. 2013;133:1904–7.
16. Nakai N, Sugiura K, Akiyama M, Katoh N. Acute generalized exanthematous pustulosis caused by dihydrocodeine phosphate in a patient with psoriasis vulgaris and a heterozygous IL36RN mutation. JAMA Dermatol. 2015;151:311–5.
17. Setta-Kaffetzi N, Navarini AA, Patel VM, et al. Rare pathogenic variants in IL36RN underlie a spectrum of psoriasis-associated pustular phenotypes. J Invest Dermatol. 2013;133:1366–9.
18. Oumeish OY, Parish JL. Impetigo herpetiformis. Clin Dermatol. 2006;24:101–4.
19. Chung J, Callis Duffin K, Takeshita J, et al. Palmoplantar psoriasis is associated with greater impairment of health-related quality of life compared with moderate to severe plaque psoriasis. J Am Acad Dermatol. 2014;71:623–32.
20. Pettey AA, Balkrishnan R, Rapp SR, Fleischer AB, Feldman SR. Patients with palmoplantar psoriasis have more physical disability and discomfort than patients with other forms of psoriasis: implications for clinical practice. J Am Acad Dermatol. 2003;49:271–5.
21. Hellgren L, Mobacken H. Pustulosis palmaris et plantaris. Prevalence, clinical observations and prognosis. Acta Derm Venereol. 1971;51:284–8.
22. Brunasso AM, Puntoni M, Aberer W, Delfino C, Fancelli L, Massone C. Clinical and epidemiological comparison of patients affected by palmoplantar plaque psoriasis and palmoplantar pustulosis: a case series study. Br J Dermatol. 2013;168:1243–51.
23. Mossner R, Frambach Y, Wilsmann-Theis D, et al. Palmoplantar pustular psoriasis is associated with missense variants in CARD14, but not with loss-of-function mutations in IL36RN in European patients. J Invest Dermatol. 2015;135:2538–41.
24. Asumalahti K, Ameen M, Suomela S, et al. Genetic analysis of PSORS1 distinguishes guttate psoriasis and palmoplantar pustulosis. J Invest Dermatol. 2003;120:627–32.
25. Mossner R, Kingo K, Kleensang A, et al. Association of TNF-238 and -308 promoter polymorphisms with psoriasis vulgaris and psoriatic arthritis but not with pustulosis palmoplantaris. J Invest Dermatol. 2005;124:282–4.
26. Mahil SK, Twelves S, Farkas K, et al. AP1S3 mutations cause skin autoinflammation by disrupting keratinocyte autophagy and up-regulating IL-36 production. J Invest Dermatol. 2016;136:2251–9.
27. Griffiths CE, Christophers E, Barker JN, et al. A classification of psoriasis vulgaris according to phenotype. Br J Dermatol. 2007;156:258–62.
28. Krieg PH, Bacharach-Buhles M, el-Gammal S, Altmeyer P. The pustule in palmoplantar psoriasis: transformed vesicle or mature microabscess? A three-dimensional study. Dermatology. 1992;185:104–12.
29. Eriksson MO, Hagforsen E, Lundin IP, Michaelsson G. Palmoplantar pustulosis: a clinical and immunohistological study. Br J Dermatol. 1998;138:390–8.
30. Murakami M, Ohtake T, Horibe Y, et al. Acrosyringium is the main site of the vesicle/pustule formation in palmoplantar pustulosis. J Invest Dermatol. 2010;130:2010–6.

31. Hagforsen E, Awder M, Lefvert AK, Nordlind K, Michaelsson G. Palmoplantar pustulosis: an autoimmune disease precipitated by smoking? Acta Derm Venereol. 2002;82:341–6.
32. Yoshizaki T, Bandoh N, Ueda S, et al. Up-regulation of CC chemokine receptor 6 on tonsillar T cells and its induction by in vitro stimulation with alpha-streptococci in patients with pustulosis palmaris et plantaris. Clin Exp Immunol. 2009;157:71–82.
33. Nozawa H, Kishibe K, Takahara M, Harabuchi Y. Expression of cutaneous lymphocyte-associated antigen (CLA) in tonsillar T-cells and its induction by in vitro stimulation with alpha-streptococci in patients with pustulosis palmaris et plantaris (PPP). Clin Immunol. 2005; 116:42–53.
34. Valdimarsson H, Thorleifsdottir RH, Sigurdardottir SL, Gudjonsson JE, Johnston A. Psoriasis—as an autoimmune disease caused by molecular mimicry. Trends Immunol. 2009;30:494–501.
35. Thorleifsdottir RH, Sigurdardottir SL, Sigurgeirsson B, et al. HLA-Cw6 homozygosity in plaque psoriasis is associated with streptococcal throat infections and pronounced improvement after tonsillectomy: a prospective case series. J Am Acad Dermatol. 2016;75:889–96.
36. Thorleifsdottir RH, Sigurdardottir SL, Sigurgeirsson B, et al. Improvement of psoriasis after tonsillectomy is associated with a decrease in the frequency of circulating T cells that recognize streptococcal determinants and homologous skin determinants. J Immunol. 2012;188:5160–5.
37. Koshiba S, Ichimiya S, Nagashima T, et al. Tonsillar crypt epithelium of palmoplantar pustulosis secretes interleukin-6 to support B-cell development via p63/p73 transcription factors. J Pathol. 2008;214:75–84.
38. Yokoyama M, Hashigucci K, Yamasaki Y. Effect of tonsillectomy in patients with pustulosis palmaris et plantaris. Acta Otolaryngol. 2004;124:1109–10.
39. Ozawa A, Ohkido M, Haruki Y, et al. Treatments of generalized pustular psoriasis: a multicenter study in Japan. J Dermatol. 1999;26:141–9.
40. Marrakchi S, Guigue P, Renshaw BR, et al. Interleukin-36-receptor antagonist deficiency and generalized pustular psoriasis. N Engl J Med. 2011;365:620–8.
41. Onoufriadis A, Simpson MA, Pink AE, et al. Mutations in IL36RN/IL1F5 are associated with the severe episodic inflammatory skin disease known as generalized pustular psoriasis. Am J Hum Genet. 2011;89:432–7.
42. Navarini AA, Simpson MA, Borradori L, Yawalkar N, Schlapbach C. Homozygous missense mutation in IL36RN in generalized pustular dermatosis with intraoral involvement compatible with both AGEP and generalized pustular psoriasis. JAMA Dermatol. 2015;151: 452–3.
43. Takahashi T, Fujimoto N, Kabuto M, Nakanishi T, Tanaka T. Mutation analysis of IL36RN gene in Japanese patients with palmoplantar pustulosis. J Dermatol. 2017;44:80–3.
44. Johnston A, Xing X, Guzman AM, et al. IL-1F5, -F6, -F8, and -F9: a novel IL-1 family signaling system that is active in psoriasis and promotes keratinocyte antimicrobial peptide expression. J Immunol. 2011;186:2613–22.
45. Blumberg H, Dinh H, Trueblood ES, et al. Opposing activities of two novel members of the IL-1 ligand family regulate skin inflammation. J Exp Med. 2007;204:2603–14.
46. Debets R, Timans JC, Homey B, et al. Two novel IL-1 family members, IL-1 delta and IL-1 epsilon, function as an antagonist and agonist of NF-kappa B activation through the orphan IL-1 receptor-related protein 2. J Immunol. 2001;167:1440–6.
47. Carrier Y, Ma HL, Ramon HE, et al. Inter-regulation of Th17 cytokines and the IL-36 cytokines in vitro and in vivo: implications in psoriasis pathogenesis. J Invest Dermatol. 2011;131:2428–37.
48. Foster AM, Baliwag J, Chen CS, et al. IL-36 promotes myeloid cell infiltration, activation, and inflammatory activity in skin. J Immunol. 2014;192:6053–61.
49. Mutamba S, Allison A, Mahida Y, Barrow P, Foster N. Expression of IL-1Rrp2 by human myelomonocytic cells is unique to DCs and facilitates DC maturation by IL-1F8 and IL-1F9. Eur J Immunol. 2012;42:607–17.

50. Tortola L, Rosenwald E, Abel B, et al. Psoriasiform dermatitis is driven by IL-36-mediated DC-keratinocyte crosstalk. J Clin Invest. 2012;122:3965–76.
51. Towne JE, Renshaw BR, Douangpanya J, et al. Interleukin-36 (IL-36) ligands require processing for full agonist (IL-36{alpha}, IL-36{beta} and IL-36{gamma}) or antagonist (IL-36Ra) activity. J Biol Chem. 2011;286:42594–602.
52. Henry CM, Sullivan GP, Clancy DM, Afonina IS, Kulms D, Martin SJ. Neutrophil-derived proteases escalate inflammation through activation of IL-36 family cytokines. Cell Rep. 2016;14:708–22.
53. Ainscough JS, Macleod T, McGonagle D, et al. Cathepsin S is the major activator of the psoriasis-associated proinflammatory cytokine IL-36gamma. Proc Natl Acad Sci U S A. 2017;114(13):E2748–57.
54. Korber A, Mossner R, Renner R, et al. Mutations in IL36RN in patients with generalized pustular psoriasis. J Invest Dermatol. 2013;133:2634–7.
55. Sugiura K, Takemoto A, Yamaguchi M, et al. The majority of generalized pustular psoriasis without psoriasis vulgaris is caused by deficiency of interleukin-36 receptor antagonist. J Invest Dermatol. 2013;133:2514–21.
56. Hussain S, Berki DM, Choon SE, et al. IL36RN mutations define a severe autoinflammatory phenotype of generalized pustular psoriasis. J Allergy Clin Immunol. 2015;135:1067–1070 e1069.
57. Setta-Kaffetzi N, Simpson MA, Navarini AA, et al. AP1S3 mutations are associated with pustular psoriasis and impaired Toll-like receptor 3 trafficking. Am J Hum Genet. 2014;94(5):790–7.
58. Robinson MS. Adaptable adaptors for coated vesicles. Trends Cell Biol. 2004;14:167–74.
59. Nakatsu F, Hase K, Ohno H. The role of the clathrin adaptor AP-1: polarized sorting and beyond. Membranes (Basel). 2014;4:747–3.
60. Jordan CT, Cao L, Roberson ED, et al. PSORS2 is due to mutations in CARD14. Am J Hum Genet. 2012;90:784–95.
61. Jordan CT, Cao L, Roberson ED, et al. Rare and common variants in CARD14, encoding an epidermal regulator of NF-kappaB, in psoriasis. Am J Hum Genet. 2012;90:796–808.
62. Berki DM, Liu L, Choon SE, et al. Activating CARD14 mutations are associated with generalized pustular psoriasis but rarely account for familial recurrence in psoriasis vulgaris. J Invest Dermatol. 2015;135:2964–70.
63. Sugiura K, Muto M, Akiyama M. CARD14 c.526G>C (p.Asp176His) is a significant risk factor for generalized pustular psoriasis with psoriasis vulgaris in the Japanese cohort. J Invest Dermatol. 2014;134:1755–7.
64. Li Q, Jin Chung H, Ross N, et al. Analysis of CARD14 polymorphisms in pityriasis rubra pilaris: activation of NF-kappaB. J Invest Dermatol. 2015;135:1905–8.
65. Fuchs-Telem D, Sarig O, van Steensel MA, et al. Familial pityriasis rubra pilaris is caused by mutations in CARD14. Am J Hum Genet. 2012;91:163–70.
66. Afonina IS, Van Nuffel E, Baudelet G, et al. The paracaspase MALT1 mediates CARD14-induced signaling in keratinocytes. EMBO Rep. 2016;17:914–27.
67. Scudiero I, Zotti T, Ferravante A, Vessichelli M, Vito P, Stilo R. Alternative splicing of CARMA2/CARD14 transcripts generates protein variants with differential effect on NF-kappaB activation and endoplasmic reticulum stress-induced cell death. J Cell Physiol. 2011;226:3121–31.
68. Howes A, O'Sullivan PA, Breyer F, et al. Psoriasis mutations disrupt CARD14 autoinhibition promoting BCL10-MALT1-dependent NF-kappaB activation. Biochem J. 2016;473:1759–68.
69. Van Nuffel E, Schmitt A, Afonina IS, Schulze-Osthoff K, Beyaert R, Hailfinger S. CARD14-mediated activation of paracaspase MALT1 in keratinocytes: implications for psoriasis. J Invest Dermatol. 2017;137:569–75.
70. Harden JL, Lewis SM, Pierson KC, et al. CARD14 expression in dermal endothelial cells in psoriasis. PLoS One. 2014;9:e111255.

71. Rossi-Semerano L, Piram M, Chiaverini C, De Ricaud D, Smahi A, Kone-Paut I. First clinical description of an infant with interleukin-36-receptor antagonist deficiency successfully treated with anakinra. Pediatrics. 2013;132:e1043–7.
72. Huffmeier U, Watzold M, Mohr J, Schon MP, Mossner R. Successful therapy with anakinra in a patient with generalized pustular psoriasis carrying IL36RN mutations. Br J Dermatol. 2014;170:202–4.
73. Viguier M, Guigue P, Pages C, Smahi A, Bachelez H. Successful treatment of generalized pustular psoriasis with the interleukin-1-receptor antagonist Anakinra: lack of correlation with IL1RN mutations. Ann Intern Med. 2010;153:66–7.
74. Skendros P, Papagoras C, Lefaki I, et al. Successful response in a case of severe pustular psoriasis after interleukin-1beta inhibition. Br J Dermatol. 2017;176:212–5.
75. Tauber M, Viguier M, Le Gall C, Smahi A, Bachelez H. Is it relevant to use an interleukin-1-inhibiting strategy for the treatment of patients with deficiency of interleukin-36 receptor antagonist? Br J Dermatol. 2014;170:1198–9.
76. Elewski BE. Infliximab for the treatment of severe pustular psoriasis. J Am Acad Dermatol. 2002;47:796–7.
77. Newland MR, Weinstein A, Kerdel F. Rapid response to infliximab in severe pustular psoriasis, von Zumbusch type. Int J Dermatol. 2002;41:449–52.
78. Johnston A, Guzman AM, Swindell WR, Wang F, Kang S, Gudjonsson JE. Early tissue responses in psoriasis to the antitumour necrosis factor-alpha biologic etanercept suggest reduced interleukin-17 receptor expression and signalling. Br J Dermatol. 2014;171:97–107.
79. Chiricozzi A, Guttman-Yassky E, Suarez-Farinas M, et al. Integrative responses to IL-17 and TNF-alpha in human keratinocytes account for key inflammatory pathogenic circuits in psoriasis. J Invest Dermatol. 2011;131:677–87.
80. Yilmaz SB, Cicek N, Coskun M, Yegin O, Alpsoy E. Serum and tissue levels of IL-17 in different clinical subtypes of psoriasis. Arch Dermatol Res. 2012;304:465–9.
81. Teraki Y, Tanaka S, Hitomi K, Izaki S. A case of generalized psoriasiform and pustular eruption induced by infliximab: evidence for skin-homing Th17 in the pathogenesis. Br J Dermatol. 2010;163:1347–51.
82. Kakeda M, Schlapbach C, Danelon G, et al. Innate immune cells express IL-17A/F in acute generalized exanthematous pustulosis and generalized pustular psoriasis. Arch Dermatol Res. 2014;306:933–8.
83. Khemis A, Cavalie M, Montaudie H, Lacour JP, Passeron T. Rebound pustular psoriasis after brodalumab discontinuation. Br J Dermatol. 2016;175:1065–6.
84. Girolomoni G, Mrowietz U, Paul C. Psoriasis: rationale for targeting interleukin-17. Br J Dermatol. 2012;167:717–4.
85. Lin AM, Rubin CJ, Khandpur R, et al. Mast cells and neutrophils release IL-17 through extracellular trap formation in psoriasis. J Immunol. 2011;187:490–500.
86. Keijsers RR, Hendriks AG, van Erp PE, et al. In vivo induction of cutaneous inflammation results in the accumulation of extracellular trap-forming neutrophils expressing RORgammat and IL-17. J Invest Dermatol. 2014;134:1276–84.
87. Taylor PR, Roy S, Leal SM Jr, et al. Activation of neutrophils by autocrine IL-17A-IL-17RC interactions during fungal infection is regulated by IL-6, IL-23, RORgammat and dectin-2. Nat Immunol. 2014;15:143–51.
88. Bohner A, Roenneberg S, Eyerich K, Eberlein B, Biedermann T. Acute generalized pustular psoriasis treated with the IL-17A antibody secukinumab. JAMA Dermatol. 2015;152(4):482–4.
89. Imafuku S, Honma M, Okubo Y, et al. Efficacy and safety of secukinumab in patients with generalized pustular psoriasis: a 52-week analysis from phase III open-label multicenter Japanese study. J Dermatol. 2016;43:1011–7.
90. Gottlieb A, Sullivan J, van Doorn M, et al. Secukinumab shows significant efficacy in palmoplantar psoriasis: results from GESTURE, a randomized controlled trial. J Am Acad Dermatol. 2017;76:70–80.
91. Yamasaki K, Nakagawa H, Kubo Y, Ootaki K, Japanese brodalumab study g. Efficacy and safety of brodalumab in patients with generalized pustular psoriasis and psoriatic erythroderma: results from a 52-week, open-label study. Br J Dermatol. 2017;176:741–51.

92. Di Meglio P, Nestle FO. The role of IL-23 in the immunopathogenesis of psoriasis. F1000 Biol Rep. 2010;2:40.
93. Langrish CL, McKenzie BS, Wilson NJ, de Waal MR, Kastelein RA, Cua DJ. IL-12 and IL-23: master regulators of innate and adaptive immunity. Immunol Rev. 2004;202:96–105.
94. Wolf J, Ferris LK. Anti-IL-36R antibodies, potentially useful for the treatment of psoriasis: a patent evaluation of WO2013074569. Expert Opin Ther Pat. 2014;24:477–9.
95. Gunther S, Sundberg EJ. Molecular determinants of agonist and antagonist signaling through the IL-36 receptor. J Immunol. 2014;193:921–30.
96. Bissonnette R, Poulin Y, Guenther L, Lynde CW, Bolduc C, Nigen S. Treatment of palmoplantar psoriasis with infliximab: a randomized, double-blind placebo-controlled study. J Eur Acad Dermatol Venereol. 2011;25:1402–8.
97. Bissonnette R, Poulin Y, Bolduc C, et al. Etanercept in the treatment of palmoplantar pustulosis. J Drugs Dermatol. 2008;7:940–6.
98. Leonardi C, Langley RG, Papp K, et al. Adalimumab for treatment of moderate to severe chronic plaque psoriasis of the hands and feet: efficacy and safety results from REACH, a randomized, placebo-controlled, double-blind trial. Arch Dermatol. 2011;147:429–36.
99. Tresh A, Smith VH, Parslew RA. Behcet's syndrome treated with infliximab, which caused a palmoplantar pustulosis, subsequently maintained on low-dose etanercept. Libyan J Med. 2012; 7.
100. Capkin E, Karkucak M, Yayli S, Aydin Capkin A, Tosun M. Infliximab-induced palmoplantar psoriasis in a patient with ankylosing spondylitis. J Clin Rheumatol. 2011;17:293–4.
101. Wermuth J, Kind F, Steuerwald M. Palmoplantar pustulosis and acrodermatitis in a patient treated with infliximab for Crohn's sacroiliitis. Clin Gastroenterol Hepatol. 2009;7:A28.
102. Ortiz Salvador JM, Cubells Sanchez L, Subiabre Ferrer D. Palmoplantar pustulosis by adalimumab in a patient with Crohn disease. Med Clin (Barc). 2016;147:565.
103. Rallis E, Korfitis C, Stavropoulou E, Papaconstantis M. Onset of palmoplantar pustular psoriasis while on adalimumab for psoriatic arthritis: a 'class effect' of TNF-alpha antagonists or simply an anti-psoriatic treatment adverse reaction? J Dermatolog Treat. 2010;21:3–5.
104. Gerdes S, Franke J, Domm S, Mrowietz U. Ustekinumab in the treatment of palmoplantar pustulosis. Br J Dermatol. 2010;163:1116–8.
105. Au SC, Goldminz AM, Kim N, et al. Investigator-initiated, open-label trial of ustekinumab for the treatment of moderate-to-severe palmoplantar psoriasis. J Dermatolog Treat. 2013;24:179–87.
106. Buder V, Herberger K, Jacobi A, Augustin M, Radtke MA. Ustekinumab in the treatment of palmoplantar pustular psoriasis—a case series of nine patients. JDDG. 2016;14:1108–13.
107. Arakawa A, Ruzicka T, Prinz JC. Therapeutic efficacy of interleukin 12/interleukin 23 blockade in generalized pustular psoriasis regardless of IL36RN mutation status. JAMA Dermatol. 2016;152:825–8.
108. Murakami M, Hagforsen E, Morhenn V, Ishida-Yamamoto A, Iizuka H. Patients with palmoplantar pustulosis have increased IL-17 and IL-22 levels both in the lesion and serum. Exp Dermatol. 2011;20:845–7.
109. Bissonnette R, Nigen S, Langley RG, et al. Increased expression of IL-17A and limited involvement of IL-23 in patients with palmo-plantar (PP) pustular psoriasis or PP pustulosis; results from a randomised controlled trial. J Eur Acad Dermatol Venereol. 2014;28:1298–305.
110. Lillis JV, Guo CS, Lee JJ, Blauvelt A. Increased IL-23 expression in palmoplantar psoriasis and hyperkeratotic hand dermatitis. Arch Dermatol. 2010;146:918–9.

Neutrophilic Eccrine Hidradenitis

12

Jean-Luc Schmutz

Neutrophilic Eccrine Hidradenitis (NEH) was initially described in 1982 by Harrist et al. [1] in a patient suffering from acute myelogenous leukemia and undergoing chemotherapy with DOXORUBICIN, CYTARABINE and VINCRISTINE. The frequency of this condition is unknown. There is a male predominance with a male to female sex ratio of 2.75:1. The mean age of diagnosis is 41 [2].

NEH may manifest clinically as tender, erythematous and purple macules, papules and nodules often coalescing into single or multiple erythematous annular plaques. Lesions can be found at injection sites. When present, an inflammatory periorbital oedema is consistent with the disease. There is no mucosal involvement. Fever can be found in two-thirds of the cases, mostly as a symptom of the underlying disease rather than of the dermatosis itself.

There are three possible clinical presentations [2]. A central form with trunk, head and neck involvement and unilateral or bilateral periorbital inflammatory oedema; a peripheral form where lesions occur on the limbs and a mixed form also called disseminated (Figs. 12.1, 12.2, and 12.3). NEH occurs in patients with an underlying cancer in 90% of cases, out of which 75% are patients suffering from acute myelogenous leukemia [3] or acute lymphoblastic leukemia [4]. In other cases the underlying disease is either a chronic lymphoid leukemia, Hodgkin's disease [5], a solid tumor (testicular carcinoma, Wilms tumor, osteosarcoma, lung cancer, breast cancer) or an infection (HIV, Serratia marcescens, Enterobacter cloacae, Staphylococcus aureus, Nocardia spp.) [6–8]. Exceptionally, NEH has been reported in patients undergoing hemodialysis for chronic renal failure, in patients with idiopathic neutropenia [9], in patients with Behcet's disease [10] or in healthy individuals [11].

J.-L. Schmutz
Dermatology and Allergology Department, CHRU Nancy–Brabois, Vandœuvre-lès-Nancy, France
e-mail: jl.schmutz@chru-nancy.fr

D. Wallach et al. (eds.), *Neutrophilic Dermatoses*,
https://doi.org/10.1007/978-3-319-72649-6_12

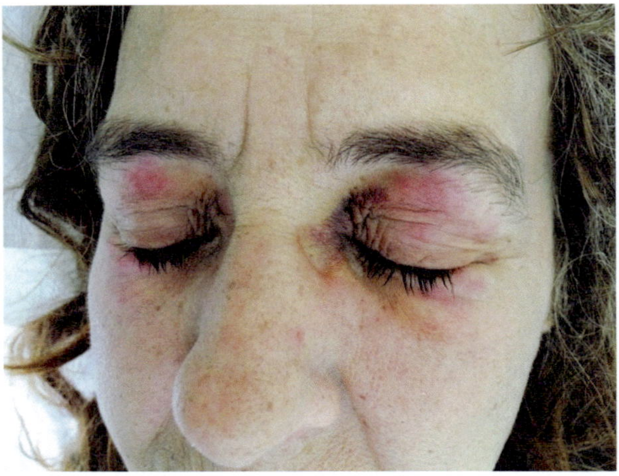

Fig. 12.1 Erythematous plaques of the eyelids

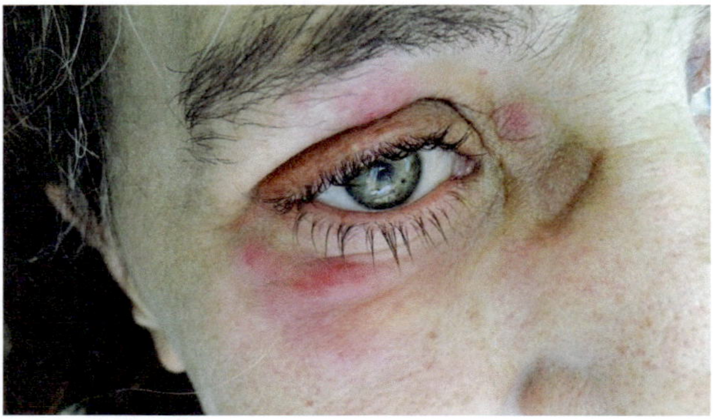

Fig. 12.2 Periorbital erythematous nodules

NEH can be considered a paraneoplastic syndrome when it precedes the cancer diagnosis or when it occurs during the cancer relapse.

The most likely responsible drugs for the induction of NEH are aracytine [12], daunorubicin, vincristine, mitoxantrone (anthracycline), bleomycin, cisplatin, cyclophosphamide, G-CSF, cetuximab [13] and imatinib [14].

NEH usually occurs within 9–12 days following the initiation of the treatment or only within 3–4 days when an anti-BRAF agent is involved (dabrafenib, vemurafenib) [15].

Without treatment symptoms usually subside within 12 days (1–4 weeks), however some authors suggest Dapsone or NSAIDs or even systemic steroid therapy. Their efficacy is however uncertain. Colchicine was also suggested for chronic presentations [16].

Relapses are possible. When the disease is induced by chemotherapy, the risk of relapse is as high as 50% when the same chemotherapy is used.

Diagnosis relies on the histolopathological examination; an oedema and a neutrophilic and lymphocytic infiltrate are found in the dermis. The eccrine glands

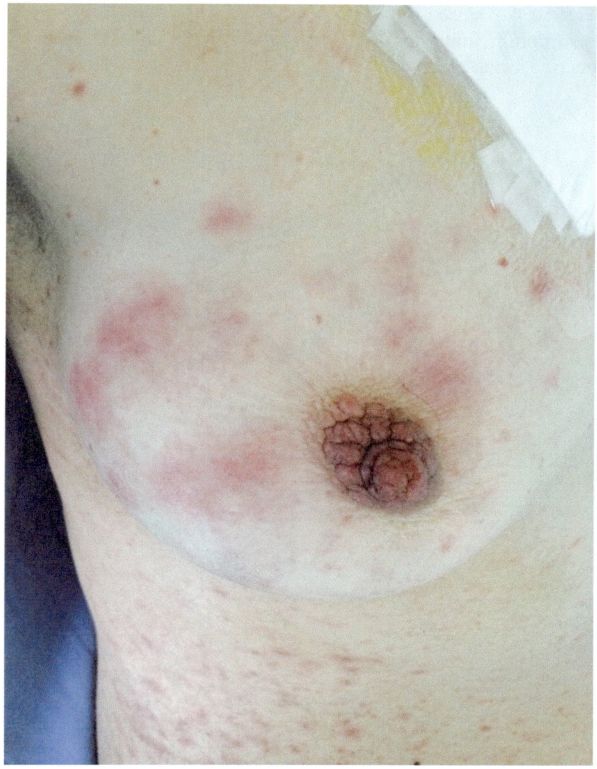

Fig. 12.3 Erythematous plaques of the left breast

are surrounded by a neutrophilic infiltrate mostly around the coiled part of the gland and the secretory part (Figs. 12.4 and 12.5). Necrosis of the eccrine epithelial cells can be found. Leukocytoclasia can be observed in the absence of vasculitis [1]. Cases of chemotherapy-induced eccrine hidradenitis without neutrophilic infiltrate have been cited [17].

The physiopathology is unknown but two possible hypotheses are considered.

The first hypothesis incriminates the toxicity of the different drugs. The accumulation of cytotoxic drugs within the eccrine sweat glands leads to necrosis which subsequently induces the release of chemotactic agents for neutrophils. The gradual clearance of the drug explains the spontaneous resolution of the lesions [18].

The second hypothesis links NEH to the broader neutrophilic dermatoses spectrum, with NEH being considered as a specific involvement of the eccrine sweat glands. Cases have been cited indeed of NEH preceding the diagnosis or the relapse of a blood disease in the absence of any possible inducing drug, thus suggesting that NEH is more likely to be caused by the underlying condition rather than by its treatment [18, 19].

However, this pathophysiological model doesn't explain the polymorphous lesions for the same drug, nor their absence on the palms and soles despite the great number of eccrine sweat glands in these areas. The palmo-plantar presentation of

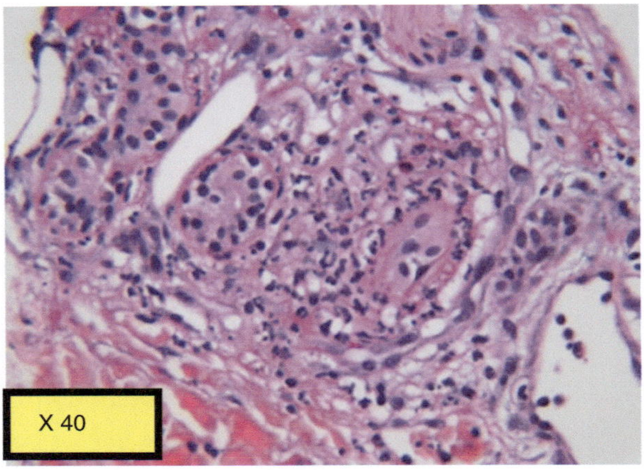

Fig. 12.4 Dense neutrophilic infiltrates of eccrine sweat glands

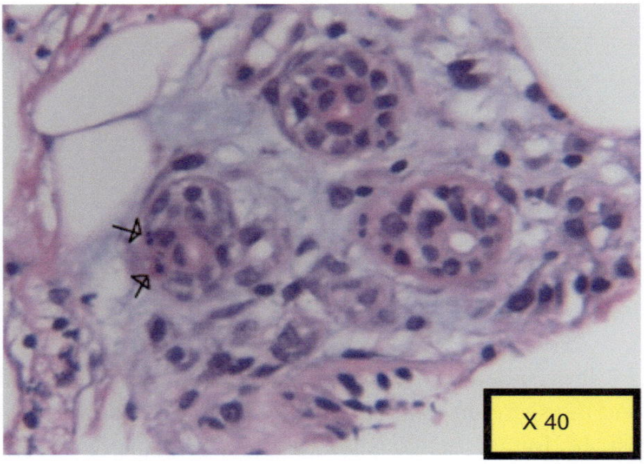

Fig. 12.5 Necrosis of glandular cells

the disease is indeed well known in pediatric patients and is considered idiopathic. It is typical in infants, teen agers and young adults. The diagnosis is clinical and histological with certain specific features: the absence of keratinizing syringometaplasia and the presence of aseptic neutrophilic abcesses [20, 21].

Differential diagnosis of NEH can be particularly difficult due to the polymorphous clinical appearance which can be found in erythema nodosum, vasculitis, urticaria or another type of neutrophilic dermatoses such as Sweet syndrome.

The clinical aspect of the face can also be found in infectious orbital cellulitis especially since fever is present in almost all of the cases and this disease occurs frequently in neutropenic patients. The absence of neutrophilia should not exclude NEH in this particular circumstance [22].

References

1. Harrist TJ, Fine JD, Berman RS, Murphy GF, Mihm MC Jr. Neutrophilic eccrines hidradenitis. A distinctive type of neutrophilic dermatosis associated with myelogenous leukemia and chemotherapy. Arch Dermatol. 1982;118(4):263–6.
2. Moisson YF, Aractingi S, Pinquier L, Reygagne P, Dubertret L. Hidradénite eccrine neutrophilique. Ann Dermatol Venereol. 1992;119(8):605–11.
3. Bonhomme A, Liegeon AL, Granel-Brocard F, Barbaud A, Schmutz JL. Hidradénite neutrophilique eccrine associée à une leucémie aiguë myéloïde. Presse Med. 2015;44(6):688–9.
4. Salik D, Kolivras A, Sass U, Huybrechts S, Dangoisse C. Hidradénite eccrine neutrophilique palmo-plantaire avec extension généralisée chez un enfant en rémission d'une leucémie aiguë lymphoblastique. Ann Dermatol Venereol. 2014;141(4):285–9.
5. Beutner KR, Packman CH, Markowitch W. Neutrophilic eccrine hidradenitis associated with Hodgkin's disease and chemotherapy. A case report. Arch Dermatol. 1986;122(7):809–11.
6. Bachmeyer C, Reygagne P, Aractingi S. Recurrent neutrophilic eccrine hidradenitis in an HIV-1 infected patient. Dermatology. 2000;200(4):328–30.
7. Combemale P, Faisant M, Azoulay-Petit C, Dupin N, Kanitakis J. Neutrophilic eccrine hidradenitis secondary to infection with Serratia marcescens. Br J Dermatol. 2000;142(4):784.8.
8. Antonovich DD, Berke A, Grant-Kels JM, Fung M. Infectious eccrine hidradenitis caused by Nocardia. J Am Acad Dermatol. 2004;50(2):315–8.
9. Keane FM, Munn SE, Buckley DA, Hopster D, Mufti GJ, de Vivier AW. Neutrophilic eccrine hidradenitis in two neutropenic patients. Clin Exp Dermatol. 2001;26(2):162–5.
10. Nijsten TE, Meuleman L, Lambert J. Chronic pruritic neutrophilic eccrine hidradenitis in a patient with Behçet's disease. Br J Dermatol. 2002;147(4):797–800.
11. Morice A, Penven K, Comoz F, Cribier B, Dompmartin A, Leroy D. Hidradénite eccrine neutrophilique chez un sujet sain. Ann Dermatol Venereol. 2005;132(8–9Pt1):686–8.
12. Flynn TC, Harrist TJ, Murphy GF, Loss RW, Moschella SL. Neutrophilic eccrine hidradenitis: a distinctive rash associated with cytarabine therapy and acute leukemia. J Am Acad Dermatol. 1984;11(4 Pt 1):584–90.
13. Turan H, Kaya E, Gurlevik Z, Erdem H, Oktay M. Neutrophilic eccrine hidradenitis induced by cetuximab. Cutan Ocul Toxicol. 2012;31(2):148–50.
14. Dib EG, Ifthikharruddin JJ, Scott GA, Partilo SR. Neutrophilic eccrine hidradenitis induced by imatinib mesylate (Gleevec) therapy. Leuk Res. 2005;29(2):233–4.
15. Herms F, Franck N, Kramkimel N, Fichel F, Delaval L, Laurent-Roussel S, Carlotti A, Avril MF. Neutrophilic eccrine hidradenitis in two patients treated with BRAF inhibitors: a new cutaneous adverse event. Br J Dermatol. 2017;176(6):1645–8. https://doi.org/10.1111/bdj.15259.
16. Belot V, Perrinaud A, Corven C, De Muret A, Lorette G, Machet L. Hidradénite eccrine neutrophilique idiopathique de l'adulte d'évolution prolongée traitée par colchicine. Presse Med. 2006;35(10):1475–8.
17. Greenbaum BH, Heymann W, Reid CS, Travis SF, Donaldson MH. Chemotherapy-associated eccrine hidradenitis: neutrophilic eccrine hidradenitis reevaluated: the role of neutrophilic infiltration. Med Pediatr Oncol. 1988;16(5):351–5.
18. Saada V, Aractingi S, Leblond V, Marinho E, Frances C, Chosidow O. Hidradénite eccrine neutrophilique associée à une rechute de leucémie aiguë myéloblastique. Ann Dermato Venereol. 1998;125(6–7):420–2.
19. Gomez Vazquez M, Peteiro C, Toribio J. Neutrophilic eccrine hidradenitis heralding the onset of classic myelogenous leukemia. J Eur Acad Dermatol Venereol. 2003;17(3):328–30.
20. Erro-Vincent T, Souillet AC, Fouilhoux A, Kanitakis J, David L. Hidradénite eccrine neutrophilique : forme plantaire idiopathique de l'enfant. Arch Pédiatr. 2001;8(3):290–3.
21. Buezo GF, Requena L, Fraga Fernandez J, Gardia Diez A, Fernandez Herrera JM. Idiopathic palmoplantar hidradenitis. Am J Dermatopathol. 1996;18(4):413–6.
22. Srivastava M, Scharf S, Meehan SA, Polsky D. Neutrophilic eccrine hidradenitis masquering as facial cellulitis. J Am Acad Dermatol. 2007;56(4):693–6.

Follicular Neutrophilic Inflammation (Hidradenitis Suppurativa)

13

Angelo Valerio Marzano, Giovanni Damiani, and Alessandro Borghi

Introduction

Follicular neutrophilic inflammation or Hidradenitis Suppurativa (HS), also known as acne inversa, is a chronic-relapsing, debilitating inflammatory disease of the hair follicle that usually presents after puberty, affecting apocrine gland-bearing skin, most commonly the axillae, inguinal regions and anogenital area [1]. It is clinically characterized by recurrent, painful, deep-seated nodules commonly ending in abscesses and sinus tracts with suppuration and hypertrophic scarring [1].

Estimates of the prevalence of HS range from less than 0.1% to 4% [2]. Treatment depends on the stage and severity of the disease, ranging from topical and systemic antibiotics for early and benign disease to biologic agents, particularly the tumour necrosis factor (TNF)-α blocker adalimumab for more severe cases; for advanced and recalcitrant lesions, complete removal by surgical excision is regarded as the most effective procedure [3, 4]. Recently, an upregulation of interleukin (IL)-1β and IL-17, which are pivotal cytokines in autoinflammation [5], has been demonstrated in the lesional skin of patients with both isolated and syndromic HS [6, 7], suggesting an important autoinflammatory component in the pathogenesis of this disease.

A. V. Marzano (✉) • G. Damiani
Dipartimento di Fisiopatologia Medico-Chirurgica e dei Trapianti, Università degli Studi di Milano, Unità Operativa di Dermatologia, IRCCS Fondazione Ca' Granda, Ospedale Maggiore Policlinico, Milano, Italy
e-mail: angelo.marzano@unimi.it

A. Borghi
Dipartimento di Scienze Mediche, Sezione di Dermatologia e Malattie Infettive, Università degli Studi di Ferrara, Ferrara, Italy
e-mail: alessandro.borghi@unife.it

D. Wallach et al. (eds.), *Neutrophilic Dermatoses*,
https://doi.org/10.1007/978-3-319-72649-6_13

Epidemiology

Although several studies have attempted to estimate the prevalence of HS in different settings, the exact prevalence of this disease remains unknown because of the difficulty in collecting and extrapolating data [8–14]. Using the medical record linkage system of the Rochester Epidemiology Project, Vazquez et al. found an overall annual age- and sex-adjusted incidence of 6.0 per 100,000 with an age adjusted incidence significantly higher in women compared with men [9]; moreover, the highest incidence was among young women aged 20–29 years (18.4 per 100,000). The same authors observed that incidence has risen over the past four decades, particularly among women. Recent American studies estimated HS prevalence to range from 0.05% to 0.2% [10, 11]. These estimations are much lower than those reported by European researchers who published a prevalence of 1–4% [12–14]. The discrepancies between European and American studies may be due to different methodologies or different diagnostic criteria but could also reflect actual differences in prevalence/incidence of HS [3].

Clinical Features

For the diagnosis of HS, the following three criteria must be met [3, 15]. First, the presence of typical lesions, such as deep-seated painful nodules, abscesses, draining sinus, bridged scars, and postinflammatory "tombstone" double-ended pseudocomedones. Usually, multiple elements are present simultaneously. The second criterion is topographical. Indeed, these elements typically occur in apocrine gland-bearing skin areas, for which HS has a predilection, namely the axillae, groin, perineal region, buttocks, and infra- and intermammary folds. Third, there must be a clear history of persistence and/or recurrence of typical HS lesions, which are hallmarks of the disease. On this regard, two disease recurrences over a period of 6 months have been arbitrarily used as a qualifier for the diagnosis of HS [3]. All these three criteria must be present for the definitive diagnosis. Family history of HS and absence of infectious agents at microbiological examination are further indicative features of HS [3]. The early lesions are solitary, painful nodules, which represent the primary lesions of HS. Subjective prodromal symptoms, including burning, stinging, pain, pruritus, heat, and hyperhidrosis, often precede the occurrence of the overt nodule [16]. The nodules may resolve spontaneously or persist for weeks or months with inflammatory recurrences or, most frequently, turn into abscesses with rupture and draining purulent material. The recurrence of inflammatory episodes may lead to chronic sinus formation, with intermittent release of serous, purulent, or bloodstained discharges and frequent foul odours from anaerobic colonization. A characteristic secondary lesion is composed of bridged, rope-like hypertrophic scars resulting from a healing process that induces marked fibrosis. Tombstone comedones involving single or multiple pores are frequently tertiary lesions. Follicular papules and pustules are observed in areas typical of HS as well as in other body areas, and they have to be considered as associated, non specific lesions. Epidermal cysts, located on external genital organs, face and thorax, are prominent in some patients.

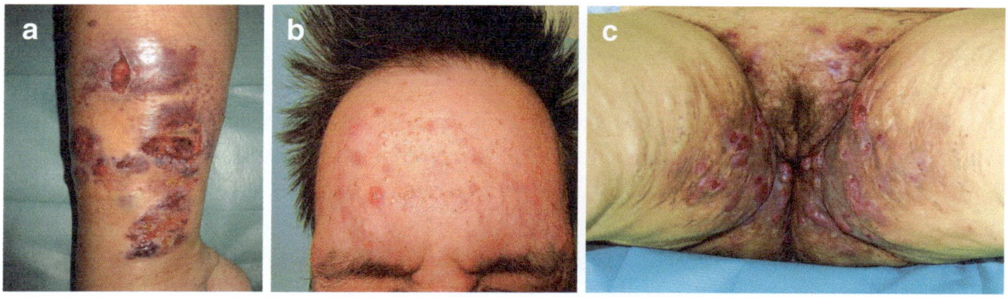

Fig. 13.1 Association of **P**yoderma gangrenosum (panel **a**), **A**cne (panel **b**) and **S**uppurative **H**idradenitis (panel **c**), christened as PASH syndrome

Although the typical patient is a young subject, mainly woman, with axillary and groin involvement, the spectrum of presentations is broad in terms of lesion appearance, sites of involvement and disease severity. Given the heterogeneity of HS, Canoui-Poitrine et al. identified three HS subgroups on the basis of demographics, medical history, and disease severity in a cohort of 618 patients [17]. In particular, the authors defined the following three phenotypes: "axillary–mammary", "follicular", and "gluteal". The "axillary–mammary" variant, comprised about half of the study population and was characterized by high prevalence of breast and armpit involvement as well as hypertrophic scars. It was more frequent in females and was consistent with the typical HS phenotype. The "follicular" class (26% of patients) was characterized by follicular lesions, most notably epidermal cysts, pilonidal sinus and comedones, as well as severe acne. The "follicular" form had higher proportions of men and smokers, and greater disease severity in comparison with the typical "axillary–mammary" variant. In the "gluteal" class, HS presented with gluteal involvement, follicular papules and pustules, with a higher proportion of smokers, lower percentage of obese and a less severe disease (despite a longer HS duration) in comparison with the "axillary–mammary" variant. Other different clinical presentations have been proposed [15], with the syndromic type deserving particular interest [6]. Patients with syndromic HS present with concomitant conditions, notably pyoderma gangrenosum (PG) and arthritis, in the context of autoinflammatory syndromes that have recently been described, such as PASH (PG, acne, and HS) [6, 18] (Fig. 13.1) and PAPASH (pyogenic arthritis, PG, acne and HS) [19]. These syndromic forms of HS are discussed in detail in another chapter within this volume.

Differential Diagnosis

HS has an extensive differential diagnosis. The appearance, age of onset, typical locations, chronicity and recurrence, poor response to antibiotics, and lack of signs of systemic sepsis can help to diagnose this condition. In spite of this, delayed diagnosis is frequent [8]. The most common differential diagnoses are follicular pyodermas. These lesions spread in a random fashion and are more pustular than HS lesions. Cutaneous Crohn's disease may be both a differential diagnosis and an associated disease. Cutaneous Crohn's disease must be differentiated from HS especially in its perianal and anogenital location; histology, that shows in Crohn's disease the typical granulomatous pattern, can help to distinguish between the two conditions [20]. Simple abscesses, which are usually single lesions, infected Bartholin's gland, infected or inflamed epidermal cysts, lymphogranuloma venereum, scrofuloderma, actinomycosis, developmental fistulae, and nodular acne are other common sources of error. Finally, HS should be differentiated from amicrobial pustulosis of the folds, a rare superficial neutrophilic dermatosis presenting with pustular lesions on the major and minor folds as well as the anogenital region [21, 22], which a chapter of this book is dedicated to.

Severity Classification Systems

In 1989, Hurley first proposed a severity classification system for HS [23] (Fig. 13.2). The author identified three different disease stages. Stage I, the most common one, is characterized by abscess formation, single or multiple, without sinus tracts and cicatrisation. Stage II is defined by recurrent abscesses, single or multiple, with tract formation and scarring and widely separated lesions. In stage III, diffuse involvement or multiple interconnected tracts and abscesses across the entire area are typically present. The Hurley classification was originally designed for selecting the appropriate treatment modality, namely medical therapy for Hurley stage I, local surgery for Hurley stage II, and wide surgical excision for Hurley stage III. This classification, albeit simple and rapid, is not a precise monitoring tool in the clinical setting, particularly for an accurate assessment of the extent of inflammation within each stage.

A more detailed and dynamic HS score for measuring clinical severity was created by Sartorius et al. and later modified [24, 25]. The parameters in the modified Sartorius score include counting of individual nodules and fistulas, measuring the longest distance between two lesions, and adding extra points to Hurley III areas, within seven anatomical regions. The Sartorius score, besides being time-consuming, may be limited in more severe cases because of the difficulty in distinguishing separate lesions, mostly when lesions become confluent and sinuses become interconnected. Nevertheless, the Sartorius score is frequently used in clinical trials.

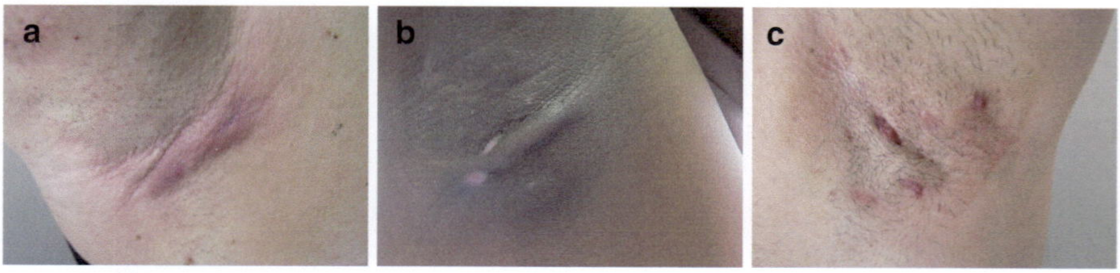

Fig. 13.2 Hidradenitis suppurativa presenting in Hurley Stage I (panel **a**), Hurley Stage II (panel **b**) and Hurley Stage III (panel **c**)

Other available clinical measures for assessing HS disease severity include HS-PGA, HSSI, HiSCR, AISI.

An anchored 6-stage, HS-specific Physician Global Assessment (HS-PGA) has been defined for objectively assessing clinical response to treatment (1, clear; 2, minimal; 3, mild-fewer; 4, moderate-fewer; 5, severe; 6, very severe) [26].

The Hidradenitis Suppurativa Severity Index (HSSI), created by Kerdel et al., incorporates categorical objective parameters with categorical subjective patient-reported parameters [27].

The Hidradenitis Suppurativa Clinical Response (HiSCR) score provides a valid and meaningful clinical endpoint for assessing HS treatment effectiveness in controlling inflammatory signs and symptoms of HS [28].

The most recently developed severity score is the Acne Inversa Severity Index (AISI), designed to include both a physician-rated assessment that considers the type of lesions occurring and the affected body sites as well as a 0–10 visual analogue scale (VAS) aimed at assessing the patient's pain, discomfort and disability due to HS [29].

These disease severity scores, while provide clinically meaningful assessments of disease severity, do not capture the influence of disease on patient's quality of life (QOL). In fact, HS affects patients' lives beyond the disease-related pain or functional impairment [30–33]. Producing malodorous discharge and affecting sensitive anatomic regions, HS can be damaging physically, emotionally and psychologically as well as can impact a vast range of life activities. Although no single QOL instrument, among the numerous ones used, captures the full extent of the disease impact [34], HS is well recognized to have a substantial adverse effect on the physical, social and emotional well-being of patients.

Sonographic Evaluation

A standardized sonographic evaluation of HS was proposed by Wortsman X et al. in 2013, when a ultrasonographic score was published, namely Sonographic Scoring (SOS)-HS [35]. Through evaluated parameters, SOS-HS set three severity categorizes: I—single fluid collection and dermal changes affecting a single body segment; II—two to four fluid collections or a single fistulous tract with dermal changes affecting up to two body segments (Fig. 13.3); III—five or more fluid collections or two or more fistulous tracts with dermal changes or involvement of three or more body segments [35]. As testify to the great importance tributed to fistulas in the SOS-HS, recently fistulas have been subdivided by sonographic morphology into three subtypes: I—low fibrotic scarring with high or low edema; II—high fibrotic scarring with low edema; III—high fibrotic scarring with high edema [36]. The high appeal of this instrumental assessment is that it detects earlier than clinics changes in the severity of lesions under treatment, since flare activity, erythema and pain are strongly correlated with ultrasound morphological changes [37].

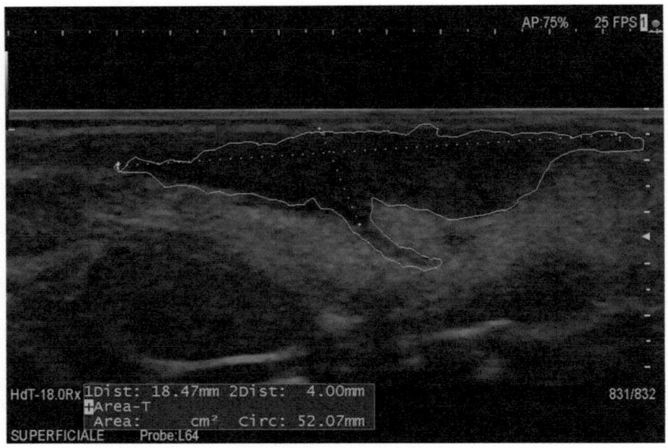

Fig. 13.3 Sonography showing an abscess with a fistulous tract (Courtesy of Dr. E. Passoni)

Comorbidities and Aggravating Factors

HS is associated with a variety of concomitant and secondary diseases, as suggested in the recent report on the new Autoinflammatory Disease Damage Index (ADDI) [38]. Overall, reported comorbidities fall into several categories, such as obesity and the metabolic syndrome, hormone-related disorders, deleterious health habits and mood, autoimmune diseases, inflammatory/autoinflammatory diseases and finally an increased risk for skin cancer, particularly squamous cell carcinoma developing on long-lasting ulcerated nodules, and sequelae of nonhealing wounds [39]. Studies to date suggest that HS is most convincingly associated with the metabolic syndrome and obesity, especially in young patients [40]. Regarding the hormonal pathogenesis, also suggested by the predilection of HS for women, the association between HS and polycystic ovary syndrome has been particularly addressed, with variable results [41]. Based on studies of prevalence, the association between cigarette smoking and HS is established, even if the etiological role of tobacco smoking is subject of much speculation [12, 42] In the systematic review of Fimmel and Zouboulis inflammatory bowel disease (IBD), and spondyloarthropathy proved to be the most common comorbid diseases in HS, in line with common dysimmune pathomechanisms [43]. HS was significantly associated with presence and risk of a new-onset IBD in a recently published study [44]. Moreover, spondyloarthritis occurs in HS patients with the prevalence in this group exceeding that in the general population, as recently demonstrated [45]. Bariatric surgery may also represent a risk factor for developing HS in a genetically predisposed individual [46]. It is uncertain whether nonmelanoma skin cancer (NMSC) has a true association with HS or it is a complication of the chronic inflammation of such condition [47]. Characteristics of comorbid NMSC in HS suggest that patients have NMSC in perineal or gluteal locations and have HS for 25 years on average before cancer development [39]. The reduced mobility of HS patients caused by contractures after healing with scarring, chronic lymphedema and anaemia are listed as other relevant complications of the disease [48].

Etiopathogenesis

The term "hidradenitis suppurativa" dates back to the original description of the disease by Verneuil [49, 50] who considered the entity as a disorder of the sweat glands based on the characteristic distribution of the apocrine glands and the anatomical coincidence with the disease process. Subsequent studies supported the view of a primary involvement of the apocrine sweat glands in HS pathogenesis [51, 52]. However, careful examination of histologic skin specimens from early and advanced HS lesions have shown that the sweat glands are not primarily or selectively inflamed. In 1952, Brunsting observed that the earliest histopathological changes consist of a folliculitis followed by severe perifolliculitis, both typical of acne, whereas apocrine gland is only secondarily involved as a consequence of the extension of the process to the deep layers of the skin [53]. In 1956, Pillsbury, Shelley and Kligman introduced the term "follicular occlusion triad" as an umbrella term for HS, dissecting cellulitis of the scalp, and acne conglobata [54]. In 1975, Plewig and Kligman added the pilonidal sinus as the fourth component of the ensemble and changed the name to "acne tetrad" [55]. Histopathologically, all four entities are identical and share the same primary pathogenetic mechanism with acne vulgaris, namely pilosebaceous follicular duct occlusion [56]. As these entities are an expression of follicular occlusion in localizations inverse to acne vulgaris, Plewig and Steger in 1989 suggested the term "acne inversa" [57]. Follicular occlusion leads to rupture of the hair follicle followed by discharge of contents, including keratin and bacteria into the surrounding dermis [58]. This sequence induces an inflammatory response that recruits neutrophils, lymphocytes and histiocytes. Various mechanisms of action and agents that may lead to follicular occlusion in HS have been proposed, in particular aberrant keratinocyte response to commensal follicular bacteria, tobacco's compounds, hormonal changes, and mechanical compression and friction [59]. About one-third of HS patients have a family history with an autosomal dominant pattern [60]. Those familial cases bear mutations in components of the γ-secretase complex, namely presenilin-1 (PSEN1), presenilin enhancer-2 (PSENEN) and nicastrin (NCSTN), which cleaves intramembrane receptors, like Notch, E-cadherin and CD44, which in turn regulate follicular keratinization [60–63]. In addition, impaired γ-secretase/Notch signaling is proposed to increase proinflammatory cytokine production including IL-1β, TNF-α and IL-23 promoting T helper (Th) 17 cell polarization [64]. Notch and toll-like receptor (TLR) signaling cross-talk has been reported where Notch signaling suppressed TLR4-triggered proinflammatory cytokine expression by macrophages [65]. Negative feedback regulation is impaired by deficient Notch signaling, leading to excessive cytokine production and release [64]. In this respect, the role of the immune system in HS is confirmed by the favourable response of the disease to tumor necrosis factor-α (TNF-α) inhibitors [4, 26, 27, 66]. Recently, an upregulation of IL-1β and IL-17 has been demonstrated in the lesional skin of patients with HS [7, 66]. Enhanced *in situ* expression of IL-17 by CD4+ T cells as well as IL-23 by dermal macrophages in HS lesional skin has been reported [5]. Aside from Th17 cells, IL-17 is produced by neutrophils, gamma/delta T cells and mast cells, which are all abundantly present in HS lesional skin [59]. Lima et al. provided evidence that IL-17+ cells are present early in perilesional skin of HS where they appear to contribute to the initiation of skin inflammation [67]. The same authors identified the lesional keratinocytes as an important source of proinflammatory molecules, namely IL-1β. In fact, they have demonstrated an upregulated expression of the inflammasome components nucleotide-binding domain, leucine-rich-containing family, pyrin domain-containing (NLRP)-3 and caspase-1 in HS lesional keratinocytes. This finding denotes activation of caspase-1 in lesional keratinocytes and suggests IL-1β production and release from the epidermis. Since IL-17-stimulated keratinocytes have been shown to secrete IL-1β through a mechanism involving the NLRP3 inflammasome [68], it has been hypothesized that IL-17 triggers the production of IL-1β by HS lesional keratinocytes. The endogenous danger-associated molecular patterns (DAMPs) S100A8 and S100A9, which are proinflammatory molecules upregulated in several chronic inflammatory diseases, are upregulated in HS lesional epidermis too [67]. Neutrophils of the HS deep infiltrate are important components of a positive feedback loop that promotes release of IL-17 and S100A8/S100A9, thereby sustaining the inflammatory process. Altogether, these data provide evidence that IL-17 releasing cells contribute to the initiation of skin inflammation via triggering the release of IL-1β by keratinocytes. The subsequently increased production of proinflammatory factors including S100A8/S100A9 and IL-1β promotes an even more massive recruitment of neutrophils, thereby amplifying and accelerating the vicious cycle, finally eliciting the clinical features of HS [5]. Although the findings reported in literature on the involvement of innate immunity in the HS pathogenesis are not univocal, most authors demonstrated an enhanced expression of the main innate immunity markers, such as TLRs, β-defensins, integrins and psoriasins [69–72]. Enhanced concentrations of TNF-α in HS patients' serum and lesional skin have been found [73–75]. Although opposite results have also been published [69, 76], the trend appears to be towards an increased expression of TNF-α in HS. Elevated levels of the anti-inflammatory cytokine IL-10 in HS skin have also been reported, this finding possibly representing a negative feedback signal against the severe proinflammatory milieu [69, 73, 74]. This scenario, involving IL-1β, IL-17 and TNF-α overexpression, innate immunity dysfunction, and inflammasome activation, suggests an important autoinflammatory component in the pathogenesis of HS, closely linking HS, neutrophilic dermatoses and autoinflammatory diseases [77–79]. The reported mutations involving a number of autoinflammatory genes, such as proline-serine-threonine phosphatase interacting protein 1(PSTPIP1), mediterranean fever (MEFV), Nucleotide-Binding Oligomerization Domain, Leucine Rich Repeat And Pyrin Domain Containing 3 (NLRP3) and nucleotide-binding oligomerization domain-containing protein 2 (NOD2), in patients with syndromic HS further support the view that HS is an autoinflammatory disease [6, 80]. The role of bacterial infection in the initiation or propagation of HS remains under investigation [81]. Bacteriology studies most frequently show a mixed growth of commensal microbes, confirming that HS is an immune-mediated condition and not a disease of primary infectious etiology [82]. Bacterial colonization of chronic-relapsing HS lesions is common [82] and may act synergistically with the hyperactive innate immunity, amplifying the autoinflammatory scenario.

Treatment

Treatment of HS can be challenging, and more than 50 interventions have been reported in the literature, often supported by only low-quality evidence. Indeed, a recent systematic review has highlighted a relative lack of high-quality evidence to guide treatment decisions in HS [83]. Until recently, HS could be characterized as an orphan disease. It has historically been treated by a great number of different specialities, like surgeons, emergency physicians, plastic surgeons, infectious disease specialists, general practitioners, and dermatologists [10]. This has resulted in a highly variable approach to HS, generally described as unsatisfactory [84]. Topical antibiotic and topical keratolytic agents have been used in the management of patients with mild HS (Hurley stage I), based on the possible pathogenesis of occlusion of follicles and the role of bacteria [85]. The European guideline in the management of HS recommended topical clindamycin as first-line therapy for patients with Hurley stage I HS [3, 86]. The action of topical clindamycin in HS treatment may be due to its antimicrobial effects, reduction of free fatty acids in the surface lipids, and suppression of leukocyte chemotaxis. No data are available on the topical use of any other antibiotics. Local hygiene may be an important factor to suppress the potential triggers of an aberrant immune response and to prevent secondary infection [85]. Antiseptics, such as silver and iodine, may potentially contribute to in the management of HS patients as well. Systemic therapies are the mainstay of treatment for patients with HS. Systemic antibiotics are the medications most often prescribed to treat HS [87]. It is likely that the efficacy of antibiotics against HS is related mainly to their anti-inflammatory properties [88]. The efficacy of a combination of rifampincin and clindamycin in the treatment of HS was documented in some modestly large case series [89–92]. A combination of rifampicin 600 mg and clindamycin 600 mg was administered in a single dose or in two divided daily doses for 10 consecutive weeks. An average of about 80% of the treated patients had some response to therapy. The use of this combination is limited by both the risk for developing an infection with *Clostridium difficile* due to clindamycin and the extensive list of possible drug interactions. Tetracycline is the only traditional systemic antibiotic that has been examined in a small randomized controlled study in the treatment of HS [93]. In particular, 46 patients with mild to moderate HS received topical clindamycin 1% twice daily or oral tetracycline 500 mg twice daily. Patients in both groups had significant improvement from baseline after 3 months of treatment, without statistically significant difference between the two treatment regimens. When surgery is indicated, a course of antibiotics beforehand may be useful to prevent infections, better delineate and identify the lesions to be excised, and effectively downsize the area to be excised. Dapsone is a sulfone antibiotic that is frequently used to treat neutrophilic and eosinophilic inflammatory dermatoses. The use of dapsone for the treatment of HS has been described in several reports with varying results [94, 95]. Efficacy is reported at doses of 25–200 mg a day. Use of high doses is often limited by symptomatic or haematological complications. Reported duration of therapy is variable (reported range, 3–48 months). Due to its relative safety, dapsone may be useful as long-term maintenance therapy for individuals with HS [87]. Evidence of the efficacy of acitretin in the treatment of HS raises from some non randomized studies [96–98]. The efficacy of acitretin is mainly due to its action in normalizing keratinocyte differentiation and proliferation. It also decreases inflammation in the dermis and epidermis by inhibiting the chemotaxis of polymorphonuclear cells and the release of proinflammatory mediators. In the available studies, patients treated with acitretin received daily doses of 0.25–0.88 mg/kg for periods of 3–12 months [3]. The response rate was high, as more than 50% of treated patients improved after treatment. The progress was maintained during the next months after the termination drug withdrawal. A study of 14 female patients with HS who were treated with low-dose (10 mg/day) alitretinoin revealed the effectiveness of such therapy [99]. Not surprisingly, isotretinoin is in contrast ineffective for HS, as this agent primarily works on sebaceous glands, which are not involved in the pathogenesis of HS [87]. Zinc gluconate, by acting on innate immunity [69, 100], may be useful in the treatment of HS at the starting dose of 90 mg/day. The daily dosage may be lowered according to results and gastrointestinal tract side effects. Zinc seems to be a suitable maintenance treatment in Hurley I and II cases [3]. There are indications that antiandrogens, such as cyproterone acetate, and estrogens improve HS [101–103] but no definitive evidence-based data exist. On the basis of the pivotal role of the immune system in HS pathophysiology, anti-inflammatory drugs have been used in the treatment of HS [104]. The use of intralesional triamcinolone acetonide 5–10 mg/mL, as both monotherapy and an adjunct to systemic therapies, has been advocated for the rapid reduction in inflammation associated with acute flares and for management of recalcitrant nodules and sinus tracts [3]. There are limited data on the use of corticosteroids in HS. Short and long-term therapy can result in rebound flare on withdrawal. Short-term, rapidly tapering therapy can provide benefit in reducing in inflammation associated with acute flares [3]. Based on the recent physiopathological evidences, biologic medications, particularly the TNF-α blocker adalimumab, have been increasingly using in the management of HS [3, 4, 26, 83, 104]. Adalimumab is a fully human therapeutic monoclonal antibody, which binds with high affinity and specificity to soluble and membrane-bound TNF-α. It is the most well-studied biologic with multiple, larger-sized, randomized, controlled studies conducted [26, 74, 104, 105]. Dosing regimens varied from 40 to 80 mg, in a frequency ranging from weekly to every other week. About 80% of treated patients showed a significant to moderate response [3, 83, 105], and adalimumab 40 mg weekly, the approved dosage regimen in HS, was found to improve patients' quality of life compared with placebo [106]. In 2016, after the publication of a two phase randomized trial demonstrating that treatment with adalimumab 40 mg weekly resulted in significantly higher clinical response, as compared with placebo [4], adalimumab obtained the registration for the management of moderate to severe HS and it is nowadays the only licensed biologic for this disease. Infliximab is a chimeric antibody composed of both human and mouse proteins targeting both soluble and transmembrane TNF-α. Several cohort studies have been published regarding the use of infliximab in patients with moderate to severe HS. Most treatments consisted of infusions of

5 mg/kg of infliximab at weeks 0, 2, and 6. Nearly all studies found that some of the patients improved with treatment [3, 105]. The only randomized, placebo-controlled trial on the use of infliximab in HS found that 26% of patients in the treatment arm experienced a ≥50% decrease in disease severity compared to 5% of patients in the placebo group [27]. In addition, DLQI, pain, and Physician Global Assessments all significantly improved from baseline in the treatment arm but not in the placebo arm. Etanercept is a fully humanized fusion protein composed of the receptor protein component of immunoglobulin G1. This protein binds to transmembrane TNF-α but does not bind to soluble TNF-α. A recent systematic review on the use of TNF-α inhibitors found that efficacy of etanercept in HS was relatively low without improvements in patients' DLQI [107]. Only one randomized, double-blind trial has been reported to date on the use of etanercept for HS [108], with no significant differences uncovered between etanercept and placebo after 12 weeks of treatment. Since it has been shown that the IL-12 /IL-23 pathway is upregulated in HS, therefore there is a rationale for the efficacy of ustekinumab, a human, anti-p40 monoclonal antibody used in the treatment of patients with psoriasis. The first results of this agent are promising [109, 110]. Anakinra is a recombinant IL-1-α receptor antagonist, that by targeting the IL-1 pathway has been successfully used for the treatment of autoinflammatory entities. HS response to anakinra on daily subcutaneous doses ranging from 100 to 200 mg has been reported in case reports [111]. Ciclosporin A is a calcineurin inhibitor with potent immunosuppressive activity. It specifically targets T lymphocytes, suppressing both the induction and proliferation of T-effector cells and inhibiting production of proinflammatory cytokines. Beneficial effects of ciclosporin A in HS are reported in limited case reports and its use should be reserved to cases not responsive to standard therapies [3, 104]. Methotrexate was reported to be ineffective in a series of three patients with severe HS [87]. In a study by Deckers et al. fumarates were found to be effective in three of seven patients whose HS was refractory to traditional therapies [112]. The proposed mechanism of action of fumarates is an anti-inflammatory effect based on the suppression of interleukins-12 and -23 and the nuclear factor kappa beta pathway. Mycophenolate mofetil, an immunosuppressant which might be theoretically effective in the treatment of HS, lacks of evidence [3, 104]. Theoretically, the future management of HS will be a tailored therapy based on the genetic and immunological profile of selected patients, blocking different physiopathological steps, namely IL-1β, IL-17 or TNF-α-mediated pathways; in refractory cases, a combined biologic treatment , such as for example an IL-1 blocker in combination with an IL-17 or TNF-α antagonist, could be considered. When the prevention of new lesions fails as well as when medical therapy of established lesions is ineffective, surgery is a valuable option [113]. The surgical treatment of HS should be individualized based on the stage and treatment history of the patient and ranges from treating individual acute lesions to complete removal of persistent disease. Five distinct surgical approaches can be considered: (1) local destruction; (2) incision and drainage; (3) mini-unroofing by punch debridement; (4) standard unroofing (deroofing) to all involved margins; and (5) surgical excision beyond all clinically apparent margins [113]. Local destruction with cryosurgery, cryoinfusion, electrosurgery, and

photodynamic therapy may be attempted for smaller and thinner individual lesions. Incision and drainage of individual suppurative lesions are aimed to empty them of pus and some semisolids. This approach provides only temporary pain relief with usual lesion recurrence. unch debridement (mini-unroofing) is a simple procedure performed using a 5- to 8-mm circular disposable biopsy punch and is aimed to eradicate the "bulge" area of the folliculo-pilosebaceous unit, which is hypothesized to be responsible for growth of HS primary lesions. This approach is indicated for the management of early or small acute or subacute inflammatory nodules. Recurrences do not occur but additional folliculo-pilosebaceous units in the treated area are at risk for new HS lesion development. Surgical unroofing, also called deroofing, can treat nodules, abscesses, and sinus tracts either individually (local unroofing) or including all lesions in an anatomic area (extensive unroofing) [114]. Under local anesthesia, the roof of each abscess, nodule, and sinus tract is removed, and all communicating cavities are exposed with scissor tips or a malleable metal probe, electrosurgery or a CO_2 laser. Patients with chronic and extensive Hurley stage III disease may be managed by wide excision of the entire affected area with surgical margins beyond the clinical borders of disease activity. Wide excision, although potentially leading to higher morbidity than local excision, has a lower recurrence rate. A retrospective analysis of 590 consecutive surgically treated cases showed that excision and unroofing procedures were effective treatments with infrequent complications and low recurrence rates [115]. To date, more surgical trials to improve HS care are needed [83]; in particular there are no randomized clinical trials investigating for the timing of surgery or type of surgical procedure. A possible comprehensive therapeutic algorithm for HS is reported in Fig. 13.4 [116].

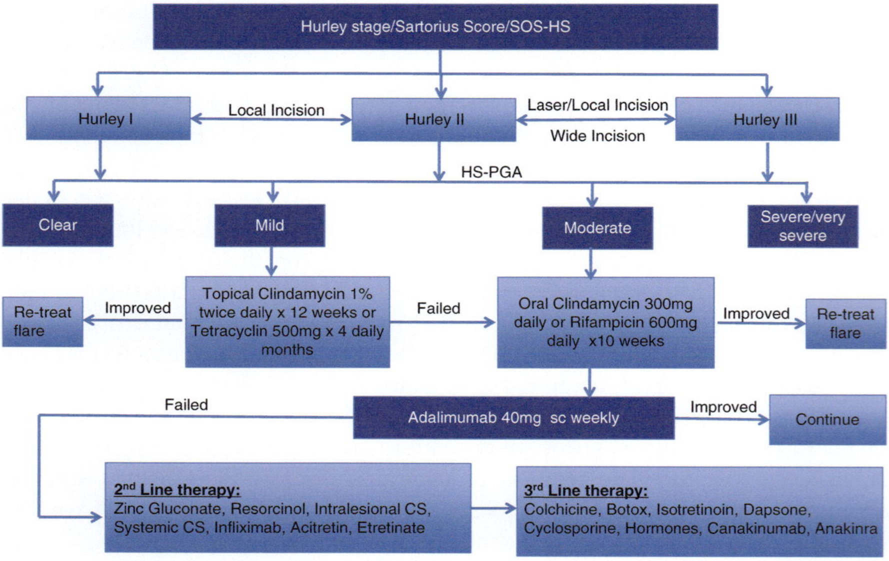

Fig. 13.4 A possible therapeutic algorithm for hidradenitis suppurativa. Modified from Gulliver W et al. [116]. *SOS-HS* sonographic scoring of hidradenitis suppurativa, *HS-PGA* hidradenitis suppurativa-physician global assessment, *SC* subcutaneous, *CS* corticosteroid

Conclusions

Based on the increasing knowledge about the pathogenesis of HS with particular respect to the involvement of the innate immune response, it seems justified to assign HS and the neutrophilic dermatoses in general, within the spectrum of which HS may be included [77, 79], to the growing family of autoinflammatory diseases. Disease-based gene discovery and basic research continue to go hand in hand in deciphering the molecular pathways that lead to excessive innate immune responses and cause the chronic autoinflammatory mechanisms underlying the HS features. Growing insights into the pathogenesis of HS will in turn provide us with novel therapeutic targets that will allow us to treat this challenging condition more effectively.

References

1. Jemec GB. Clinical practice. Hidradenitis suppurativa. N Engl J Med. 2012;366:158–64.
2. Miller IM, McAndrew RJ, Hamzavi I. Prevalence, risk factors, and comorbidities of hidradenitis suppurativa. Dermatol Clin. 2016;34:7–16.
3. Zouboulis CC, Desai N, Emtestam L, et al. European S1 guideline for the treatment of hidradenitis suppurativa/acne inversa. J Eur Acad Dermatol Venereol. 2015;29(4):619–44.
4. Kimball AB, Okun MM, Williams DA, et al. Two phase 3 trials of adalimumab for hidradenitis suppurativa. N Engl J Med. 2016;375:422–34.
5. Schlapbach C, Hänni T, Yawalkar N, Hunger RE. Expression of the IL-23/Th17 pathway in lesions of hidradenitis suppurativa. J Am Acad Dermatol. 2011;65:790–8.
6. Marzano AV, Ceccherini I, Gattorno M, et al. Association of pyoderma gangrenosum, acne, and suppurative hidradenitis (PASH) shares genetic and cytokine profiles with other autoinflammatory diseases. Medicine (Baltimore). 2014;93:e187.
7. Feldmeyer L, Werner S, French LE, Beer HD. Interleukin-1, inflammasomes and the skin. Eur J Cell Biol. 2010;89:638–44.
8. Jemec GB, Kimball AB. Hidradenitis suppurativa: epidemiology and scope of the problem. J Am Acad Dermatol. 2015;73(5 Suppl 1):S4–7.
9. Vazquez BG, Alikhan A, Weaver AL, et al. Incidence of hidradenitis suppurativa and associated factors: a population-based study of Olmsted County, Minnesota. J Invest Derm. 2013;133:97–103.
10. Sung S, Kimball AB. Counterpoint: analysis of patient claims data to determine the prevalence of hidradenitis suppurativa in the United States. J Am Acad Dermatol. 2013;69:818–9.
11. Cosmatos I, Matcho A, Weinstein R, et al. Analysis of patient claims data to determine the prevalence of hidradenitis suppurativa in the United States. J Am Acad Dermatol. 2013;68:412–9.
12. Revuz JE, Canoui-Poitrine F, Wolkenstein P, et al. Prevalence and factors associated with hidradenitis suppurativa: results from two case-control studies. J Am Acad Dermatol. 2008;59:596–601.
13. Jemec GB, Heidenheim M, Nielsen NH. The prevalence of hidradenitis suppurativa and its potential precursor lesions. J Am Acad Dermatol. 1996;35:191–4.
14. Jemec GB. The symptomatology of hidradenitis suppurativa in women. Br J Dermatol. 1988;119:345–50.
15. van der Zee HH, Jemec GB. New insights into the diagnosis of hidradenitis suppurativa: clinical presentations and phenotypes. J Am Acad Dermatol. 2015;73:S23–6.
16. Revuz J. Hidradenitis suppurativa. Presse Med. 2010;39:1254–64.

17. Canoui-Poitrine F, Le Thuaut A, Revuz JE, et al. Identification of three hidradenitis suppurativa phenotypes: latent class analysis of a cross-sectional study. J Invest Dermatol. 2013;133:1506–11.
18. Braun-Falco M, Kovnerystyy O, Lohse P, Ruzicka T. Pyoderma gangrenosum, acne, and suppurative hidradenitis (PASH)—a new autoinflammatory syndrome distinct from PAPA syndrome. J Am Acad Dermatol. 2012;66:409–15.
19. Marzano AV, Trevisan V, Gattorno M, et al. Pyogenic arthritis, pyoderma gangrenosum, acne, and hidradenitis suppurativa (PAPASH): a new autoinflammatory syndrome associated with a novel mutation of the PSTPIP1 gene. JAMA Dermatol. 2013;149:762–4.
20. Marzano AV, Borghi A, Stadnicki A, et al. Cutaneous manifestations in patients with inflammatory bowel diseases: pathophysiology, clinical features, and therapy. Inflamm Bowel Dis. 2014;20:213–27.
21. Marzano AV, Ramoni S, Caputo R. Amicrobial pustulosis of the folds. Report of 6 cases and a literature review. Dermatology. 2008;216:305–11.
22. Marzano AV, Tavecchio S, Berti E, et al. Cytokine and chemokine profile in amicrobial pustulosis of the folds: evidence for autoinflammation. Medicine (Baltimore). 2015;94:e2301.
23. Hurley H. Axillary hyperhidrosis, apocrine bromhidrosis, hidradenitis suppurativa, and familial benign pemphigus: surgical approach. In: Roenigh RRH, editor. Dermatologic surgery. New York: Marcel Dekker; 1989. p. 729–39.
24. Sartorius K, Lapins J, Emtestam L, Jemec GB. Suggestions for uniform outcome variables when reporting treatment effects in hidradenitis suppurativa. Br J Dermatol. 2003;149:211–3.
25. Sartorius K, Emtestam L, Jemec GB, Lapins J. Objective scoring of hidradenitis suppurativa reflecting the role of tobacco smoking and obesity. Br J Dermatol. 2009;161:831–9.
26. Kimball AB, Kerdel F, Adams D, et al. Adalimumab for the treatment of moderate to severe hidradenitis suppurativa: a parallel randomized trial. Ann Intern Med. 2012;18:846–55.
27. Grant A, Gonzalez T, Montgomery MO, et al. Infliximab therapy for patients with moderate to severe hidradenitis suppurativa: a randomized, double-blind, placebo-controlled crossover trial. J Am Acad Dermatol. 2010;62:205–17.
28. Kimball AB, Jemec GB, Yang M, et al. Assessing the validity, responsiveness and meaningfulness of the Hidradenitis Suppurativa Clinical Response (HiSCR) as the clinical endpoint for hidradenitis suppurativa treatment. Br J Dermatol. 2014;171:1434–42.
29. Chiricozzi A, Faleri S, Franceschini C, et al. AISI: a new disease severity assessment tool for hidradenitis suppurativa. Wounds. 2010;27:258–64.
30. Smith HS, Chao JD, Teitelbaum J. Painful hidradenitis suppurativa. Clin J Pain. 2010;26:435–44.
31. Matusiak L, Bieniek A, Szepietowski JC. Hidradenitis suppurativa markedly decreases quality of life and professional activity. J Am Acad Dermatol. 2010;62:706–8.
32. Wolkenstein P, Loundou A, Barrau K, et al. Quality of life impairment in hidradenitis suppurativa: a study of 61 cases. J Am Acad Dermatol. 2007;56:621–3.
33. Kurek A, Peters EM, Chanwangpong A, et al. Profound disturbances of sexual health in patients with acne inversa. J Am Acad Dermatol. 2012;67:e1.
34. Gooderham M, Papp K. The psychosocial impact of hidradenitis suppurativa. J Am Acad Dermatol. 2015;73:S19–22.
35. Wortsman X, Moreno C, Soto R, et al. Ultrasound in-depth characterization and staging of hidradenitis suppurativa. Dermatol Surg. 2013;39:1835–42.
36. Wortsman X, Castro A, Figueroa A. Color Doppler ultrasound assessment of morphology and types of fistulous tracts in hidradenitis suppurativa (HS). J Am Acad Dermatol. 2016;75:760–7.
37. Zarchi K, Yazdanyar N, Yazdanyar S, et al. Pain and inflammation in hidradenitis suppurativa correspond to morphological changes identified by high-frequency ultrasound. J Eur Acad Dermatol Venereol. 2015;29:527–32.
38. Damiani G, Della Valle V, Iannone M, et al. Autoinflammatory Disease Damage Index (ADDI): a possible newborn also in hidradenitis suppurativa daily practice. Ann Rheum Dis. 2017;76(8):e25. pii: annrheumdis-2016-210901.

39. Kohorst JJ, Kimball AB, Davis MD. Systemic associations of hidradenitis suppurativa. J Am Acad Dermatol. 2015;73:S27–35.
40. Sabat R, Chanwangpong A, Schneider-Burrus S, et al. Increased prevalence of metabolic syndrome in patients with acne inversa. PLoS One. 2012;7:e31810.
41. Shlyankevich J, Chen AJ, Kim GE, Kimball AB. Hidradenitis suppurativa is a systemic disease with substantial comorbidity burden: a chart-verified case-control analysis. J Am Acad Dermatol. 2014;71:1144–50.
42. Kromann CB, Deckers IE, Esmann S, et al. Risk factors, clinical course and long-term prognosis in hidradenitis suppurativa: a cross-sectional study. Br J Dermatol. 2014;171:819–24.
43. Fimmel S, Zouboulis CC. Comorbidities of hidradenitis suppurativa (acne inversa). Dermatoendocrinology. 2010;2:9–16.
44. Egeberg A, Jemec GB, Kimball AB, et al. Prevalence and risk of inflammatory bowel disease in patients with hidradenitis suppurativa. J Invest Dermatol. 2017;137(5):1060–4. pii: S0022-202X(17)30011-3018.
45. Richette P, Molto A, Viguier M, et al. Hidradenitis suppurativa associated with spondyloarthritis—results from a multicenter national prospective study. J Rheumatol. 2014;41:490–4.
46. Marzano AV, Ishak RS, Colombo A, et al. Pyoderma gangrenosum, acne and suppurative hidradenitis syndrome following bowel bypass surgery. Dermatology. 2012;225:215–9.
47. Lapins J, Ye W, Nyrén O, Emtestam L. Incidence of cancer among patients with hidradenitis suppurativa. Arch Dermatol. 2001;137:730–4.
48. Meixner D, Schneider S, Krause M, et al. Acne inversa. J Dtsch Dermatol Ges. 2008;6:189–96.
49. Verneuil A. Études sur les tumeurs de la peau; des quelques maladies des glandes sudoripares. Arch Gen Med. 1854;IV:447–68.
50. Verneuil A. De l'hidrosadénite phlegmoneuse et des abcés sudoripares. Arch Gén Méd. 1864;2:537–57.
51. Shelley WB, Cahn MM. The pathogenesis of hidradenitis suppurativa in man. Arch Dermatol. 1955;72:562.
52. Brunsting HA. Hidradenitis suppurativa; abscess of the apocrine sweat glands. Arch Derm Syphilol. 1939;39:108–20.
53. Brunsting HA. Hidradenitis and other variants of acne. Arch Derm Syphilol. 1952;65:303–15.
54. Pillsbury DM, Shelley WB, Kligman AM. Bacterial infections of the skin. In: Pillsbury DM, Shelley WB, Kligman AM, editors. Dermatology. 1st ed. Philadelphia: Saunders; 1956. p. 459–98.
55. Plewig G, Kligman AM. Acne morphogenesis and treatment. Berlin: Springer; 1975. p. 192.
56. Yu CC-W, Cook MG. Hidradenitis suppurativa: a disease of follicular epithelium, rather than apocrine glands. Br J Dermatol. 1990;122:763–9.
57. Plewig G, Steger M. Acne inversa (alias acne triad, acne tetrad or hidradenitis suppurativa). In: Marks R, Plewig G, editors. Acne and related disorders. London: Martin Dunitz; 1989. p. 345–57.
58. Jemec GB, Hansen U. Histology of hidradenitis suppurativa. J Am Acad Dermatol. 1996;34:994–9.
59. Prens E, Deckers I. Pathophysiology of hidradenitis suppurativa: an update. J Am Acad Dermatol. 2015;73:S8–S11.
60. Wang B, Yang W, Wen W, et al. Gamma-secretase gene mutations in familial acne inversa. Science. 2010;330:1065.
61. Pink AE, Simpson MA, Desai N, et al. Mutations in the gamma-secretase genes NCSTN, PSENEN, and PSEN1 underlie rare forms of hidradenitis suppurativa (acne inversa). J Invest Dermatol. 2012;132:2459–61.
62. Pink AE, Simpson MA, Brice GW, et al. PSENEN and NCSTN mutations in familial hidradenitis suppurativa (Acne Inversa). J Invest Dermatol. 2011;131:1568–70.
63. Radtke F, Fasnacht N, Macdonald HR. Notch signaling in the immune system. Immunity. 2010;32:14–27.
64. Melnik BC, Plewig G. Impaired Notch-MKP-1 signalling in hidradenitis suppurativa: an approach to pathogenesis by evidence from translational biology. Exp Dermatol. 2013;22:172–7.

65. Gentle ME, Rose A, Bugeon L, et al. Noncanonical notch signaling modulates cytokine responses of dendritic cells to inflammatory stimuli. J Immunol. 2012;189:1274–84.
66. Miller I, Lynggaard CD, Lophaven S, et al. A double-blind placebo-controlled randomized trial of adalimumab in the treatment of hidradenitis suppurativa. Br J Dermatol. 2011;165:391–8.
67. Lima AL, Karl I, Giner T, et al. Keratinocytes and neutrophils are important sources of proinflammatory molecules in hidradenitis suppurativa. Br J Dermatol. 2016;174:514–21.
68. Cho KA, Suh JW, Lee KH, et al. IL-17 and IL-22 enhance skin inflammation by stimulating the secretion of IL-1b by keratinocytes via the ROS-NLRP3-caspase-1 pathway. Int Immunol. 2012;24:147–58.
69. Dréno B, Khammari A, Brocard A, et al. Hidradenitis suppurativa: the role of deficient cutaneous innate immunity. Arch Dermatol. 2012;148:182–6.
70. Hofmann SC, Saborowski V, Lange S, et al. Expression of innate defense antimicrobial peptides in hidradenitis suppurativa. J Am Acad Dermatol. 2012;66:966–74.
71. Hunger RE, Surovy AM, Hassan AS, et al. Toll-like receptor 2 is highly expressed in lesions of acne inversa and colocalizes with C-type lectin receptor. Br J Dermatol. 2008;158:691–7.
72. Schlapbach C, Yawalkar N, Hunger RE. Human beta-defensin-2 and psoriasin are overexpressed in lesions of acne inversa. J Am Acad Dermatol. 2009;61:58–65.
73. van der Zee HH, de Ruiter L, van den Broecke DG, et al. Elevated levels of tumour necrosis factor (TNF)-α, interleukin (IL)-1β and IL-10 in hidradenitis suppurativa skin: a rationale for targeting TNF-α and IL-1β. Br J Dermatol. 2011;164:1292–8.
74. Kurayev A, Ashkar H, Saraiya A, Gottlieb AB. Hidradenitis suppurativa: review of the pathogenesis and treatment. J Drugs Dermatol. 2016;15:1017–22.
75. van der Zee HH, Laman JD, de Ruiter L, et al. Adalimumab (antitumour necrosis factor-α) treatment of hidradenitis suppurativa ameliorates skin inflammation: an in situ and ex vivo study. Br J Dermatol. 2012;166:298–305.
76. Alikhan A, Lynch PJ, Eisen DB. Hidradenitis suppurativa: a comprehensive review. J Am Acad Dermatol. 2009;60:539–61.
77. Marzano AV, Borghi A, Meroni PL, Cugno M. Pyoderma gangrenosum and its syndromic forms: evidence for a link with autoinflammation. Br J Dermatol. 2016;175:882–91.
78. Marzano AV, Menicanti C, Crosti C, Trevisan V. Neutrophilic dermatoses and inflammatory bowel diseases. G Ital Dermatol Venereol. 2013;148:185–96.
79. Marzano A, Damiani G, Ceccherini I, et al. Autoinflammation in pyoderma gangrenosum and its syndromic form PASH. Br J Dermatol. 2016;176(6):1588–98. https://doi.org/10.1111/bjd.15226.
80. Matusiak L, Bieniek A, Szepietowski JC. Increased serum tumour necrosis factor-alpha in hidradenitis suppurativa patients: is there a basis for treatment with anti-tumour necrosis factor-alpha agents? Acta Derm Venereol. 2009;89:601–3.
81. Satoh TK, Mellett M, Contassot E, French LE. Are neutrophilic dermatoses autoinflammatory disorders? Br J Dermatol. 2016. https://doi.org/10.1111/bjd.15105. [Epub ahead of print].
82. Nikolakis G, Join-Lambert O, Karagiannidis I, et al. Bacteriology of hidradenitis suppurativa/acne inversa: a review. J Am Acad Dermatol. 2015;73(5 Suppl 1):S12–8.
83. Ingram JR, Woo PN, Chua SL, et al. Interventions for hidradenitis suppurativa: a Cochrane systematic review incorporating GRADE assessment of evidence quality. Br J Dermatol. 2016;174:970–8.
84. Saunte DM, Boer J, Stratigos A, et al. Diagnostic delay in hidradenitis suppurativa is a global problem. Br J Dermatol. 2015;173:1546–9.
85. Alavi A, Kirsner RS. Local wound care and topical management of hidradenitis suppurativa. J Am Acad Dermatol. 2015;73:S55–61.
86. Clemmensen OJ. Topical treatment of hidradenitis suppurativa with clindamycin. Int J Dermatol. 1983;22:325–8.
87. Alhusayen R, Shear NH. Scientific evidence for the use of current traditional systemic therapies in patients with hidradenitis suppurativa. J Am Acad Dermatol. 2015;73:S42–6.
88. Sapadin AN, Fleischmajer R. Tetracyclines: nonantibiotic properties and their clinical implications. J Am Acad Dermatol. 2006;54:258–65.

89. Mendonça CO, Griffiths CE. Clindamycin and rifampicin combination therapy for hidradenitis suppurativa. Br J Dermatol. 2006;154:977–8.
90. Gener G, Canoui-Poitrine F, Revuz JE, et al. Combination therapy with clindamycin and rifampicin for hidradenitis suppurativa: a series of 116 consecutive patients. Dermatology. 2009;219:148–54.
91. van der Zee HH, Boer J, Prens EP, Jemec GB. The effect of combined treatment with oral clindamycin and oral rifampicin in patients with hidradenitis suppurativa. Dermatology. 2009;219:143–7.
92. Bettoli V, Zauli S, Borghi A, et al. Oral clindamycin and rifampicin in the treatment of hidradenitis suppurativa-acne inversa: a prospective study on 23 patients. J Eur Acad Dermatol Venereol. 2014;28:125–6.
93. Jemec GB, Wendelboe P. Topical clindamycin versus systemic tetracycline in the treatment of hidradenitis suppurativa. J Am Acad Dermatol. 1998;39:971–4.
94. Kaur MR, Lewis HM. Hidradenitis suppurativa treated with dapsone: a case series of five patients. J Dermatolog Treat. 2006;17:211–3.
95. Yazdanyar S, Boer J, Ingvarsson G, et al. Dapsone therapy for hidradenitis suppurativa: a series of 24 patients. Dermatology. 2011;222:342–6.
96. Hogan DJ, Light MJ. Successful treatment of hidradenitis suppurativa with acitretin. J Am Acad Dermatol. 1988;19:355–6.
97. Boer J, Nazary M. Long-term results of acitretin therapy for hidradenitis suppurativa. Is acne inversa also a misnomer? Br J Dermatol. 2011;164:170–5.
98. Matusiak L, Bieniek A, Szepietowski JC. Acitretin treatment for hidradenitis suppurativa: a prospective series of 17 patients. Br J Dermatol. 2014;171:170–4.
99. Verdolini R, Simonacci F, Menon S, Pavlou P, Mannello B. Alitretinoin: a useful agent in the treatment of hidradenitis suppurativa, especially in women of child-bearing age. G Ital Dermatol Venereol. 2015;150:155–62.
100. Brocard A, Dreno B. Innate immunity: a crucial target for zinc in the treatment of inflammatory dermatosis. J Eur Acad Dermatol Venereol. 2011;25:1146–52.
101. Sawers RS, Randall VA, Ebling FJ. Control of hidradenitis suppurativa in women using combined antiandrogen (cyproterone acetate) and oestrogen therapy. Br J Dermatol. 1986;115:269–74.
102. Stellon AJ, Wakeling M. Hidradenitis suppurativa associated with use of oral contraceptives. BMJ. 1989;298:28–9.
103. Mortimer PS, Dawber RP, Gales MA, et al. A double-blind controlled cross-over trial of cyproterone acetate in females with hidradenitis suppurativa. Br J Dermatol. 1986;115:263–8.
104. Blok JL, van Hattem S, Jonkman MF, Horváth B. Systemic therapy with immunosuppressive agents and retinoids in hidradenitis suppurativa: a systematic review. Br J Dermatol. 2013;168:243–52.
105. Lee RA, Eisen DB. Treatment of hidradenitis suppurativa with biologic medications. J Am Acad Dermatol. 2015;73:S82–8.
106. Basra MK, Salek MS, Camilleri L, et al. Determining the minimal clinically important difference and responsiveness of the Dermatology Life Quality Index (DLQI): further data. Dermatology. 2015;230:27–33.
107. Gisondi P, Girolomoni G. Impact of TNF-α antagonists on the quality of life in selected skin diseases. G Ital Dermatol Venereol. 2013;148:243–8.
108. Adams DR, Yankura JA, Fogelberg AC, Anderson BE. Treatment of hidradenitis suppurativa with etanercept injection. Arch Dermatol. 2010;146:501–4.
109. Gulliver WP, Jemec GB, Baker KA. Experience with ustekinumab for the treatment of moderate to severe hidradenitis suppurativa. J Eur Acad Dermatol Venereol. 2012;26:911–4.
110. Sharon VR, Garcia MS, Bagheri S, et al. Management of recalcitrant hidradenitis suppurativa with ustekinumab. Acta Derm Venereol. 2012;92:320–1.
111. Zarchi K, Dufour DN, Jemec GB. Successful treatment of severe hidradenitis suppurativa with anakinra. JAMA Dermatol. 2013;149:1192–4.
112. Deckers IE, van der Zee HH, Balak DM, Prens EP. Fumarates, a new treatment option for therapy-resistant hidradenitis suppurativa: a prospective open-label pilot study. Br J Dermatol. 2015;172:828–9.

113. Danby FW, Hazen PG, Boer J. New and traditional surgical approaches to hidradenitis suppurativa. J Am Acad Dermatol. 2015;73:S62–5.
114. van Hattem S, Spoo JR, Horváth B, et al. Surgical treatment of sinuses by deroofing in hidradenitis suppurativa. Dermatol Surg. 2012;38:494–7.
115. Kohorst JJ, Baum CL, Otley CC, et al. Surgical management of hidradenitis suppurativa: outcomes of 590 consecutive patients. Dermatol Surg. 2016;42:1030–40.
116. Gulliver W, Zoubolis CC, Prens E, et al. Evidence-based approach to the treatment of hidradentis suppurativa/acne inversa, based on the European guidelines for hidradenitis suppurativa. Rev Endocr Metab Disord. 2016;17:343–51.

PAPA and Related Syndromes

14

Angelo Valerio Marzano, Alessandro Borghi,
and Massimo Cugno

Introduction

Pyoderma gangrenosum (PG) is a prototypical neutrophilic dermatosis that usually manifests itself in the form of cutaneous ulcers with undermined erythematous-violaceous borders. It may be isolated or associated with systemic conditions (i.e. inflammatory bowel diseases, rheumatological disorders and lymphoproliferation), or occur in the context of autoinflammatory syndromes such as PAPA (pyogenic arthritis, PG and acne) [1], PASH (PG, acne and suppurative hidradenitis) [2–4] or other more recently described syndromes such as PAPASH (pyogenic arthritis, acne, PG and suppurative hidradenitis) [5]. Autoinflammatory diseases (AIDs) are characterised by apparently unprovoked episodes of systemic inflammation in the absence of the typical features of autoimmunity, such as autoantibodies or antigen-specific T lymphocytes [6]. All of the autoinflammatory syndromes described here have the shared characteristic of skin involvement, hallmarked by an accumulation of neutrophils. Inflammatory conditions characterised by infiltrates mainly

A. V. Marzano (✉)
Dipartimento di Fisiopatologia Medico-Chirurgica e dei Trapianti, Università degli Studi di Milano, Unità Operativa di Dermatologia, IRCCS Fondazione Ca' Granda, Ospedale Maggiore Policlinico, Milan, Italy
e-mail: angelo.marzano@unimi.it

A. Borghi
Dipartimento di Scienze Mediche, Sezione di Dermatologia e Malattie Infettive, Università degli Studi di Ferrara, Ferrara, Italy
e-mail: alessandro.borghi@unife.it

M. Cugno
Medicina Interna, Dipartimento di Fisiopatologia Medico-Chirurgica e dei Trapianti, Università degli Studi di Milano, IRCCS Fondazione Ca' Granda, Ospedale Maggiore Policlinico, Milan, Italy
e-mail: massimo.cugno@unimi.it

D. Wallach et al. (eds.), *Neutrophilic Dermatoses*,
https://doi.org/10.1007/978-3-319-72649-6_14

consisting of mature neutrophils without infection are defined as neutrophilic dermatoses. Originally, the main forms of neutrophilic dermatoses included prototypical conditions such as PG, Sweet's syndrome, subcorneal pustular dermatosis, and erythema elevatum diutinum [7], but this list was subsequently extended to other diseases, including syndromic entities. From a pathophysiological point of view, these neutrophilic dermatoses present high levels of the same pro-inflammatory cytokines, chemokines and tissue damage effector molecules as those found in AIDs [8, 9]. Taken together, these aspects suggest that autoinflammatory syndromes and neutrophilic dermatoses have the common pathological mechanisms of an over-activated innate immune system leading to the increased production of the IL-1 family and "sterile" neutrophil-rich cutaneous inflammation. The autoinflammatory syndromes characterised by neutrophilic dermatoses therefore represent a model of integration between two conditions that can probably be considered "innate immune disorders" [6, 9].

Pathophysiology

Autoinflammatory syndromes are pathophysiologically characterised by a dysregulated innate immune response. A number of the mutations associated with autoinflammatory disorders occur in the IL-1β pathway [10]. IL-1β is mainly produced by macrophages, T lymphocytes, endothelial cells, fibroblasts, and activated keratinocytes, and can induce tissue damage when its levels reach a critical threshold [11]. Its over-expression is usually related to the dysregulation of inflammasome function. Inflammasome activation begins with the presence of the molecules associated with cell damage (damage associated molecular patterns, DAMPs) or pathogen infections (pathogen associated molecular patterns, PAMPs) in the extracellular environment that are recognised by specific receptors [12]. Mutations affecting the proteins of the inflammasome complex or the proteins that regulate inflammasome function are associated with autoinflammatory disorders [13]. The overproduction of IL-1β triggers the release of proinflammatory cytokines, such as TNF-α and IFN-γ, and chemokines, notably IL-8 and RANTES, which are responsible for the recruitment and activation of neutrophils that lead to neutrophil-mediated inflammation [14–16]. Furthermore, neutrophils are themselves an important source of IL-1β, which suggests they play a role in amplifying and maintaining inflammation [17–19]. It has also been shown that IL-1β directly induces anti-apoptotic effects in neutrophils, and so it may amplify neutrophil-mediated inflammation by prolonging the lifespan of neutrophils [20]. An important contributory role in autoinflammation is played by IL-17 which is also a leading actor in neutrophil recruitment and activation [21]. IL-17 amplifies the recruitment of neutrophils and monocytes by increasing the local production of chemokines [22], and acting in synergy with various other cytokines, particularly TNF-α [23]. It has recently been demonstrated that the ratio between T regulatory cells and T helper-17 cells is decreased in the peripheral blood and lesioned skin of patients with isolated PG, which also contributes to the autoinflammatory process [24]. Neutrophil-derived proteases such as cathepsin G, elastase and proteinase-3, activate IL-36, a cytokine belonging to the IL-1 family that recruits neutrophils to the skin [25]. This suggests that neutrophils are key players in amplifying IL-36-mediated inflammation. Pro-inflammatory cytokines (mainly IL-17, but also IL-1 and TNF-α) also induce the production of metalloproteinases (MMPs) [26], a family of endopeptidases that includes the so-called gelatinases MMP-2 and MMP-9. It is known that the inappropriate activity of the MMPs synthesised by inflammatory cells, particularly neutrophils, cause tissue destruction by degrading the components of the extracellular matrix and influence the production of chemokines by promoting transendothelial neutrophil migration [16].

Pyogenic Arthritis, Pyoderma Gangrenosum and Acne (PAPA) Syndrome

First reported in 1997 [27], PAPA syndrome is a rare autosomal dominant disease that is characterised by aseptic inflammation of the skin and joints, particularly the elbows, knees and ankles [28]. Painful, recurrent, sterile monoarticular arthritis with a prominent neutrophilic infiltrate usually occurs in childhood, and may be the presenting sign of this disease [29]. The episodes of arthritis may be precipitated by traumatic events, but recurrences can also occur spontaneously. Persistent disease can cause joint erosions and destruction, although joint symptoms tend to decrease and skin symptoms become more prominent in young adults. Cutaneous involvement varies. Pathergy is frequent, and pustule formation followed by ulceration may be induced early in life upon minimal trauma. Severe nodulocystic acne and PG tend to develop around puberty, and may persist into adulthood [30]. In the context of PAPA syndrome, PG has a clinicopathological aspect that is closely similar to that of the classical presentation of its isolated form [31]. Acne is a clinically polymorphic inflammatory disease affecting the pilosebaceous units, and consists of open comedones (blackheads), closed comedones (whiteheads) and inflammatory lesions such as papules, pustules and nodules. Its complex pathophysiology includes disordered keratinisation with abnormal sebaceous stem cell differentiation. It has recently been demonstrated that an autoinflammatory component induced by *Propionibacterium acnes* via inflammasome activation is also involved [32–34], thus linking acne to classic AIDs. In PAPA syndrome, the inflammatory aspects of acne tend to predominate, but retentional elements are also present. Other dermatological manifestations described in the setting of PAPA include psoriasis and rosacea. Standard laboratory findings reflect systemic inflammation with leukocytosis and high levels of acute phase reactants, but are otherwise non-diagnostic. The high production of IL-1β and TNF-α in peripheral blood leukocytes has been reported [35, 36]. PAPA syndrome is a result of various mutations on chromosome 15q that affect the PSTPIP1 gene, which encodes proline–serine–threonine phosphatase interacting protein 1 [36, 37], and has an extended Fes-CIP4 homology domain, also known as F-BAR (F refers to the Fer-CIP4 homology domain) at the N-terminal end [38, 39], and a SH3 domain at the C-terminal end [40]. Both domains have the ability to interact with poly-Pro motifs. The F-BAR domain binds to the C-terminal homology domain (CTH) poly-Pro motif of rich in proline (P), glutamic acid (E), serine (S), and threonine (T) residue-type (PEST) phosphatases, such as protein-tyrosine phosphatase (PTP)-PEST (PTP-PEST) [41], and to CD2 [42]; the SH3 domain binds the Wiskott-Aldrich syndrome protein (WASP) [43], tyrosine kinase c-Abl (ABL) [44] and CD2 [45] poly-Pro motifs. Mutations in PSTPIP1 may interfere with its ability to phosphorylate targets including pro-inflammation pyrin domains [30, 46]. The PAPA mutations originally identified in PSTPIP1, A230T and E250Q, are located in the F-BAR domain [1, 47] and abolish the interaction of PSTPIP1 with PTP-PEST, thus leading to the hyperphosphorylation of PSTPIP1 that has been suggested to cause the assembly and activation of the inflammasome and consequent IL-1β release [30]. Pyrin loses its inhibitory effect on the NALP3 inflammasome-driven and caspase 1-mediated pro-inflammatory signalling pathway that cleaves pro-IL-1β into active IL-1β. The consequent overproduction of IL-1β triggers neutrophil-mediated inflammation. Other PSTPIP1 adaptor functions may also play a role in the pathogenesis of PAPA syndrome, including WASP (Wiskott–Aldrich syndrome protein) and PTP-PEST (protein tyrosine phosphatase – proline, glutamic acid, serine and threonine sequence), which regulate the cytoskeleton, podosome formation and cell migration [48–50]. As podosomes also have extracellular matrix-degrading capabilities due to the activity of MMPs [51], a PSTPIP1 R405C mutation that has been recently identified in a patient with aggressive PG regulates a transition from podosome to filopodia formation in macrophages that, in its turn, regulates invasive macrophage migration and increased matrix degradation [52]. Interestingly, two recently reported cases of PAPA syndrome with a E250K mutation in PSTPIP1 had a number of similarities, such as bleeding diathesis with epistaxis during childhood, splenomegaly, and recurrent serious skin and lung infections that persisted into adulthood [46]. Although it is not clear whether the E250K mutation can account for the additional features seen in these two cases, it is possible that the clinical spectrum of PAPA syndrome is wider than currently thought and is at least partially conditioned by different gene mutations.

Pyoderma Gangrenosum, Acne and Suppurative Hidradenitis (PASH)

It has recently been suggested that the clinical triad of PASH (PG, acne and suppurative hidradenitis) is an autoinflammatory syndrome [2, 4] that can be distinguished from PAPA by the absence of pyogenic sterile arthritis. Both PG and hidradenitis suppurativa (HS), also known as suppurative hidradenitis, are prototypical neutrophilic dermatoses that are themselves currently considered to be autoinflammatory in origin [53–55]. HS is a chronic-relapsing, debilitating inflammatory disease of the hair follicles that usually presents after puberty and affects apocrine gland-bearing skin, most frequently the axillae, inguinal and anogenital regions. It is clinically characterised by recurrent, painful, deep-seated nodules that usually end in abscesses and sinus tracts with suppuration and hypertrophic scarring [56, 57]. The subjects affected by PASH so far described in the literature are young adults with a very early onset of the syndrome's clinical features, especially acne [2–4, 58, 59]. Three patterns of skin lesions have been described: ulcers and ulcerated nodules, sometimes with the vegetating aspects typical of PG (Fig. 14.1a, b); papulopustular lesions, abscesses, and fistulae evolving into draining sinuses and scars that are consistent with HS (Fig. 14.1c); and mild to severe facial acne (Fig. 14.1d), including acne fulminans. Concurrent rheumatological symptoms and inflammatory bowel diseases have also been reported [4]. Patients with PASH syndrome have a significantly impaired quality of life due to the extensive cutaneous involvement, the chronicity of the skin manifestations, their disfiguring sequelae, and the limited available treatment options. For the first two reported PASH cases, it was suggested that the presence of alleles

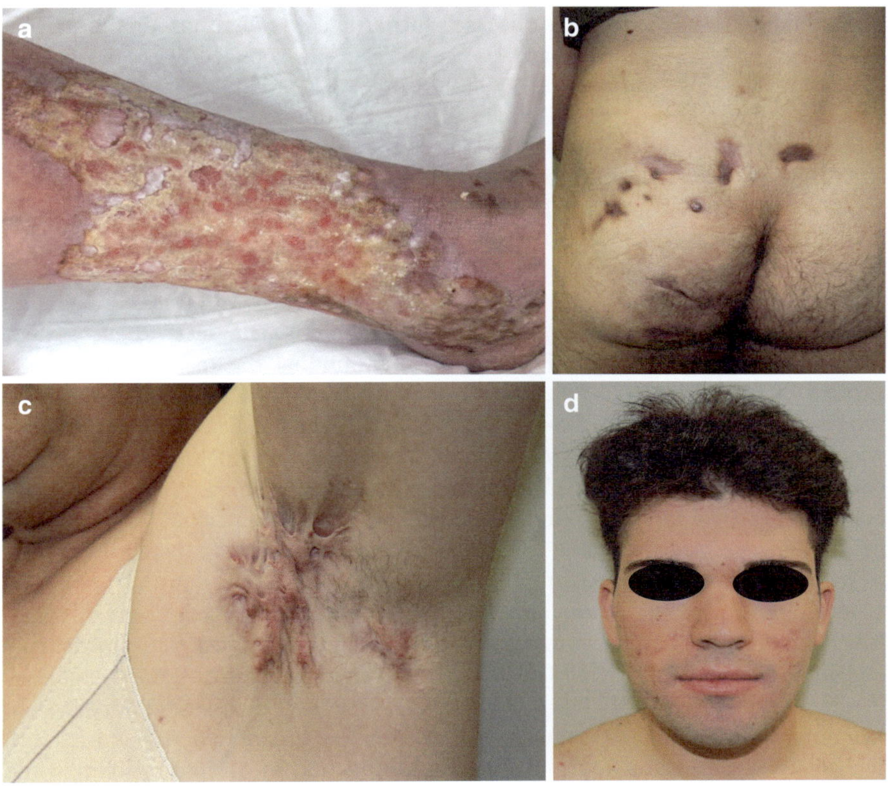

Fig. 14.1 Clinical features of pyoderma gangrenosum, acne and suppurative hidradenitis (PASH): (**a**) ulcerative pyoderma gangrenosum on the leg; (**b**) ulcerated plaques with vegetating aspect, which were histologically diagnosed as pyoderma gangrenosum; (**c**) hypertrophic scars and multiple interconnected tracts of hidradenitis suppurativa involving the axillary fold; (**d**) polymorphic acne of the face

carrying a higher number of CCTG motif repeats close to the PSTPIP1 promoter deregulated PSTPIP1 expression and predisposed the patients to forms of neutrophilic inflammation such as aseptic abscesses with/without Crohn's disease [2]. This microsatellite may therefore be involved as a modifier gene, although it is probably not causal [60]. It was initially hypothesised that, like PAPA syndrome, PASH was a monogenic disorder involving pleiotropic mutations in a single gene that led to the clinical manifestations, but there is now evidence of its polygenic autoinflammatory nature [4, 9]. A recent observational study of five patients with PASH syndrome [4] found that their nine gene mutations had already been entered in the single-nucleotide polymorphism (dbSNP) database (http://www.ncbi.nlm.nih.gov/snp/), and that seven were in the registry of hereditary autoinflammatory disorder mutations (INFEVERS; http://fmf.igh.cnrs.fr/ISSAID/infevers/). Four of these five patients had genetic alterations typical of well known AIDs, including inflammatory bowel diseases, and the only patient without any genetic changes had clinically evident Crohn's disease. In particular, mutations of the MEFV (Mediterranean fever) gene have previously been associated with the typical symptoms of recessive familial Mediterranean fever (FMF) and mutations of the NOD2 (nucleotide-binding oligomerisation domain-containing protein 2) gene are intermittently associated with susceptibility to Crohn's disease [26, 61]. A loss-of-function mutation in the γ-secretase gene, nicastrin (NCSTN), has been found in one PASH patient [59]. The nature and location of this mutation does not distinguish it from the reported HS mutations [62], thus supporting a close relationships between isolated HS and PASH. A recent study has analysed the expression of cytokines, chemokines and other effector molecules in the lesional skin and peripheral blood of PASH patients using a protein array method and ELISA [4]. As in the case of isolated PG [16], the main finding was the cutaneous over-expression of IL-1β and its receptors. In line with its pivotal role in promoting the production and release of pro-inflammatory cytokines and chemokines, TNF-α was also found to be over-expressed in the PG lesions, together with a number of chemokines such as IL-8, CXCL 1/2/3, CXCL16, and RANTES [4]. The cutaneous over-expression of IL-17 and its receptor was also documented, thus confirming the hypothesised role of this T-helper 17-related cytokine in the pathophysiology of the whole spectrum of neutrophilic dermatoses [4, 16]. Two further important systems, the Fas/Fas L system and the CD40/CD40 ligand system, both of which belong to the TNF/TNF receptor superfamily, seem to contribute to tissue damage and inflammation in PASH. The Fas/FasL system is the best-known pathway mediating apoptosis [63]. The CD40/CD40L system is a co-stimulatory system that amplifies the immune response and can promote inflammation by up-regulating adhesion molecules and inducing the production of various cytokines and chemokines [64]. Taken together, these findings show that PASH has the same profile of cytokines and other effector molecules as those previously found in non-syndromic PG and other AIDs [15, 16]. In peripheral blood, the serum levels of the main proinflammatory cytokines (such as IL-1β, TNF-α, and IL-17) are within the normal range, suggesting that the inflammatory process is mainly localised to the skin in patients with PASH syndrome [4].

Synovitis, Acne, Pustulosis, Hyperostosis and Osteitis (SAPHO)

SAPHO is an acronym for synovitis, acne, pustulosis, hyperostosis and osteitis. The most frequently mentioned diagnostic criteria for this entity are those proposed by Kahn and Khan, as (1) multifocal osteitis with or without skin symptoms; (2) sterile acute/chronic joint inflammation with either pustules or psoriasis of the palms/soles, or acne or HS; and (3) sterile osteitis and any one of the above skin manifestations, with any one of the criteria being sufficient for the diagnosis [65]. SAPHO syndrome is generally considered to be a rare condition, possibly due to being underdiagnosed. Clinical features occur mostly in young and middle-aged persons, and a slight female predominance has been noted in some series [66, 67]. The disease is mostly self-limiting, lasting about 4–5 years on average. Female sex, elevated erythrocyte sedimentation rate and C-reactive protein values, anterior chest wall involvement, peripheral synovitis and skin involvement at the onset are associated with a chronic course [68]. The clinical features are heterogeneous and overlap with other disease entities. In general, the association of noninfectious, inflammatory osteitis with palmoplantar pustulosis (PPP) is a finding of key importance for diagnosis. Skin and bone lesions may present at different times. The most common cutaneous manifestation is PPP, including pustular psoriasis, representing 50–75% of all dermatological manifestations and affecting close to 60% of patients [69]. Psoriasis vulgaris may also be included among the dermatological manifestations of SAPHO. Severe acne, namely acne conglobate and fulminans, affects approximately one-quarter of patients with SAPHO syndrome, with men clearly predominating [66, 67]. Men also predominate among the cases of SAPHO syndrome that have been reported in association with HS. African Americans appear to be particularly susceptible [66, 67, 70]. Other rare cutaneous manifestations of SAPHO syndrome include PG, Sweet syndrome and Sneddon–Wilkinson disease [66–71]. Associations of SAPHO syndrome and IBD seem not to be rare, especially in Crohn disease [72]. There are no laboratory tests that are diagnostic of SAPHO. They can be normal or may show elevated inflammatory markers and elevated levels of components of complements C3 and C4. Mild leukocytosis and mild anaemia have also been reported. Compared with healthy controls, patients can have elevated levels of IgA [73]. Concerning its pathogenesis, there is increasing understanding that SAPHO shares similarities with other AIDs. Indeed, proinflammatory cytokines, such as IL-1β and TNF-α, as well as the chemokine IL-8, are regarded as relevant in the pathogenesis of SAPHO [73–75]. Impaired gene expression of IL-10, with consequent disruption of both the pro- and anti-inflammatory cytokine balance and immunologic homeostasis which result in enhanced proinflammatory responses, has also been reported [76]. The dysregulation of the P2X7–IL-1β axis is hypothesized to lead to an increased release of IL-1β, as found in other AIDs [77]. Increasing evidence points to P2X7R as a main player in Th17 differentiation and IL-17 secretion [78]. In line with these findings, Th17 cells were recently found to be increased in the peripheral blood of patients with SAPHO [79]. The hereditary basis of SAPHO has been supported by the finding of familial clustering cases [80], but no specific mutations have been found. PSTPIP2, which is involved in macrophage activation, neutrophil motility and osteoclast differentiation, has recently been supposed to play a role in innate immunity and development of autoinflammatory bone disorders, including SAPHO syndrome. Other genes potentially involved in SAPHO syndrome, both located on chromosome 18, are LPIN2 and NOD2 [81]. LPIN2 encodes lipin 2, which is involved in modulating apoptosis of polymorphonuclear cells. Mutations of the NOD2 gene may lead to an abnormal immune response to bacterial peptidoglycans via activation of the proinflammatory transcription factor NF-kB [82]. Furthermore, SAPHO syndrome is supposed to be associated with mutations of IL1RN, causing deficiency of the interleukin-1 receptor antagonist. This defect is responsible for the severe, early-onset autosomal recessive autoinflammatory syndrome DIRA, which clinically manifests as generalized pustular psoriasis associated with osteoarticular and central nervous system involvements [83]. A genetic association reported for the SAPHO syndrome is with the T309G allele and the GG genotype of the Mdm2-gene, a negative regulator of p53 [84]. The tumour suppressor protein p53 regulates the transcription factor NF-kB, which is central for a variety of proinflammatory pathways. Both of the alleles with increased frequencies in patients with SAPHO syndrome have been associated with ineffective p53 responses. Therefore, the lack of inhibitory effects of p53/Mdm2 axis on NF-kB-induced proinflammatory pathways may be particularly relevant. Finally, different types of pathogens have been isolated from different bone sites as well as from pustular lesions in the skin, mostly *P. acnes* [85, 86]. However, in a vast majority of patients, cultures are negative, even when tested with polymerase chain reaction employing universal primers for eubacterial and mycobacterial genes [87, 88], and efficacy of antibiotics is controversial. In the current view, an infectious state which involves *P. acnes* may be an antigenic trigger for proinflammatory/autoinflammatory responses. These induce a sclerotic and hyperostotic reaction as well as neutrophilic skin disorders.

Pyogenic Arthritis, Acne, Pyoderma Gangrenosum and Suppurative Hidradenitis (PAPASH) and Other Syndromic Forms

In 2012, Bruzzese reported the case of a patient with the simultaneous presence of PG, acne conglobata, HS, and axial spondyloarthritis, a condition that differed from PASH (in which arthritis is absent), and PAPA syndrome (in which HS is absent). The author suggested that the simultaneous development of these four pictures may represent a distinct syndrome, which he called PASS syndrome [89]. Two other research teams independently described two new entities among the autoinflammatory syndromes, both of which were christened PAPASH syndrome [5, 90]. Marzano et al. described the case of a 16-year-old female with pyogenic arthritis, PG, acne and HS [5], in whom genetic studies evaluating exons 10 and 11 of the PSTPIP1 gene revealed a previously unreported p.E277D missense mutation. On the other hand, Garzorz et al. proposed using the same acronym PAPASH to define the association of PG, acne, psoriasis, arthritis and HS observed in a 39-year-old woman

[90]. Neutrophil activation by the Th-17/TNF-α axis, which is involved in the pathogenesis of psoriasis, acne, HS, arthritis and PG, was suggested to be the molecular key feature in this patient. Finally, it has been suggested that the concomitant diagnosis of psoriatic arthritis (PsA), PG, acne and HS described in a 50-year-old man represent a new syndrome known as PsAPASH [91].

Management

Given the rarity of these syndromic entities, no randomised, controlled clinical trials have yet investigated the efficacy of individual therapies. Medications targeting IL-1 and TNFα are usually successful in managing the manifestations of PAPA syndrome. The most consistent responses have been observed with the anti-TNFα antagonists etanercept, adalimumab and infliximab [92–94]. The response to the anti-IL-1 agent anakinra varies [95, 96], but it seems to be more effective in managing joint manifestations than cutaneous disease. Joint disease is also responsive to corticosteroids, but they may exacerbate acne. Joint effusions may also be surgically managed by means of drainage and/or intra-articular steroid injections. Topical and systemic retinoids have been shown to be effective in the management of the most severe forms of acne. The treatment of PASH patients can be challenging. Classic immunosuppressive regimens such as systemic glucocorticosteroids and azathioprine, as well as dapsone and isotretinoin, may fail to control the disease satisfactorily [2]. In line with the pathological mechanisms of PASH syndrome, it has been found that TNF-α blockers infliximab and adalimumab remarkably improve the cutaneous picture of PG and acne lesions [2–4, 97, 98], and anakinra (possibly combined with cyclosporin) can also be very beneficial [2, 4, 99]. Antiseptic preparations and topical immunosuppressants, such as tacrolimus ointment, can be used for local treatment. Intra-articular or systemic corticosteroids are effective in the majority of patients affected with SAPHO [100]. Disease-modifying antirheumatic drugs (DMARDs) such as methotrexate, sulfasalazine, ciclosporin and leflunomide have been widely used, giving inconstant results [69, 101]. Considering the hypothesized role of *P. acnes* in the pathogenesis of SAPHO syndrome, antibiotic treatment, in particular with doxycycline, can be another treatment option [66, 67, 69]. Nonetheless, only a part of patients responds, and the effect is often partial and lost after treatment withdrawal. Bisphosphonates, especially pamidronate, which act by inhibiting bone resorption and turnover, and by possible anti-inflammatory activity, have rapid but transient activity of pain relief in some of these patients, and may lead to partial or complete sustained remission over time [102]. However, they have no effect on skin lesions. Various case series and reports stated the use of anti-TNF-α agents as a therapeutic option for SAPHO cases unresponsive or refractory to conventional drugs, demonstrating their efficacy for bone, skin and joints manifestations at standard doses and achieving complete remission in most of cases [82, 103–105]. For patients with disease worsening or unresponsive to anti-TNF-α, anakinra can be considered as an alternative option, as it has been proven effective in a small number of published SAPHO patients [106, 107].

Table 14.1 Genetic and immunologic alterations in pyoderma gangrenosum (PG) and its syndromic forms PAPA (pyogenic arthritis, pyoderma gangrenosum and acne), PASH (pyoderma gangrenosum, acne and suppurative hidradenitis), SAPHO (synovitis, acne, pustulosis, hyperostosis and osteitis), and PAPASH (pyogenic arthritis, pyoderma gangrenosum, acne and suppurative hidradenitis)

	Genetic alterations	Immunologic alterations	Source
PG	R52Q mutation in the PSTPIP1 gene	Not evaluated	Newman et al. [108]
	G258A and R52Q mutations in the PSTPIP1 gene	Not evaluated	Nesterovitch et al. [109]
	Not evaluated	Increased skin IL-23	Guenova et al. [110]
	Not evaluated	Increased skin IL-1-beta, IL-1RI, IL-1RII, TNF-alpha, TNFRI, TNFRII, IL-17, IL-17R, L-selectin, IL-8, CXCL 1/2/3, CXCL 16, RANTES, MMP-2, MMP-9, TIMP-1, TIMP-2, Siglec 5, Siglec 9, Fas, FasL, CD40 and CD40L.	Marzano et al. [16]
PAPA	E250Q and A230T mutations in the PSTPIP1 gene	Not evaluated	Wise et al. [1]
	E250K in the PSTPIP1 gene	Increased serum IL-1 beta	Demidowich et al. [36]
PASH	Increased CCTG microsatellite repeats in the PSTPIP1 gene	Not evaluated	Braun-Falco et al. [2]
	p.I591T, p.M694 V, p.V726A mutations in the MEFV gene; p.R702W and p.G908R in the NOD2 gene; p.Q703K in NLRP3 gene; p.A106T in the IL1RN gene; p.E277D in the PSTPIP1 gene; and p.G8R in the PSMB8 gene	Increased skin IL-1-beta, IL-1RI, IL-1RII, TNF-alpha, TNFRI, TNFRII, IL-17, IL-17R, L-selectin, IL-8, CXCL 1/2/3, CXCL 16, RANTES, MMP-2, MMP-9, TIMP-1, TIMP-2, Siglec 5, Siglec 9, Fas, FasL, CD40 and CD40L.	Marzano et al. [4]
SAPHO	1082G single-nucleotide polymorphism in the IL-10 promoter region	susceptibility to infections and autoimmunity	Hamal et al. [111]
	T309G allele and the GG genotype of the Mdm2-gene	NF-kB-induced proinflammatory pathways	Assmann et al. [84]
	Not evaluated	Increased expression of both the inflammasome constituent ASC and P2X7R	Colina et al. [107]
PAPASH	p.E277D missense mutation in the PSTPIP1 gene	Not evaluated	Marzano et al. [5]

PSTPIP1 proline-serine-threonine phosphatase-interacting protein 1; *MEFV* mediterranean fever; *NOD2* nucleotidebinding oligomerization domain-containing protein 2; *NLRP3* NOD-like receptor family, pyrin domain containing 3; *IL1RN* interleukin 1 receptor antagonist; *PSMB8* proteasome [prosome, macropain] subunit, beta type, 8; *CD40* cluster of differentiation 40; *CD40 L* CD40 ligand, *CXCL* C-X-C motif ligand; *E-selectin* endothelial selectin; *IL* interleukin; *Lselectin* leukocyte selectin; *MMP* matrix metalloproteinase; *RANTES* regulated on activation, normal T cell expressed and secreted; *Siglec* sialic acid-binding immunoglobulin-type lectin; *TIMP* tissue 1 inhibitor of metalloproteinase; *TNF* tumor necrosis factor; *NF-kB* nuclear factor kappa-light-chain-enhancer of activated B cells; *ASC* apoptosis-associated speck-like protein containing a carboxy-terminal CARD; *P2X7R* purinergic receptor P2X7 receptor

Conclusions

PAPA, PASH, SAPHO and the other more recently described autoinflammatory syndromes such as PAPASH can be seen as belonging to a spectrum of polygenic autoinflammatory conditions caused by innate immunity dysfunction. Although they have distinctive features and specific diagnostic criteria, these syndromic conditions also have many overlapping clinical, pathogenetic, histological and genetic aspects. In particular, they are pathogenetically characterised by the over-activation of innate immune signalling pathways. This leads to the dysregulation of neutrophil homeostasis causing excessive skin inflammation, neutrophil granulocyte infiltration, and subsequent tissue damage. The cutaneous manifestations of this process are typically polymorphic and are related to those of neutrophilic dermatoses. As these distressing autoinflammatory entities are all associated with the over-expression of IL-1 and TNF-α, biological agents specifically targeting these cytokines are currently the most effective treatments but, given the emerging pathogenetic role of IL-17, IL-17 antagonists may represent the future management of these syndromes (Table 14.1).

References

1. Wise CA, Gillum JD, Seidman CE, Lindor NM, Veile R, Bashiardes S, Lovett M. Mutations in CD2BP1 disrupt binding to PTP PEST and are responsible for PAPA syndrome, an autoinflammatory disorder. Hum Mol Genet. 2002;11:961–9.
2. Braun-Falco M, Kovnerystyy O, Lohse P, Ruzicka T. Pyoderma gangrenosum, acne, and suppurative hidradenitis (PASH) - a new autoinflammatory syndrome distinct from PAPA syndrome. J Am Acad Dermatol. 2012;66:409–15.
3. Marzano AV, Ishak RS, Colombo A, Caroli F, Crosti C. Pyoderma gangrenosum, acne and suppurative hidradenitis syndrome following bowel bypass surgery. Dermatology. 2012;225:215–9.
4. Marzano AV, Ceccherini I, Gattorno M, Fanoni D, Caroli F, Rusmini M, Grossi A, De Simone C, Borghi OM, Meroni PL, Crosti C, Cugno M. Association of pyoderma gangrenosum, acne, and suppurative hidradenitis (PASH) shares genetic and cytokine profiles with other autoinflammatory diseases. Medicine (Baltimore). 2014;93:e187.
5. Marzano AV, Trevisan V, Gattorno M, Ceccherini I, De Simone C, Crosti C. Pyogenic arthritis, pyoderma gangrenosum, acne, and hidradenitis suppurativa (PAPASH): a new autoinflammatory syndrome associated with a novel mutation of the PSTPIP1 gene. JAMA Dermatol. 2013;149:762–4.
6. Navarini AA, Satoh TK, French LE. Neutrophilic dermatoses and autoinflammatory diseases with skin involvement--innate immune disorders. Semin Immunopathol. 2016;38:45–56.
7. Wallach D. Les dermatoses neutrophiliques. (Editorial). Presse Med. 1991;20:105–7.
8. Prat L, Bouaziz JD, Wallach D, Vignon-Pennamen MD, Bagot M. Neutrophilic dermatoses as systemic diseases. Clin Dermatol. 2014;32:376–88.
9. Marzano AV, Borghi A, Meroni PL, Cugno M. Pyoderma gangrenosum and its syndromic forms: evidence for a link with autoinflammation. Br J Dermatol. 2016;175:882–91.
10. Dinarello CA. Interleukin-1 in the pathogenesis and treatment of inflammatory diseases. Blood. 2011;117:3720–32.
11. Dinarello CA. Immunological and inflammatory functions of the interleukin-1 family. Annu Rev Immunol. 2009;27:519–50.
12. Saïd-Sadier N, Ojcius DM. Alarmins, inflammasomes and immunity. Biomed J. 2012;35:437–49.
13. Strowig T, Henao-Mejia J, Elinav E, Flavell R. Inflammasomes in health and disease. Nature. 2012;481:278–86.

14. Dinarello CA. A clinical perspective of IL-1β as the gatekeeper of inflammation. Eur J Immunol. 2011;41:1203–17.
15. Marzano AV, Cugno M, Trevisan V, Fanoni D, Venegoni L, Berti E, et al. Role of inflammatory cells, cytokines and matrix metalloproteinases in neutrophil-mediated skin diseases. Clin Exp Immunol. 2010;162:100–7.
16. Marzano AV, Fanoni D, Antiga E, Quaglino P, Caproni M, Crosti C, Meroni PL, Cugno M. Expression of cytokines, chemokines and other effector molecules in two prototypic autoinflammatory skin diseases, pyoderma gangrenosum and Sweet's syndrome. Clin Exp Immunol. 2014;178:48–56.
17. Mankan AK, Dau T, Jenne D, et al. The NLRP3/ASC/Caspase-1 axis regulates IL-1beta processing in neutrophils. Eur J Immunol. 2012;42:710–5.
18. Chen KW, Gross CJ, Sotomayor FV, et al. The neutrophil NLRC4 inflammasome selectively promotes IL-1beta maturation without pyroptosis during acute Salmonella challenge. Cell Rep. 2014;8:570–82.
19. Guma M, Ronacher L, Liu-Bryan R, et al. Caspase 1-independent activation of interleukin-1beta in neutrophil-predominant inflammation. Arthritis Rheum. 2009;60:3642–50.
20. Mitroulis I, Kourtzelis I, Kambas K, et al. Regulation of the autophagic machinery in human neutrophils. Eur J Immunol. 2010;40:1461–72.
21. Lima AL, Karl I, Giner T, Poppe H, Schmidt M, Presser D, Goebeler M, Bauer B. Keratinocytes and neutrophils are important sources of proinflammatory molecules in hidradenitis suppurativa. Br J Dermatol. 2016;174:514–21.
22. Isailovic N, Daigo K, Mantovani A, Selmi C. Interleukin-17 and innate immunity in infections and chronic inflammation. J Autoimmun. 2015;60:1–11.
23. Donetti E, Cornaghi L, Gualerzi A, Baruffaldi Preis FW, Prignano F. An innovative three-dimensional model of normal human skin to study the proinflammatory psoriatic effects of tumor necrosis factor-alpha and interleukin-17. Cytokine. 2014;68:1–8.
24. Caproni M, Antiga E, Volpi W, Verdelli A, Venegoni L, Quaglino P, et al. The Treg/Th17 cell ratio is reduced in the skin lesions of patients with pyoderma gangrenosum. Br J Dermatol. 2015;73:275–8.
25. Foster AM, Baliwag J, Chen CS, et al. IL-36 promotes myeloid cell infiltration, activation, and inflammatory activity in skin. J Immunol. 2014;192:6053–61.
26. Agarwal S, Misra R, Aggarwal A. Interleukin 17 levels are increased in juvenile idiopathic arthritis synovial fluid and induce synovial fibroblasts to produce proinflammatory cytokines and matrix metalloproteinases. J Rheumatol. 2008;35:515–9.
27. Lindor NM, Arsenault TM, Solomon H, et al. A new autosomal dominant disorder of pyogenic sterile arthritis, pyoderma gangrenosum and acne: PAPA syndrome. Mayo Clin Proc. 1997;72:611–5.
28. Naik HB, Cowen EW. Autoinflammatory pustular neutrophilic diseases. Dermatol Clin. 2013;31:405–25.
29. Tallon B, Corkill M. Peculiarities of PAPA syndrome. Rheumatology. 2006;45:1140–3.
30. Smith EJ, Allantaz F, Bennett L, et al. Clinical, molecular, and genetic characteristics of PAPA syndrome: a review. Curr Genomics. 2010;11:519–27.
31. Callen JP. Pyoderma gangrenosum. Lancet. 1996;351:581–5.
32. Kistowska M, Gehrke S, Jankovic D, et al. IL-1β drives inflammatory responses to Propionibacterium acnes in vitro and in vivo. J Invest Dermatol. 2014;134:677–85.
33. Qin M, Pirouz A, Kim MH, et al. Propionibacterium acnes induces IL-1β secretion via the NLRP3 inflammasome in human monocytes. J Invest Dermatol. 2014;134:381–8.
34. Li ZJ, Choi DK, Sohn KC, et al. Propionibacterium acnes activates the NLRP3 inflammasome in human sebocytes. J Invest Dermatol. 2014;134:2747–56.
35. Cortis E, De Benedetti F, Insalaco A, et al. Abnormal production of the tumour necrosis factor alpha and clinical efficacy of the TNF inhibitor etanercept in a patient with PAPA syndrome. J Pediatr. 2004;145:851–5.
36. Demidowich AP, Freeman AF, Kuhns DB, et al. Brief report: genotype, phenotype, and clinical course in five patients with PAPA syndrome (pyogenic sterile arthritis, pyoderma gangrenosum, and acne). Arthritis Rheum. 2012;64:2022–7.

37. Shoham NG, Centola M, Mansfield E, et al. Pyrin binds the PSTPIP1/CD2BP1 protein, defining familial Mediterranean fever and PAPA syndrome as disorders in the same pathway. Proc Natl Acad Sci U S A. 2003;100:13501–6.
38. Shimada A, Niwa H, Tsujita K, Suetsugu S, Nitta K, Hanawa-Suetsugu K, Akasaka R, Nishino Y, Toyama M, Chen L, et al. Curved EFC/F-BAR-domain dimers are joined end to end into a filament for membrane invagination in endocytosis. Cell. 2007;129:761–72.
39. Henne WM, Kent HM, Ford MG, Hegde BG, Daumke O, Butler PJ, Mittal R, Langen R, Evans PR, McMahon HT. Structure and analysis of FCHo2 F-BAR domain: a dimerizing and membrane recruitment module that effects membrane curvature. Structure. 2007;15:839–52.
40. Marcos T, Ruiz-Martín V, de la Puerta ML, Trinidad AG, Rodríguez Mdel C, de la Fuente MA, Sánchez Crespo M, Alonso A, Bayón Y. Proline-serine-threonine phosphatase interacting protein 1 inhibition of T-cell receptor signaling depends on its SH3 domain. FEBS J. 2014;281:3844–54.
41. Cote JF, Chung PL, Theberge JF, Halle M, Spencer S, Lasky LA, Tremblay ML. PSTPIP is a substrate of PTP-PEST and serves as a scaffold guiding PTP-PEST toward a specific dephosphorylation of WASP. J Biol Chem. 2002;277:2973–86.
42. Badour K, Zhang J, Shi F, McGavin MK, Rampersad V, Hardy LA, Field D, Siminovitch KA. The Wiskott-Aldrich syndrome protein acts downstream of CD2 and the CD2AP and PSTPIP1 adaptors to promote formation of the immunological synapse. Immunity. 2003;18:141–54.
43. Wu Y, Spencer SD, Lasky LA. Tyrosine phosphorylation regulates the SH3-mediated binding of the Wiskott-Aldrich syndrome protein to PSTPIP, a cytoskeletal-associated protein. J Biol Chem. 1998;273:5765–70.
44. Cong F, Spencer S, Cote JF, Wu Y, Tremblay ML, Lasky LA, Goff SP. Cytoskeletal protein PSTPIP1 directs the PEST-type protein tyrosine phosphatase to the c-Abl kinase to mediate Abl dephosphorylation. Mol Cell. 2000;6:1413–23.
45. Li J, Nishizawa K, An W, Hussey RE, Lialios FE, Salgia R, Sunder-Plassmann R, Reinherz EL. A cdc15-like adaptor protein (CD2BP1) interacts with the CD2 cytoplasmic domain and regulates CD2-triggered adhesion. EMBO J. 1998;17:7320–36.
46. Lindwall E, Singla S, Davis WE, Quinet RJ. Novel PSTPIP1 gene mutation in a patient with pyogenic arthritis, pyoderma gangrenosum and acne (PAPA) syndrome. Semin Arthritis Rheum. 2015;45:91–3.
47. Yeon HB, Lindor HM, Seidman JG, Seidman CE. Pyogenic arthritis, pyoderma gangrenosum, and acne syndrome maps to chromosome 15q. Am J Hum Genet. 2000;66:1443–8.
48. Wang D, Höing S, Patterson HC, et al. Inflammation in mice ectopically expressing human pyogenic arthritis, pyoderma gangrenosum, and acne (PAPA) syndrome-associated PSTPIP1 A230T mutant proteins. J Biol Chem. 2013;288:4594–601.
49. Dovas A, Gevrey J-C, Grossi A, et al. Regulation of podosome dynamics by WASp phosphorylation: implication in matrix degradation and chemotaxis in macrophages. J Cell Sci. 2009;122:3873–82.
50. Monypenny J, Chou H-C, Banon-Rodriguez I, et al. Role of WASP in cell polarity and podosome dynamics of myeloid cells. Eur J Cell Biol. 2011;90:198–204.
51. Gawden-Bone C, Zhou Z, King E, et al. Dendritic cell podosomes are protrusive and invade the extracellular matrix using metalloproteinase MMP-14. J Cell Sci. 2010;123:1427–37.
52. Starnes TW, Bennin DA, Bing X, et al. The F-BAR protein PSTPIP1 controls extracellular matrix degradation and filopodia formation in macrophages. Blood. 2014;123:2703–14.
53. Marzano AV, Ishak RS, Saibeni S, et al. Autoinflammatory skin disorders in inflammatory bowel diseases, pyoderma gangrenosum and Sweet's syndrome: a comprehensive review and disease classification criteria. Clin Rev Allergy Immunol. 2013;45:202–10.
54. Almeida de Jesus A, Goldbach-Mansky R. Monogenic autoinflammatory diseases: concept and clinical manifestations. Clin Immunol. 2013;147:155–74.
55. Wollina U, Haroske G. Pyoderma gangrenosum. Curr Opin Rheumatol. 2011;23:50–6.
56. Dessinioti C, Katsambas A, Antoniou C. Hidradenitis suppurativa (acne inversa) as a systemic disease. Clin Dermatol. 2014;32:397–408.
57. Jemec GB. Clinical practice. Hidradenitis suppurativa. N Engl J Med. 2012;366:158–64.

58. Duchatelet S, Miskinyte S, Join-Lambert O, Ungeheuer MN, Francès C, Nassif A, et al. First nicastrin mutation in PASH (pyoderma gangrenosum, acne and suppurative hidradenitis) syndrome. Br J Dermatol. 2015;173:610–2.
59. Calderón-Castrat X, Bancalari-Diaz D, Román-Curto C, Romo-Melgar A, Amorós-Cerdán D, Alcaraz-Mas L, et al. PSTPIP1 Gene mutation in a pyoderma gangrenosum, acne and suppurative hidradenitis (PASH) syndrome. Br J Dermatol. 2016;175:194–8.
60. André MF, Aumaître O, Grateau G, Chamaillard M, Costedoat-Chalumeau N, Cardoso MC, et al. Longest form of CCTG microsatellite repeat in the promoter of the CD2BP1/PSTPIP1 gene is associated with aseptic abscesses and with Crohn disease in French patients. Dig Dis Sci. 2010;55:1681–8.
61. Hampe J, Grebe J, Nikolaus S, Solberg C, Croucher PJ, Mascheretti S, et al. Association of NOD2 (CARD 15) genotype with clinical course of Crohn's disease: a cohort study. Lancet. 2002;359:1661–5.
62. Pink AE, Simpson MA, Desai N, Trembath RC, Barker JN. γ-Secretase mutations in hidradenitis suppurativa: new insights into disease pathogenesis. J Invest Dermatol. 2012;133:601–7.
63. Wehrli P, Viard L, Bullani R, Tschopp J, French LE. Death receptors in cutaneous biology and disease. J Invest Dermatol. 2000;115:141–8.
64. Danese S, Sans M, Fiocchi C. The CD40/CD40L costimulatory pathway in inflammatory bowel disease. Gut. 2004;53:1035–43.
65. Kahn MF, Khan MA. The SAPHO syndrome. Baillieres Clin Rheumatol. 1994;8:333–62.
66. Nguyen MT, Borchers A, Selmi C, et al. The SAPHO syndrome. Semin Arthritis Rheum. 2012;42:254–65.
67. Carneiro S, Sampaio-Barros PD. SAPHO syndrome. Rheum Dis Clin N Am. 2013;39:401–18.
68. Kundu BK, Naik AK, Bhargava S, Srivastava D. Diagnosing the SAPHO syndrome: a report of three cases and review of literature. Clin Rheumatol. 2013;32:1237–43.
69. Colina M, Govoni M, Orzincolo C, Trotta F. Clinical and radiologic evolution of synovitis, acne, pustulosis, hyperostosis, and osteitis syndrome: a single center study of a cohort of 71 subjects. Arthritis Rheum. 2009;61:813–21.
70. Richette P, Molto A, Viguier M, et al. Hidradenitis suppurativa associated with spondyloarthritis – results from a multicentre national prospective study. J Rheumatol. 2014;41:490–4.
71. Claudepierre P, Clerc D, Cariou D, et al. SAPHO syndrome and pyoderma gangrenosum: is it fortuitous? J Rheumatol. 1996;23:400–2.
72. Naves JE, Cabré E, Mañosa M, et al. A systematic review of SAPHO syndrome and inflammatory bowel disease association. Dig Dis Sci. 2013;58:2138–47.
73. Rukavina I. SAPHO syndrome: a review. J Child Orthop. 2015;9:19–27.
74. Assmann G, Simon P. The SAPHO syndrome – are microbes involved? Best Pract Res Clin Rheumatol. 2011;25:423–34.
75. Hurtado-Nedelec M, Chollet-Martin S, Nicaise-Roland P, et al. Characterization of the immune response in the synovitis, acne, pustulosis, hyperostosis, osteitis (SAPHO) syndrome. Rheumatology (Oxford). 2008;47:1160–7.
76. Hofmann SR, Morbach H, Schwarz T, Rosen-Wolff A, Girschick HJ, Hedrich CM. Attenuated TLR4/MAPK signaling in monocytes from patients with CRMO results in impaired IL-10 expression. Clin Immunol. 2012;145:69–76.
77. Lopalco G, Cantarini L, Vitale A, et al. Interleukin-1 as a common denominator from autoinflammatory to autoimmune disorders: premises, perils, and perspectives. Mediat Inflamm. 2015;2015:194864.
78. Killeen ME, Ferris L, Kupetsky EA, et al. Signaling through purinergic receptors for ATP induces human cutaneous innate and adaptive Th17 responses: implications in the pathogenesis of psoriasis. J Immunol. 2013;190:4324–36.
79. Firinu D, Barca MP, Lorrai MM, et al. TH17 cells are increased in the peripheral blood of patients with SAPHO syndrome. Autoimmunity. 2014;47:389–94.
80. Golla A, Jansson A, Ramser J, et al. Chronic recurrent multifocal osteomyelitis (CRMO): evidence for a susceptibility gene located on chromosome 18q21.3–18q22. Eur J Hum Genet. 2002;10:217–21.

81. Hurtado-Nedelec M, Chollet-Martin S, Chapeton D, et al. Genetic susceptibility factors in a cohort of 38 patients with SAPHO syndrome: a study of PSTPIP2, NOD2, and LPIN2 genes. J Rheumatol. 2010;37:401–9.
82. Burgemeister LT, Baeten DL, Tas SW. Biologics for rare inflammatory diseases: TNF blockade in the SA PHO syndrome. Neth J Med. 2012;70:444–9.
83. Jesus AA, Goldbach-Mansky R. IL-1 blockade in autoinflammatory syndromes. Annu Rev Med. 2014;65:223–44.
84. Assmann G, Wagner AD, Monika M, Pfoehler C, Pfreundschuh M, Tilgen W, et al. Single-nucleotide polymorphisms p53 G72C and Mdm2 T309G in patients with psoriasis, psoriatic arthritis, and SAPHO syndrome. Rheumatol Int. 2010;30:1273–6.
85. Assmann G, Kueck O, Kirchhoff T, Rosenthal H, Voswinkel J, Pfreundschuh M, et al. Efficacy of antibiotic therapy for SAPHO syndrome is lost after its discontinuation: an interventional study. Arthritis Res Ther. 2009;11:R140.
86. Govoni M, Colina M, Massara A, Trotta F. SAPHO syndrome and infections. Autoimmun Rev. 2009;8:256–9.
87. Girschick HJ, Huppertz HI, Harmsen D, Krauspe R, Müller-Hermelink HK, Papadopoulos T. Chronic recurrent multifocal osteomyelitis in children: diagnostic value of histopathology and microbial testing. Hum Pathol. 1999;30:59–65.
88. Job-Deslandre C, Krebs S, Kahan A. Chronic recurrent multifocal osteomyelitis: five-year outcomes in 14 pediatric cases. Joint Bone Spine. 2001;68:245–51.
89. Bruzzese V. Pyoderma gangrenosum, acne conglobata, suppurative hidradenitis, and axial spondyloarthritis: efficacy of anti-tumor necrosis factor α therapy. J Clin Rheumatol. 2012;18:413–5.
90. Garzorz N, Papanagiotou V, Atenhan A, Andres C, Eyerich S, Eyerich K, et al. Pyoderma gangrenosum, acne, psoriasis, arthritis and suppurative hidradenitis (PAPASH)-syndrome: a new entity within the spectrum of autoinflammatory syndromes? J Eur Acad Dermatol Venereol. 2016;30:141–3.
91. Saraceno R, Babino G, Chiricozzi A, Zangrilli A, Chimenti S. PsAPASH: a new syndrome associated with hidradenitis suppurativa with response to tumor necrosis factor inhibition. J Am Acad Dermatol. 2015;72:e42–4.
92. Stichweh DS, Punaro M, Pascual V. Dramatic improvement of pyoderma gangrenosum with infliximab in a patient with PAPA syndrome. Pediatr Dermatol. 2005;22:262–5.
93. Tofteland ND, Shaver TS. Clinical efficacy of etanercept for treatment of PAPA syndrome. J Clin Rheumatol. 2010;16:244–5.
94. Lee H, Park SH, Kim SK, Choe JY, Park JS. Pyogenic arthritis, pyoderma gangrenosum, and acne syndrome (PAPA syndrome) with E250K mutation in CD2BP1 gene treated with the tumor necrosis factor inhibitor adalimumab. Clin Exp Rheumatol. 2012;30:452.
95. Brenner M, Ruzicka T, Plewig G, Thomas P, Herzer P. Targeted treatment of pyoderma gangrenosum in PAPA (pyogenic arthritis, pyoderma gangrenosum and acne) syndrome with the recombinant human interleukin-1 receptor antagonist anakinra. Br J Dermatol. 2009;161:1199–201.
96. Dierselhuis MP, Frenkel J, Wulffraat NM, Boelens JJ. Anakinra for flares of pyogenic arthritis in PAPA syndrome. Rheumatology (Oxford). 2005;44:406–8.
97. Staub J, Pfannschmidt N, Strohal R, Braun-Falco M, Lohse P, Goerdt S, et al. Successful treatment of PASH syndrome with infliximab, cyclosporine and dapsone. J Eur Acad Dermatol Venereol. 2015;29:2243–7.
98. Scheinfeld N. Diseases associated with hidradenitis suppurativa: part 2 of a series on hidradenitis. Dermatol Online J. 2013;19:18558.
99. Dinarello CA, van der Meer JW. Treating inflammation by blocking interleukin-1 in humans. Semin Immunol. 2013;25:469–84.
100. Jung J, Molinger M, Kohn D, et al. Intra-articular glucocorticosteroid injection into sternocostoclavicular joints in patients with SAPHO syndrome. Semin Arthritis Rheum. 2012;42:266–70.
101. Hayama K, Inadomi T, Fujisawa D, Terui T. A pilot study of medium-dose cyclosporine for the treatment of palmoplantar pustulosis complicated with pustulotic arthro-osteitis. Eur J Dermatol. 2010;20:758–62.

102. Amital H, Applbaum YH, Aamar S, et al. SAPHO syndrome treated with pamidronate: an open-label study of 10 patients. Rheumatology (Oxford). 2004;43:658–61.
103. Firinu D, Murgia G, Lorrai MM, Barca MP, Peralta MM, Manconi PE, et al. Biological treatments for SAPHO syndrome: an update. Inflamm Allergy Drug Targets. 2014;13:199–205.
104. Olivieri I, Padula A, Ciancio G, Salvarani C, Niccoli L, Cantini F. Successful treatment of SAPHO syndrome with infliximab: report of two cases. Ann Rheum Dis. 2002;61:375–6.
105. Wagner AD, Andresen J, Jendro MC, Hulsemann JL, Zeidler H. Sustained response to tumor necrosis factor alpha-blocking agents in two patients with SAPHO syndrome. Arthritis Rheum. 2002;46:1965–8.
106. Wendling D, Prati C, Aubin F. Anakinra treatment of SAPHO syndrome: short-term results of an open study. Ann Rheum Dis. 2012;71:1098–100.
107. Colina M, Pizzirani C, Khodeir M, Falzoni S, Bruschi M, Trotta F, et al. Dysregulation of P2X7 receptor-inflammasome axis in SAPHO syndrome: successful treatment with anakinra. Rheumatology (Oxford). 2010;49:1416–8.
108. Newman B, Cescon D, Domenchini A, et al. CD2BP1 and CARD15 mutations are not associated with pyoderma gangrenosum in patients with inflammatory bowel disease. J Invest Dermatol. 2004;122:1054–6.
109. Nesterovitch AB, Hoffman MD, Simon M, et al. Mutations in the PSTPIP1 gene and aberrant splicing variants in patients with pyoderma gangrenosum. Clin Exp Dermatol. 2011;36:889–95.
110. Guenova E, Teske A, Fehrenbacher B, et al. Interleukin 23 expression in pyoderma gangrenosum and targeted therapy with ustekinumab. Arch Dermatol. 2011;147:1203–5.
111. Hamel J, Paul D, Gahr M, Hedrich CM. Pilot study: possible association of IL10 promoter polymorphisms with CRMO. Rheumatol Int. 2012;32:555–6.

Part II

Pathology, Internal Medicine, Pathophysiology, Therapy

An Histological Approach to the Diagnosis of Neutrophilic Dermatoses

15

Marie-Dominique Vignon-Pennamen

An analysis of histological lesions delineate the history of the neutrophilic dermatoses (ND). In all steps of the description of these diseases, the cutaneous biopsy has been essential to ascertain their specificity. Moreover some of them have been distinguished in accordance with their histological presentation, for example, the subcorneal pustular dermatosis of Sneddon and Wilkinson, the neutrophilic eccrine hidradenitis or the Ig A pemphigus. The cutaneous biopsy has also been one of the major criteria to group dermatoses that are clinically completely different with the common denominator of an aseptic infiltration by neutrophils. The prototypic ND are Sweet's syndrome (SS) and pyoderma gangrenosum (PG) [1]. However many other dermatoses characterized by a cutaneous infiltration by neutrophils have been recognized later and linked to this group. Skin biopsy plays a pivotal role in the diagnosis and classification of these rare dermatoses. For a better comprehension of these ND, we have proposed in 2006 a simple classification [2]. In this way, ND are grouped into three categories—superficial, dermal and deep dermatoses—that allows a comprehensive approach for clinicians. For each category, many differential diagnoses and pitfalls may be encountered. Neutrophils are the key for diagnosis, but sometimes other cellular partners may be seen and make the diagnosis obscure. A clinical pathological correlation is therefore always needed.

Superficial Neutrophilic Dermatoses

In this group of dermatoses the infiltrate is predominantly epidermal with collections of neutrophils located at different levels in the epidermis.

M.-D. Vignon-Pennamen, M.D.
Pathology Department, APHP Hôpital Saint Louis, Paris, France
e-mail: dominique.vignon-pennamen@wanadoo.fr

D. Wallach et al. (eds.), *Neutrophilic Dermatoses*,
https://doi.org/10.1007/978-3-319-72649-6_15

General Diagnosis

Collections of neutrophils in the epidermis can occur in a large variety of conditions (Table 15.1). Identification of the associated epidermal or dermal patterns help differenciate these conditions from one another.

The pustules can be subcorneal, intraepidermal or sub and intraepidermal. Some of them can relate to the follicles with neutrophis filling the ostia.

The pustules are unique or multiple.

They may be unilocular or associated with spongiosis and hence referred as "spongiform pustule of Kogog".

The epidermis can be normal or acanthotic. Rarely necrosis or balooning degeneration may be seen. The epidermal pustules may be outlined by acantholytic keratinocytes.

The dermal infiltrate is superficial, sparse or more abundant, composed of neutrophils admixed with lymphocytes and histiocytes. Eosinophils are sometimes associated with neutrophils.

Finally histochemical stains, mainly PAS are very usefull to exclude infections.

Table 15.1 Dermatoses with intraepidermal pustules

Subcorneal pustules
Unilocular
Subcorneal pustular dermatosis
Scabies
Fungal infections
With spongiosis
Pustular psoriasis
Pustulosis of main folds
Acute generalized exanthematous pustulosis
Scabies
Impetigo
Fungal infections
Intraepidermal pustules
Intra and subepidermal
Bullous pyoderma gangrenosum
Unilocular
Palmo-plantar pustulosis
Follicular
Crohn's disease
Behçet's disease
With acantholysis
Pemphigus
Impetigo
With balooning degeneration
Herpes

Epidermal/Superficial ND

Subcorneal pustular dermatosis of Sneddon and Wilkinson. It is the prototypic superfical ND. The dermatosis is clinically characterized by flat pustules. On biopsy there is an epidermal infiltration with neutrophils that are grouped in an unique unilocular cavity located under the stratum corneum (Fig. 15.1). Usually, there is no acantholysis. The epidermis is normal and there are very few inflammatory cells in the superficial dermis [3].

The Ig A pemphigus is very close to the subcorneal pustular dermatosis [4]. The collections of neutrophils can be subcorneal or intraepidermal with or without acantholysis and there is a more or less dense dermal inflammation with neutrophils. Most importantly there are intraepidermal Ig A deposits on direct immunofluorescence.

The superficial and bullous variant of PG is very difficult to diagnose and requires a clinical pathological discussion [5]. It is characterized by a large intraepidermal and/or subepidermal pustule associated with a dense superficial dermal neutrophilic infiltrate (Fig. 15.2). Sometimes subepidermal pustules resemble autoimmune bullous dermatoses such as Ig A linear dermatosis or dermatitis herpetiformis. Direct immunofluorescence is always needed.

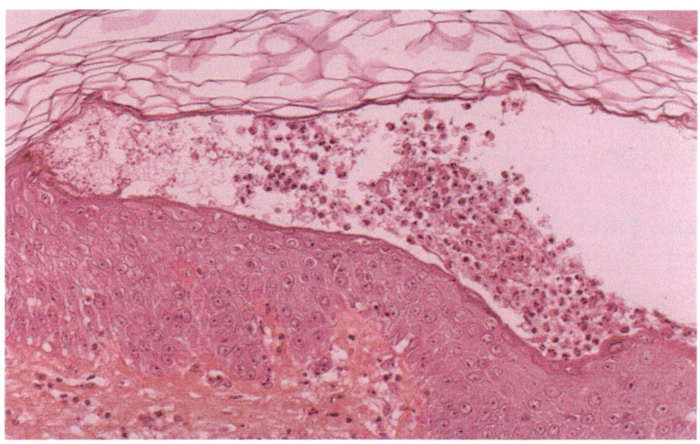

Fig. 15.1 Subcorneal pustulosis (subcorneal pustular dermatosis) HE ×200

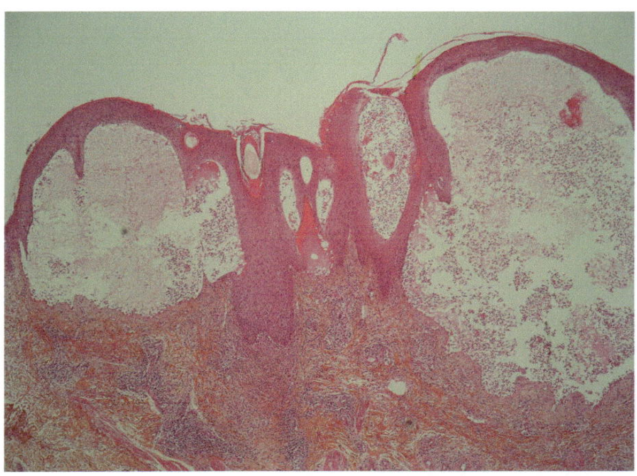

Fig. 15.2 Subepidermal pustule (superficial bullous PG) HE ×100

In the pustulosis of main folds, pustules are smaller, mutilocular, close to the pattern seen in pustular psoriasis [6].

The vesiculo-pustular eruption of colitis, especially of Crohn's disease presents tense pustules with an inflammatory border. On biopsy these pustules are frequently follicular with an ostial accumulation of neutrophils and/or a dense dermal infiltrate that replaces the follicular sheat. It is also considered by some pathologists as a pustular variant of PG [7]. Similar follicular pustules have been described in association with rheumatoid arthritis, Behçet's disease and some myeloproliferative disorders. They have also been observed in the bowell by pass syndrome.

Pustular psoriasis. For a long time, pustular psoriasis has been considered as a differential diagnosis of subcorneal pustular dermatosis. It is currently admitted that it belongs to the same group of autoinflammatory diseases as do the other ND [8]. Under the microscope, neutrophilic collections occurring in the stratum corneum are associated with spongiosis (Fig. 15.3). As they ascend the epidermis these pustules become more compact and present as Munro's microabcesses. The epidermis is slightly acanthotic with regular papillomatosis and the dermal infiltrate is sparse located in the papilla, composed of lymphocytes and neutrophils.

In palmo-plantar pustulosis, also considered as a variant of pustular psoriasis, the epidermal pustule is large overall unilocular, with few neutrophils dispersed between keratinocytes outlining the cavity.

Differential Diagnosis

Infectious dermatoses are the main differential diagnosis of the superficial ND. Histochemical stains such as PAS and Gram are always performed to exclude fungal infections or impetigo. Morphologicals alterations in keratinocytes make the

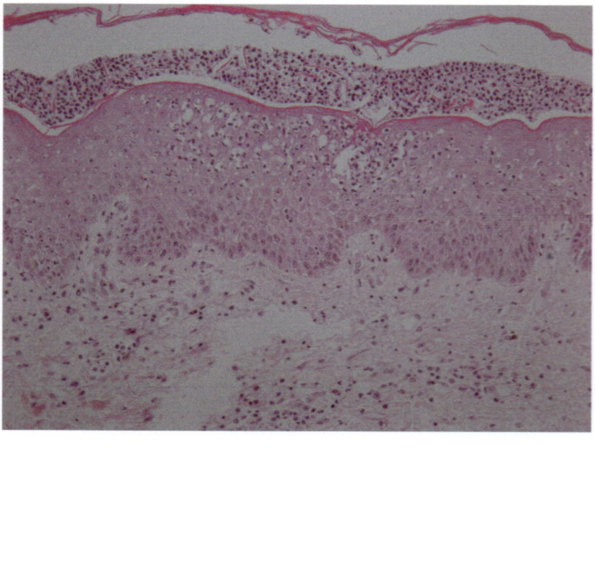

Fig. 15.3 Spongiform pustule (pustular psoriasis) HE ×200

diagnosis of herpes virus infection. When they are subtle, immunohistochemical studies may be applied. The diagnosis of scabies requires a clinical information because mites are not always observed in the stratum corneum.

Bullous autoimmune diseases. When acantholysis is seen in an intraepidermal pustule or when the picture is that of neutrophilic spongiosis, direct immunofluorescence is warranted to eliminate pemphigus.

Drug eruptions. Intraepidermal pustules along with spongiosis is found in acute generalized exanthematous pustulosis. The dermal infiltrate is polymorphous rich in lymphocytes sometimes, atypical. The diagnosis is clinical. Intraepidermal pustules located in an hyperplastic epidermis may be seen in haloderma. However the pustules contain eosinophils in addition to neutrophils.

Dermal Neutrophilic Dermatoses

This group of dermatoses is characterized by a dermal infiltrate. Clinically they present as papules, plaques and nodules.

General Diagnosis

The pattern of the cellular infiltrate can be classified into five mains types.

- Superficial perivascular infiltrate
- Superficial and deep perivascular and periadnexal infiltrate
- Diffuse dermal infiltrate
- Bandlike infiltrate in the upper dermis with or without nodular tendency and perivascular and periadnexal infiltrate in the lower dermis
- Abcess-like collection of neutrophils and nuclear dust in the upper dermis

The density of the cellular infiltrate can be mild, moderate or severe. Within these main patterns, some cases present a predominantly follicular involvement, a prominent eccrine glands involvement or vascular damages. More rarely the infiltrate is palisaded, organized around collagen alterations with necrosis.

Composition of the Cellular Infiltrate

The mature neutrophil is the typical and most frequent inflammatory cell in dermal ND. Yet, lymphocytes or histiocytes may be present in the inflammatory infiltrate. In addition, eosinophils can be noted in the cutaneous lesions. In cases occurring in patients with myeloid hemopathies, there is sometimes the concurrent presence of abnormal neutrophils and normal mature neutrophils within the same lesion.

The Prototypic Dermal Neutrophilic Dermatosis: Sweet's Syndrome

The pathologic features of SS characteristically involve the dermis. Typically, in addition to edema of the papilla and papillary dermis, there is an infilrate of mature neutrophils in the superficial dermis (Fig. 15.4). The distribution of the inflammatory cells within the upper dermis is usually dense and diffuse. Less commonly, it has been noted to be perivascular [9]. Swelling of endothelial cells, dilatation of small blood vessels and fragmentation of neutrophils nuclei (referred as leukocytoclasia or karyorrhexis) are also frequently present [9]. Usually, neither fibrin deposition nor neutrophils are present in the vessel wall and the overlying epidermis is normal. Several authors have observed the presence of leukocytoclastic vasculitis [10]. It is now hypothesized that the vascular changes are occurring as an epiphenomenon and do not represent a primary vasculitis [11].

Although the dermis is the typical site of the inflammatory infiltrate in SS, neutrophils may migrate into the overlying epidermis. The location of the infiltrate

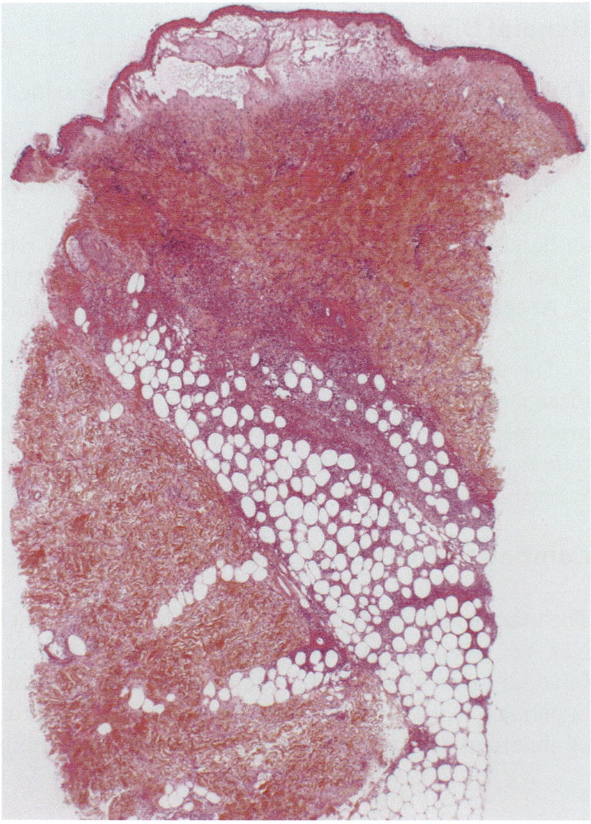

Fig. 15.4 Dermal neutrophilic infiltrate with edema (SS) HE ×100

determines wether the lesions appear as neutrophilic spongiotic vesicles or subcorneal pustules. Neutrophils may also migrate into the underlying adipose tissue with usually a partial involvement [12].

Other Dermal Neutrophilic Neutrophilic Dermatoses

Other ND are characterized by a dermal neutrophilic inflammation.

Neutrophilic Eccrine Hidradenitis

It is most commonly observed in the induction phase of chemotherapy for acute myeloid leukemia. It consists of variable infiltration of the eccrine coil by neutrophils sometimes with necrosis of the secretory epithelium and squamous metaplasia of eccrine ducts [13]. In plantar hidradenitis, described in children, with no association to myeloid hemopathies, the histopathologic picture is similar without syringosquamous metaplasia.

Rheumatoid Neutrophilic Dermatitis

This condition resulting in plaque-like neutrophilic infiltrates is observed in patients with rheumatoid arthritis. The histology is very similar to that seen in SS [14]. Perivascular and interstitial neutrophilic infiltrates are present within the upper and midreticular dermis. Overt leukocytoclastic vasculitis is absent. Papillary dermal edema is less extensive that in SS. Spongiotic intraepidermal vesicles and subepidermal vesicles are occasionnally seen.

Bowel-Associated Dermatosis-Arthritis Syndrome

The histopathologic findings are similar to those seen in SS. Perivascular and nodular infiltrates of varying density composed largely of neutrophils and nuclear dust are present within an edematous papillary and superficial dermis. Although most vessels do not show changes of leukocytoclastic vasculitis, occasional ones have fibrin deposition within their walls.

Erythema Elevatum Diutinum

The histopathologic changes depend on the age of lesions [15]. Early papules display leukocytoclastic vasculitis with a wedge-shaped infiltrate and fibrin deposition in and around the blood vessels walls. Around the vessels are neutrophils, leukocytoclastic debris, lymphocytes, macrophages, histiocytes and rare eosinophils. Papillary edema can be present and may lead to vesiculation in extreme cases. The number of neutrophils in the dermis exceeds that seen in most other forms of leukocytoclastic vasculitis bearing a ressemblance to SS and PG. More developed nodular lesions show a storiform proliferation of dermal spindle cells with fibrosis and sometimes multinuclear giant cells, ressembling dermatofibroma. Foci of neutrophils or neutrophilic vasculitis can be seen in the the dermal fibrosis, a feature unique to erythema elevatum diutinum (Fig. 15.5).

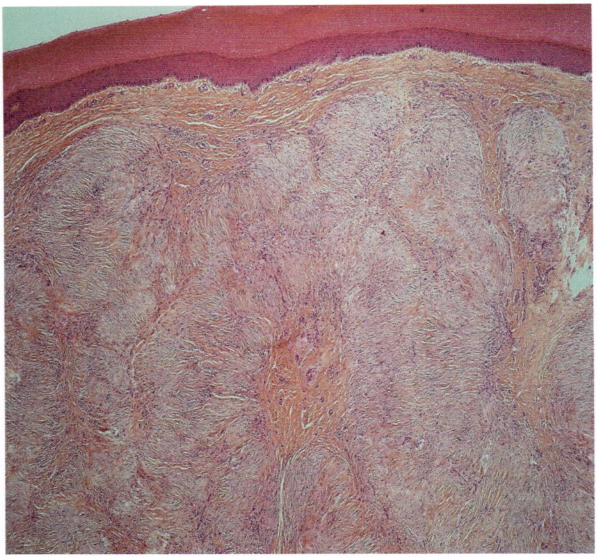

Fig. 15.5 Late fibrous stage of erythema elevatum diutinum HE ×100

Pyoderma Gangrenosum Granulomatous Variant

In this variant of PG, the infiltrate is predominantly dermal. It is diffuse and massive. It is polymorphous associating neutrophils, lymphocytes, plasma cells, and macrophages with multinucleated giants cells [16]. It is easily confused with infectious dermatoses.

Differential Diagnosis and Pitfalls

Many differential diagnoses can be discussed under the microscope. They can be related to the pattern of the infiltrate and to the composition of the inflammatory infiltrate.

Differential Diagnoses Related to the Pattern of the Infiltrate (Table 15.2)

1. When the infiltrate is superficicial and perivascular with neutrophils filling the dermal papilla, direct immunofluorescence is required to exclude bullous autoimmune disorders such as linear IgA dermatosis, dermatitis herpetiformis or bullous lupus erythematosus.
2. Superficial and deep perivascular infiltrates, mostly when there are accompanied with vessel damage need to be differenciated from leukocytoclastic vasculitis, Behçet's disease, and bowel by pass syndrome [17].
3. Moderate and interstitial neutrophilic infiltrates characterize neutrophilic urticarial dermatosis [18]. They are also observed in Still's disease or in mediterranean fever [19]. In erysipelas, rarely analysed on biopsy, the neutrophilic infiltrate is sparse located in the whole dermis without vasculitis.

Table 15.2 Differential diagnosis in dermal neutrophilic dermatoses related to the pattern of the infiltrate

Superficial infiltrates
Bullous autoimmune diseases
Superficial and deep perivascular infiltrates
Leukocytoclastic vasculitis
Behçet's disease
Bowel by-pass syndrome
Mild and interstitial infiltrates
Neutrophilic urticarial dermatosis
Urticarial vasculitis
Still's disease
Mediteranean fever
Erysipela
Dense and diffuse infiltrates
Infections
Palissaded infiltrates
Palissaded neutrophilic and granulomatous dermatitis

4. Dense and diffuse neutrophilic infiltrates are observed in different kinds of bacterial, mycobacterial and fungal infections. Histochemical stains and cultures are recommanded [20, 21].

   On the opposite, morphologic mimickers of microorganisms mainly cryptococcus have recently emerged as a novel histopathologic pitfall. Five cases have been reported describing acutely ill patients with a massive and diffuse neutrophilic inflammation [22–24]. Among the inflammatory infiltrate are numerous polymorphous atypical acellular bodies surrounded by capsule-like vacuolated spaces hightly suggestive of cryptococcal yeasts forms. In all cases fungal work-up, including cultures and multiple stains are negative. In some cases, transmission electron microscopy has been performed to definitively rule out fungal infection. The acellular bodies appear compatible with residual degenerated nuclei of cells having undergone autolysis and can be considered as a unique form of cell death. The recognition of this microscopic pitfall is essential to prevent unecessary delay of appropriate therapy.
5. Even more rarely, the dermal infiltrate may be palissaded, characterized by small areas of basophilic degeneration of collagen surrounded by neutrophils, nuclear dust and lymphocytes. These areas show some similarity to classic flame figures described with eosinophilic infiltates in Well's syndrome. This histologic picture is reported under the denomination of palissaded neutrophilic and granulomatous dermatitis [25, 26]. It is mainly observed in connective tissue diseases, anti-neutrophil cytoplasmic antibody-associated vasculitis (such as granulomatosis with polyangeitis or eosinophilic granulomatosis with polyangeitis) and drug reactions [27, 28].

Differential Diagnoses Related to the Composition of the Cellular Infiltrate (Table 15.3)

The mature neutrophil is the typical inflammatory cell in dermal ND. However, other inflammatory cells may be encountered, sometimes predominant leading to misdiagnosed situation and delay in the appropriate diagnosis.

1. The presence of eosinophils may range from rare to abundant and is not always related to the use of medication [29]. A mixed perivascular infiltrate composed of lymphocytes, histiocytes and numerous eosinophils is typically observed in arthropod bites reactions. However, in some cases of arthropode bite reactions the inflammatory infiltrate is mostly composed of neutrophils mimicking lesions of SS [30]. The same mixed infiltrate with lymphocytes, histiocytes, neutrophils and eosinophils is observed in granuloma faciale [31]. In addition there is evidence of small vessel vasculitis such as fibrin deposition and neutrophilic nuclear dust in and around the walls of veinules. Later lesions show concentric fibrosis around veinules with an increase in the number of histiocytes as seen in erythema elevatum diutinum.
2. Some dense and diffuse inflammatory infiltrates are composed of prominent neutrophils admixed with a variable number of lymphocytes. This picture is classicaly observed in SS. It is also described in connective tissue diseases, especially in lupus erythematosus [32, 33]. The most important clues for the diagnosis of lupus are the presence of interface dermatitis and mucin deposition in the dermis. However these features are not seen in all cases making the diagnosis extremely difficult. Although most of the case reports have a history of lupus before biopsy, the diagnosis of lupus is not established in some of them. It is therefore very important for clinicians and pathologists to be aware of the broad histologic spectrum that mat be encountered in lupus erythematosus-associated neutrophilic dermatosis.

Table 15.3 Differential diagnosis and pitfalls in dermal neutrophilic dermatoses related to the composition of the inflammatory infiltrate

Mixed infiltrates with eosinophils
Arthropods bites reactions
Granuloma faciale
Mixed infiltrates with neutrophils and lymphocytes
Neutrophilic lupus erythematosus
Connective tissue diseases
Mixed infiltrates with granuloma
Infections
Crohn's disease
Lymphocytic infiltrates
Lymphocytis SS
Histiocytic-Histiocytoid infiltrates
Histiocytoid SS
Leukemia cutis
Myelodysplasia cutis

3. Mixed infiltrates with granulomatous reaction are reported in the superficial granulomatous variant of PG. As discussed previously the main differential diagnosis is infection which can be ruled out with histochemical stains and cultures. Sometimes the dermal infiltrate is composed of sheets of neutrophils involving the entire dermis associated with areas of epithelioid histiocytes and multinucleated cells allowing the diagnosis of Crohn's disease.
4. Lymphocytic infiltrates are not usually discussed in a chapter devoted to the histology of ND. Nevertherless in a few case reports and small series of SS, the inflammatory infiltrate has been reported as lymphocyte rich without neutrophils [34, 35]. The histological picture is observed in patients with a chronic relapsing form of SS (Fig. 15.6). The clinical presentation is characteristic with raised tender plaques sometimes with an annular configuration. All patients have constitutional symptoms including fever, sweats, general malaise and arthralgia. On initial biopsies the infiltrate is mostly composed of lymphocytes and later, after numerous relapses, it is made of neutrophils. On closer examination some unusual mononuclear cells, myeloperoxydase positive on immunohistochemical stains, are present. For most patients a diagnosis of myelodysplastic syndrome has been made concomittantly or many months or years following the diagnosis of SS.

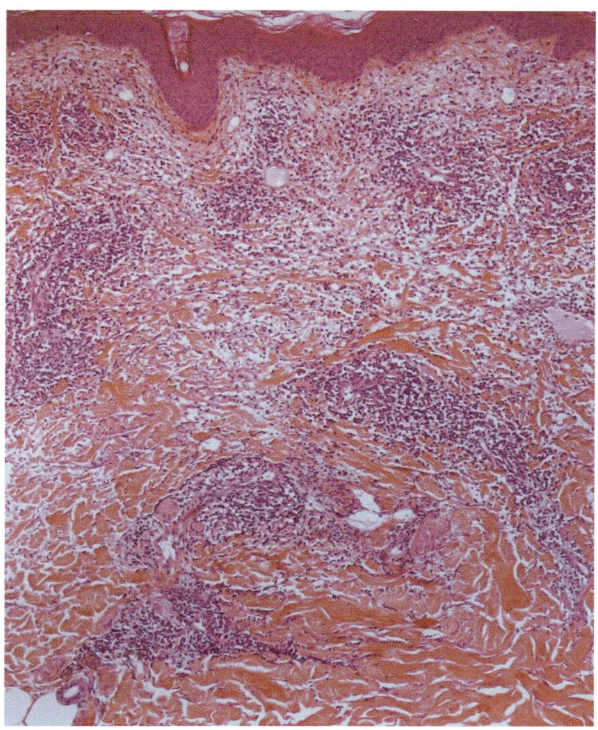

Fig. 15.6 Lymphocytic SS HE ×100

5. Histiocytoid SS is a new histological variant. It refers to an infiltrate of immature myeloid cells with an histiocytoid appearance which may be misinterpreted as histiocytes [36]. In 1989 in an histopathological study of 37 patients, one author proposed that lesions of SS pass through lymphocytic, neutrophilic and histiocytic stages depending on the age of lesions [9]. Two years later, another report indicated that there was no relationship between the duration of the lesions and the composition of the cellular infiltrate [37]. In most cases from this study the infiltrate consisted mainly of histiocytes or was composed of an equal number of neutrophils and histiocytes. The histiocytes are described with small elongated twisted nuclei or with a large and oval nucleus mimicking neutrophils. One can consider that the authors were the first to describe the histiocytoid variant of SS. Diagnostic criteria for histiocytoid SS represent a challenge. It must be differenciated from leukemia cutis. The infiltrate is usually dense extended to the whole dermis, separated from the epidermis by a edema as in classic SS (Fig. 15.7a). It is composed of few mature neutrophils and mostly mononuclear cells with a scant slightly eosinophilic cytoplasm and small size oval elongated kidney-shape or twisted nuclei (Fig. 15.7b). These mononuclear cells ressemble histiocytes but they express markers of myeloid lineage (CD68/KP1, myeloperoxydase). They represent immature myeloid cells or abnormal neutrophils which are hyposegmented, a morphologic anomaly described in myelodysplastic syndromes as a pseudo Pelger-Huet anomaly [38]. In their initial report Requena and coll fail to demonstrate an association with myeloid hemopathy and follow-up of their patient rules out this possibility. In further case reports and small series, histiocytoid SS has been described in association with underlying hemopathies [39–44]. Among them, myelodysplastic syndromes were the most common

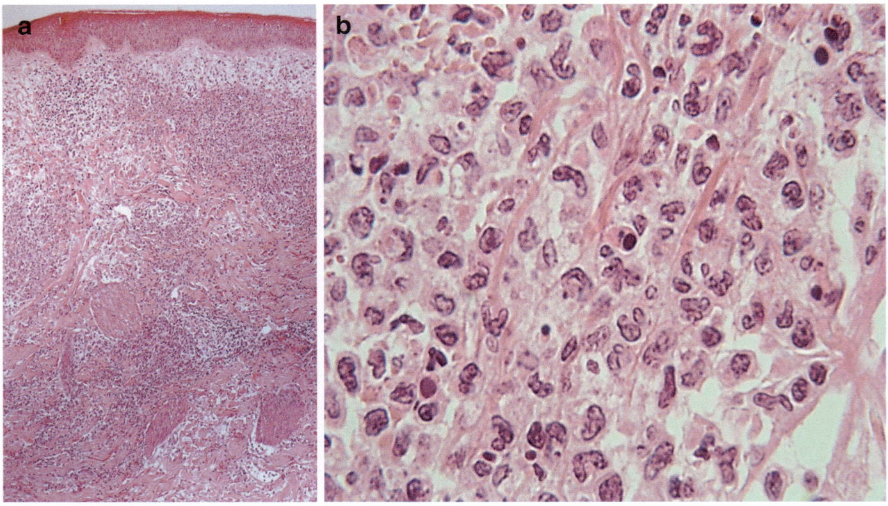

Fig. 15.7 (**a**) Histiocytoid SS. (**b**) Abnormal hyposegmented neutrophils in histiocytoid SS HE ×400

disorders. For most authors, the association of histiocytoid SS and myeloid hemopathies appears to support the premise that some exemples of histiocytoid SS are in fact a form of leukemia cutis. In a recent case series of 33 patients, the investigators confirme that histiocytoid SS is composed of immature myeloid cells associated with a minor component of authentic histiocytes and that it is not an infiltrate of M2 macrophages as previously reported [45]. They consider that histiocytoid SS is not more frequently related to hematologic malignancies than classic neutrophilic SS and conclude that the infiltrate should not be interpreted as leukemia cutis. In a work published in 2015, Osio and coll, indicate that infiltrates observed in histiocytoid SS can be interpreted as abnormal neutrophils with pseudo Pelger-Huet anomaly, a specific myelodysplastic marker on blood smears [46]. They conclude that histiocytoid SS in patients having myelodysplastic syndrome is in fact a myelodysplasia cutis. When compared with leukemia cutis they have identified different clinical morphological discriminating features that have translational value, given the far better prognosis of myelodysplasia cutis. However, approximately 50% of histiocytoid SS reported cases have shown no association with myeloid hemopathies. Histiocytoid SS is actually a biological heterogeneous group of disorders requiring further work and research.

In some case reports and small series, FISH analysis has been performed on skin biopsy specimens with a diagnosis of SS or PG and concomitant myeloid hemopathy [47–49]. It shows that chromosomal abnormality can be identified in the neutrophilic infiltrate, confirming the neutrophilic infiltrate to be clonaly related to the underlying myeloid malignancy. With the same FISH analysis, it has been shown that the skin infiltrate of histiocytoid SS can be also clonal, exhibiting the same chromosomal abnormality than in bone marrow [46]. In our opinion, these cases should not be interpretated as leukemia cutis and we suggest that they represent a complete or incomplete differenciation of malignant myeloid cells [46, 48].

6. Other pitfalls.

In some rare elastic tissue disorders such as acquired cutis laxa or mid-dermal elastolysis lesions may be preceded by erythema and/or urticaria. The biopsy of the inflammatory lesional skin can reveal an interstitial diffuse neutrophilic infiltrate with a normal pattern of elastic tissue ressembling SS [50]. The course of disease and subsequent biopies make the diagnosis.

Loss of elastic fibers determining cutis laxa after the acute neutrophilic stage is reported mainly in children as a variant of SS also called Marshall's syndrome [51]. It is very important to know this peculiar presentation because of the association with cardiac disease.

Deep Neutrophilic Dermatoses

In these dermatoses the infiltrates are deeply located in the dermis and subcutaneous tissue. Clinically patients present with ulcerations, nodules, cellulitis and abcesses.

General Diagnosis

The inflammatory infiltrate is massive and diffuse replacing normal adnexal structures and fat tissue. Among the neutrophilic inflammation vessel walls may be damaged with necrosis and thrombosis. The infiltrate is suppurative with collagen necrosis.

The Prototypic Deep Neutrophilic Dermatosis: Pyoderma Gangrenosum

Although histological lesions are not considered specific, a biopsy is always required to confirm neutrophilic inflammation and to exclude other causes of ulceration and misdiagnosis [52]. Histopathogic features differ according to the age of the lesions and site of the biopsy that need to be carefully selected. It is recommended to take an elliptic specimen including the margin and the floor of the ulcer. In early lesions and on the peripheral extension area, there is a perivascular and/or perifollicular infiltrate composed of lymphocytes and histiocytes with a variable proportion of neutrophils and endothelial swelling. On a large and deep enough biopsy, the dermis and subcutaneous fat are massively infiltrated by a suppurative inflammation that contains neutrophils, hemorrhages and necrosis (Fig. 15.8). The infiltrates destroy preexisting structures. Vessels can be necrotic and thrombotic, these alterations beeing secondary to the neutrophilic inflammation. All these features are in favor of classic PG after exclusion of an infection. It is not unusual to see sheets of epithelioid histiocytes and multinucleated cells in chronic ulcerations of classic PG. Histochemical stains and cultures are always needed for microbiological identification.

Other Deep Neutrophilic Dermatoses

Neutrophilic Panniculitis

Neutrophilic panniculitis encompasses an heterogeneous group of disorders, some of them belonging to the spectrum of ND. Some authors prefer the denomination of subcutaneous SS [53]. In this deep variant of SS, lesions demonstrate pathologic changes that are located either entirely or only partially in the subcutaneous fat. The most common pattern is that neutrophilic lobular panniculitis, although a predominantly septal pattern has also been reported in few cases (Fig. 15.9) [54]. Mild fat necrosis may be seen. As in classic SS, the neutrophilic infiltrate demonstrates leukocytoclasia and may be admixed with scattered eosinophils. Interestingly histiocytoid subcutaneous SS has been described and also cases with nuclear hypersegmentation or hyposegmentation of neutrophils in patients with myeloid disorders especially with myelodysplastic syndromes [55, 56]. The blood vessels lack fibrinoid necrosis and other evidence of vasculitis.

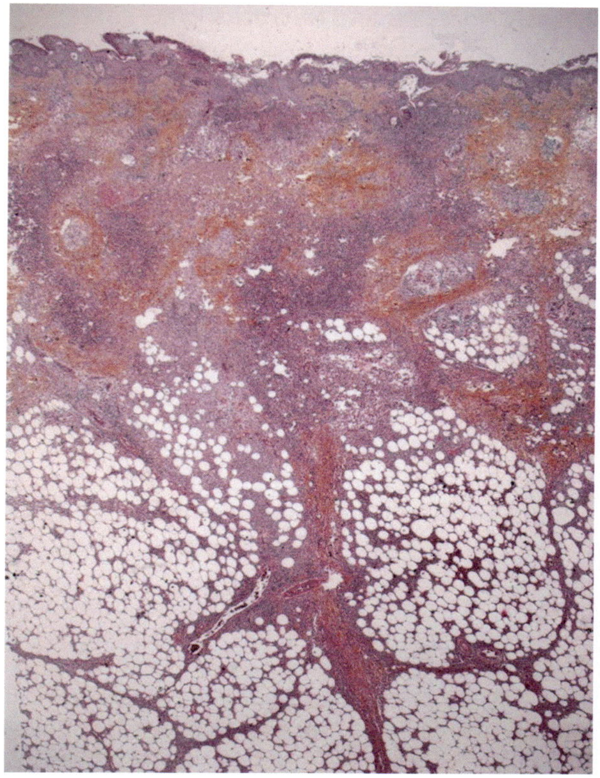

Fig. 15.8 Diffuse neutrophilic infiltration in the dermis and fat tissue (PG) HE ×100

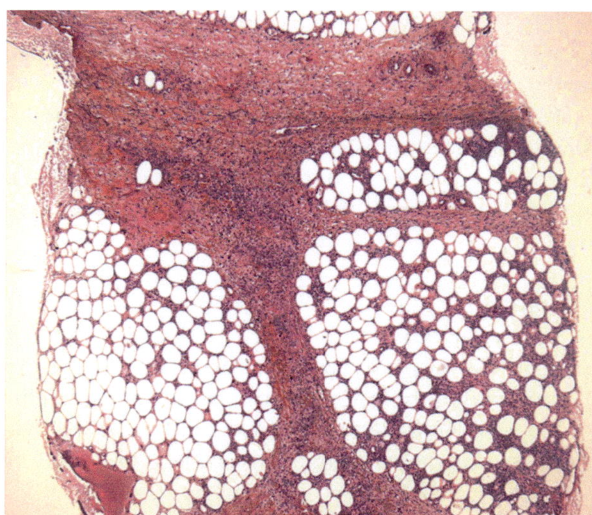

Fig. 15.9 Neutrophilic septal and lobular infiltration HE ×100

Aseptic Abcesses and Necrotizing SS

In these rare presentations of neutrophilic dermatoses, there is an extensive neutrophilic infiltration and necrosis of the subcutaneous fat, fascia and skeletal muscles [57].

Differential Diagnosis

Infections

The main differential diagnosis of all variants of deep neutrophilic dermatoses is infection that will be ruled out by histochemical stains and cultures. On biopsy there is an extensive involvement of the dermis and fat lobules and frequently of the septa by an heavy neutrophilic infiltrate. Abcesses may be present. The infiltrate is associated with basophilic debris giving a dirty appearance at low magnification. Another key feature is vascular damage, including necrotizing vasculitis and thrombosis.

Other Causes of Neutrophilic Panniculitis

They frequently display fat necrosis whose type may serve as an important diagnostic clue [56].

In pancreatic panniculitis, the histopathogical hallmark is the presence of "ghost cells" referring to necrotic adipocytes transformed into an amorphous to granular blue-gray substance in the process of saponification.

In alpha-1 antitrypsine deficiency panniculitis, the affected fat lobules are necrotic and replaced with an intense neutrophilic infiltrate. The lesions tend to be focal and sharply delineated, juxtaposed with large areas of relatively normal fat.

Facticial panniculitis is diagnosed by exclusion of others. The histopathology is hightly variable depending on the type of injury and the injected substance. There is usually fat necrosis, membranous fat necrosis and hemorrhage. Foreign materials may be seen under polarized light.

It may be difficult to differenciate erythema nodosum from subcutaneous SS when inflammation is limited to the septa. Miescher radial granuloma referring to small aggregates of histiocytes and neutrophils surrounding a central cleft of stellate or banana shape may be used as a diagnostic clue for erythema nodosum.

Conclusion

Neutrophilic dermatoses are rare diseases with a significant systemic component. The diagnosis is often difficult requiring an experienced clinical evaluation and carefull exclusion of other causes of neutrophilic inflammation. Cutaneous biopsy plays a pivotal role in the diagnosis. It provides essential informations to make an appropriate diagnosis and help to classify heterogeneous and very exciting dermatoses.

References

1. Wallach D, Vignon-Pennamen MD. Pyoderma gangrenosum and Sweet syndrome: the prototypic neutrophilic dermatoses. Br J Dermatol. 2015. https://doi.org/10.1111/bjd.13955.
2. Wallach D, Vignon Pennamen MD. From acute febrile neutrophilic dermatosis to neutrophilic disease: forty years of clinical research. J Am Acad Dermatol. 2006;55:1066–71.
3. Cheng S, Edmonds E, Ben-Gashir M, Yu RC. Subcorneal pustular dermatosis: 50 years on. Clin Exper Dermatol. 2008;33:229–33.
4. Wallach D. Intraepidermal IgA pustulosis. J Am Acad Dermatol. 1992;27:993–1000.
5. Koester G, Tarnower A, Levisohn D, Burgdorf W. Bullous pyoderma gangrenosum. J Am Acad Dermatol. 1993;29:875–8.
6. Boms S, Gambichler T. Review of literature on amicrobial pustulosis of the folds associated with autoimmune disorders. Am J Clin Dermatol. 2006;7:369–74.
7. Shangar S, Sterling JC, Rytina E. Pustular pyoderma gangrenosum. Clin Exper Dermatol. 2003;28:600–3.
8. Naik HB, Cowen EW. Autoinflammatory pustular neutrophilic diseases. Dermatol Clin. 2013;31:405–25.
9. Jordaan HF. Acute febrile neutrophilic dermatosis. A histopathological study of 37 patients and review of the literature. Am J Dermatopathol. 1989;11:99–11.
10. Ratzinger G, Burgdorf W, Zelger BG, Zelger B. Acute febrile neutrophilic dermatosis: a histopathologic study of 31 cases with review of literature. Am J Dermatopathol. 2007;29:125–33.
11. Malone JC, Slone SP, Wills-Frank LA, Fearneyhough PK, Lear SC, Jane Goldsmith L, Hood AF, Callen JP. Vascular inflammation (vasculitis) in Sweet syndrome. A clinicopathologic study of 28 biopsy specimens from 21 patients. Arch Dermatol. 2002;138:345–9.
12. Cohen PR, Kurzrock R. Sweet's syndrome revisited: a review of disease concepts. Int J Dermatol. 2003;42:761–78.
13. Bachmeyer C, Aractingi S. Neutrophilic eccrine hidradenitis. Clin Dermatol. 2000;18:319–30.
14. Magro CM, Crowson AN. The spectrum of cutaneous lesions in rheumatoid arthritis: a clinical and pathological study of 43 patients. J Cutan Pathol. 2003;30:1–10.
15. Leboit PE, Yen TSB, Wintroub B. The evolution of lesions in erythemaelevatum diutinum. Am J Dermatopathol. 1986;8:392–402.
16. Wilson-Jones E, Winkelmann RK. Superficial granulomatous pyoderma: a localized vegetative form of pyoderma gangrenosum. J Am Acad Dermatol. 1988;18:511–21.
17. Karadogan SK, Baskan EB, Alkan G, Saricaoglu H, Tunali S. Generalized Sweet syndrome lesions associated with Behçet disease: a true association or simply co-morbidity? Am J Clin Dermatol. 2009;10:331–5.
18. Kieffer C, Cribier B, Lipsker D. Neutrophilic urticaial dermatosis: a variant of neutrophilic urticaria strongly associated with systemic disease. Report of 9 new cases and review of the literature. Medicine (Baltimore). 2009;88:23–31.
19. Larson AR, Laga AC, Granter SR. The spectrum of histopathologic findings in cutaneous lesions in patients with Still disease. Am J Clin Pathol. 2015;144:945–51.
20. Wilkerson A, King R, Googe PB, Page RN, Fulk CS. Sweet's syndrome-like blastomycosis. Am J Dermatopathol. 2003;25:152–4.
21. Haydee Chacon A, Farooq U, Shiman MI, Nolan B, Elgart GW. Cutaneous aspergillosis masquerading as Sweet's syndrome in a patient with acute myelogenous leukemia. J Cutan Pathol. 2013;40:66–8.
22. Ko JS, Fernandez AP, Anderson KA, Burdick LM, Billings SD, Procop GW, McMahon JT, Bergfeld WF, Piliang MP. Morphologic mimickers of Cryptococcus occurring within inflammatory infiltrates in the setting of neutrophilic dermatitis: a series of three cases highlighting clinical dilemmas associated with a novel histopathologic pitfall. J Cutan Pathol. 2013;40:38–45.

23. Byekova YA, Shedd AD, Schiro JA, Barrett TL, Lewin MR. An additional case of neutrophilic dermatosis histopathogically mimicking *Cryptococcus* in a patient with Sweet's syndrome. J Cutan Pathol. 2014;41:972–4.
24. Wilson TC, Stone MS, Swick BL. Histiocytoid Sweet syndrome with haloed myeloid cells masquerading as a cryptococcal infection. Am J Dermatopathol. 2014;36:264–9.
25. Gulati A, Paige D, Yaqoob M, Proby CM, Cerio R, Harwood CA. Palisaded neutrophilic granulomatous dermatitis associated with systemic lupus erythematosus presenting with the burning rope sign. J Am Acad Dermatol. 2009;61:711–4.
26. de Unamuno Bustos B, Rabasco AG, de Miquel VA. Palisaded neutrophilic and granulomatous dermatitis associated with ankylosing spondylitis. Am J Dermatopathol. 2013;35:847–50.
27. Hu CH, O'Loughlin S, Winkelmann RK. Cutaneous manifestations of Wegener granulomatosis. Arch Dermatol. 1977;113:175–82.
28. Stephenson SR, Campbell SM, Drew GS, Magro CM. Palisaded neutrophilic and granulomatous dermitis presenting in a patient with rheumatoid arthritis on adalimumab. J Cutan Pathol. 2011;38:644–8.
29. Rochael MC, Pantaleao L, Guedes Vilar EA, Zacaron LH, Quelhas Spada E, Xavier MH, Strong Rodrigues KS. Sweet's syndrome; study of 73 cases emphasizing histopathological findings. An Bras Dermatol. 2011;86:278–83.
30. Battistella M, Bourrat E, Fardet L, Saada V, Janin A, Vignon-Pennamen MD. Sweet-like reaction due to arthropod bites: a histopathologic pitfall. Am J Dermatopathol. 2012;34:442–5.
31. Ortonne N, Wechsler J, Bagot M, Grosshans E, Cribier B. Granuloma faciale: a clinicopathologic study of 66 patients. J Am Acad Dermatol. 2005;53:1002–9.
32. Larson AR, Granter SR. Systemic lupus erythrmatosus-associated neutrophilic dermatosis. An underrecognized neutrophilic dermatosis in patients with systemic lupus erythematosus. Hum Pathol. 2014;45:598–605.
33. Hau E, Vignon Pennamen MD, Battistella M, Saussine A, Bergis M, Cavelier-Balloy B, Janier M, Cordoliani F, Bagot M, Rybojad M, Bouaziz JD. Neutrophilic skin lesions in autoimmune connective tissue diseases. 9 cases and a literature review. Medicine. 2014;93:e346.
34. Vignon Pennamen MD, Juillard C, Rybojad M, Wallach D, Daniel MT, Morel P, Verola O, Janin A. Chronic recurrent lymphocytic Sweet syndrome as a predictive marker of myelodysplasia. Arch Dermatol. 2006;142:1170–6.
35. Kulasekararaj AG, Kordasti S, Basu T, Salisbury JR, Mufti GJ, du Vivier AWP. Chronic relapsing remitting Sweet syndrome – a harbinger of myelodysplastic syndrome. Br J Haematol. 2015;170:649–56.
36. Requena L, Kutzner H, Palmedo G, Pascual M, Fernandez-Herrera J, Fraga J, Garcia-Diez A, Sanchez Yus E. Histiocytoid Sweet syndrome. A dermal infiltration of immature neutrophilic granulocytes. Arch Dermatol. 2005;141:834–42.
37. Delabie J, De Wolf-Peeters C, Morren M, Marien K, Roskams T, Desmet V. Histiocytes in Sweet's syndrome. Br J Dermatol. 1991;124:348–53.
38. Morioka N, Otsuka F, Nogita T, Igisu K, Urabe A, Ishibashi Y. Neutrophilic dermatosis with myelodysplastic syndrome: nuclear segmentation anomalies of neutrophils in the skin lesion and in peripheral blood. J Am Acad Dermatol. 1990;23:247–9.
39. Chow S, Pasternak S, Green P, Tremaine R, Reardon M, Murray S, Northgrave S, Walsh N. Histiocytoid neutrophilic dermatoses and panniculitides: variations on a theme. Am J Dermatopathol. 2007;29:334–41.
40. Chavan RN, Cappel MA, Ketterling RP, Wada DA, Rochet NM, Knudson R, Gibson LE. Histiocytoid Sweet syndrome may indicate leukemia cutis: a novel application of fluorescent in situ hybridization. J Am Acad Dermatol. 2014;70:1021–7.
41. Magro CM, Momtahen S, Nguyen GH, Wang X. Histiocytoid Sweet's syndrome: a localized cutaneous proliferation of macrophages frequently associated with chronic myeloproliferative disease. Eur J Dermatol. 2015;25:335–41.
42. Peroni A, Colato C, Schena D, Rongioletti F, Girolomoni G. Histiocytoid Sweet syndrome is infiltrated predominantly by M2-like macrophages. J Am Acad Dermatol. 2015;72:131–9.

43. Bush JW, Wick MR. Cutaneous histiocytoid Sweet syndrome and its relationship to hematological diseases. J Cutan Pathol. 2016;43:394–9.
44. Ghoufi L, Ortonne N, Ingen-Housz-Oro S, Barhoumi W, Begon E, Haioun C, Pautas C, Beckerich F, Robin C, Wolkenstein P, Cordonnier C, Chosidow O, Toma A. Histiocytoid Sweet syndrome is more frequently associated with myelodysplastic syndromes than the classical neutrophilic variant. A comparative series of 62 patients. Medicine. 2016;95:e3033.
45. Alegria-Landa V, Rodriguez-Pinilla SM, Santos-Briz A, Rodriguez-Peralto JL, Alegre V, Cerroni L, Kutzner H, Requena L. Clinicopathologic, immunohistochemical, and molecular features of histocytoid Sweet syndrome. JAMA Dermatol. 2017;153:651–9.
46. Osio A, Battistella M, Feugeas JP, Cuccuini W, Petrella T, Raffoux E, Janin A, Vignon Pennamen MD. Myelodysplasia cutis versus leukemia cutis. J Invest Dermatol. 2015;135:2321–4.
47. Van Loon K, Gill RM, McMahon P, Chigurupati R, Siddiqi I, Fox L, Damon L, McCalmont TH, Jordan R, Wolf J. 20q-clonality in a case of oral Sweet syndrome and myelodysplasia. Am J Clin Pathol. 2012;137:310–5.
48. Sujobert P, Cuccuini W, Vignon-Pennamen D, Martin-Garcia N, Albertini AF, Uzunov M, Redjoul R, Dombret H, Raffoux E. Evidence of differenciation in myeloid malignancies associated neutrophilic dermatosis: a fluorescent *in situ* hybridization study of 14 patients. J Invest Dermatol. 2013;133:1111–4.
49. Haga N, Iwata H, Yamaguchi Y, Shirato T, Nishimura K, Yamane N, Shinkuma S, Natsuga K, Kondo T, Shimizu H. Mucocutaneous pyoderma gangrenosum due to trisomy 8 neutrophilic infiltrates in a patient with myelodysplastic syndrome. Br J Dermatol. 2016;174:239–41.
50. Lewis KG, Dill SW, Wilkel CS, Robinson-Bostom L. Mid-dermal elastolysis preceded by acute neutrophilic dermatosis. J Cutan Pathol. 2004;31:72–6.
51. Webb K, Hlela C, Jordaan HF, Sulimlan S, Scriba T, Lipsker D, Scott C. A review and proposal approach to the neutrophilic dermatoses of childhood. Pediatr Dermatol. 2015;32:437–46.
52. Weening RH, Davis MD, Dahl PR, Su WP. Skin ulcers misdiagnosed as pyoderma gangrenosum. N Engl J Med. 2002;347:1412–8.
53. Cohen PR. Subcutaneous Sweet's syndrome: a variant of acute febrile neutrophilic dermatosis that is included in the histopathologic differantial diagnosis of neutrophilic panniculitis. J Am Acad Dermatol. 2005;52:927–8.
54. Sutra-Loubet C, Carlotti A, Guillemette J, Wallach D. Neutrophilic panniculitis. J Am Acad Dermatol. 2004;50:280–5.
55. Becherer K, Golda N, Feldman M, Diaz-Arias A, Caldwell C. Neutrophilic panniculitis associated with myelodysplastic syndrome with abnormal nuclear forms. J Cutan Pathol. 2009;36:1024–6.
56. Chan MP, Duncan LM, Nazarian RM. Subcutaneous Sweet syndrome in the setting of myeloid disorders: a case series and review of the literature. J Am Acad Dermatol. 2013;68:1006–15.
57. Andre M, Piette JC, Kemeny JL, Ninet J, Jego P, Delevaux I, Wechsler B, Weiller PJ, Frances C, Bletry O, Wismans PJ, Rousset H, Colombel JF, Aumaître O, French Study Group on Aseptic Abscesses. Aseptic abscesses: a study of 30 patients with or without inflammatory bowel disease and review of the literature. Medicine. 2007;86:145–61.

The Extra-cutaneous Localizations of the Neutrophilic Disease

16

Didier Bessis

Abbreviations

CRMO	Chronic recurrent multifocal osteomyelitis
CT	Computer tomography
DIRA	Deficiency of interleukin-1 receptor
EED	Erythema elevatum diutinum
GPP	Generalized pustular psoriasis
ND	Neutrophilic disease
NIO	Non-infectious osteomyelitis
PG	Pyoderma gangrenosum
SAPHO	Synovitis, acne, pustulosis, hyperostosis and osteitis
SPD	Subcorneal pustular dermatosis
SwS	Sweet syndrome

In 1991, Vignon-Pennamen and Wallach proposed a unifying and prescient concept of "neutrophilic disease" (ND) in the light of clinical observations: (1) numerous reports of clinicopathological symptoms overlapping the typical forms of ND, including subcorneal pustular dermatosis (SPD; Sneddon-Wilkinson disease); Sweet's syndrome (SwS); pyoderma gangrenosum (PG) and erythema elevatum diutinum (EED); (2) extracutaneous manifestations of neutrophilic disease; (3) non fortuitous association with systemic diseases and (4) usual therapeutic response to corticosteroid and/or dapsone [1]. In their article, they reviewed and argued the rare cases of various organ involvement suspected to be related to ND and previously

D. Bessis
Department of Dermatology, St Eloi Hospital, University of Montpellier Cedex 5, France
e-mail: d-bessis@chu-montpellier.fr

D. Wallach et al. (eds.), *Neutrophilic Dermatoses*,
https://doi.org/10.1007/978-3-319-72649-6_16

reported, generally one or two observations for each organ, including bones, liver, lymph nodes, spleen, lung and kidney. Almost a quarter century later, a large number of extracutaneous manifestations of ND have been reported and allow a clarification on the risk of organ involvement depending on type of neutrophilic diseases, mostly Sweet syndrome and pyoderma gangrenosum, and their treatment (Table 16.1).

Table 16.1 Summary of organ involvement in neutrophilic dermatoses

Organ	Neutrophilic dermatoses	Organ involvement	Main clinical symptoms[a]
Lung	Sweet syndrome (≈40 cases) Pyoderma gangrenosum (≈30 cases) Generalized pustular psoriasis (≈10 cases)	Interstitial pneumonia	Dry cough Dyspnea Chest pain Hemoptysis
Bone	Palmoplantar pustulosis +++ Nonpalmoplantar pustulosis Pyoderma gangrenosum (≈10 cases) Sweet syndrome (exceptional, Majeed syndrome)	CRMO SAPHO Focal aseptic osteitis (pyoderma gangrenosum only)	Bone pain Swelling and tenderness over affected bones
Joints	Sweet syndrome (31–62%) Pyoderma gangrenosum (19–56%) Erythema elevatum diutinum (5–25%)	Seronegative destructive polyarthritis Seronegative nondestructive polyarthritis Monoarthritis	Arthralgia
Muscle	Sweet syndrome (10%) Pyoderma gangrenosum	Neutrophilic myositis (rare)	Myalgias Muscle weakness (rare)
Central nervous system	Sweet syndrome (≈70 cases)	Encephalitis	Disturbing of consciousness Headache Memory disorders
Intraabdominal viscera			
Liver	Pyoderma gangrenosum (<10 cases) Sweet syndrome (rare) Generalized pustular psoriasis	Abscess (pyoderma gangrenosum only) Neutrophilic cholangitis (psoriasis) Liver tests abnormalities	Epigastric pain Jaundice

Table 16.1 (continued)

Organ	Neutrophilic dermatoses	Organ involvement	Main clinical symptoms[a]
Spleen	Pyoderma gangrenosum (≈10 cases) Sweet syndrome (3 cases) Pustular subcorneal dermatosis (1 case)	Abscess	Abdominal pain
Pancréas	Pyoderma gangrenosum (2 cases) Sweet syndrome (1 case)	Acute pancreatitis	Abdominal pain
Heart	Sweet syndrome (<10 cases)	Myopericarditis Acute valvulitis Aneurysms and chronic valvulitis (elastolysis, in children only)	Dyspnea Chest pain Heart failure
Eye	Sweet syndrome (20–30%) Pyoderma gangrenosum (34 cases) Erythema elevatum diutinum (<10 cases) Generalized pustular psoriasis (rare)	Periorbital and orbital inflammation Dacryoadenitis, conjunctivitis, episcleritis, scleritis, keratitis, iritis, choroiditis, glaucoma and limbal nodules	Ocular inflammation Vision impairment
Kidney1	Sweet syndrome (rare) Pyoderma gangrenosum (exceptional)	Glomerulonephritis	Asymptomatic
Fallopian tube	Pyoderma gangrenosum (1 case)	Aseptic pyosalpinx	Abdominal pain

Abreviations: *CRMO* chronic recurrent multifocal osteomyelitis, *SAPHO* synovitis, acne, pustulosis, hyperostosis and osteitis
[a]Excluding general signs

Lung

Pulmonary manifestations are rarely reported in the context of ND, mostly in patients with SwS or PG [2]. Most patients had fever and non-specific pulmonary symptoms including dry cough, dyspnea, chest pain or hemoptysis, but asymptomatic chest radiological discoveries have also been reported. In any case and in the absence of pathognomonic laboratory tests, chest radiological characteristics or specific pathologic changes, lung diseases such as pulmonary infections, malignancy or vasculitis (granulomatosis with polyangiitis) need to be excluded before the diagnosis of lung neutrophilic disease can be done [3]. Almost 40 cases of SwS with pulmonary involvement have been reported, the most recent review of the literature in 2012 recording 34 cases [4]. The male/female ratio was 1:1 and the age average 57 years old (±14 years, range 25–82 years old). Skin lesions appeared before pulmonary involvement in almost one case in two, whereas skin and pulmonary manifestations were simultaneous in one-third of the cases. No clinical or histological signs of cutaneous lesions of SwS appears clinically predictive of lung involvement. SwS with pulmonary involvement seems to be more frequently associated with hematologic disorders than classical (or idiopathic) SwS, in almost half of cases. The main symptoms of pulmonary involvement are progressive dyspnea, dry cough and fever. Chest radiograph (X-ray or computer tomography (CT) scan) confirms pulmonary lesions, disclosing almost consistently unilateral or bilateral interstitial infiltrates, more rarely unique or multiple opacities and/or pleural effusion. Videobronchoscopy is usually normal. When bronchoalveolar lavage is performed, it shows a predominance of neutrophils (>50%) and open-lung biopsy or transbronchial biopsy discloses interstitial inflammation, edema and intra-alveolar dense infiltration by neutrophils [5]. More than 30 cases of PG with pulmonary involvement have been described, the most recent review of the literature in 2015 recording 29 cases, including 3 pediatric cases [6]. In adult PG, the female/male ratio was 1.6 and the age average 31.5 years old (range 17–82 years old). PG with pulmonary involvement seems to be more frequently associated with hematologic disorders, in almost 28% of cases. Skin lesions appeared before or simultaneously with pulmonary involvement in more than two-thirds of the cases. The most frequent radiological lung alterations in PG are quite similar with SwS with pulmonary involvement with the exception of infiltrates with cavitation, which appears more frequent in pulmonary PG (one-third of cases) (Fig. 16.1). Prognosis of SwS and PG associated with pulmonary lesions is good and treatment relies on systemic corticosteroids, usually after failure of empirical antimicrobial and/or antifungal therapy.

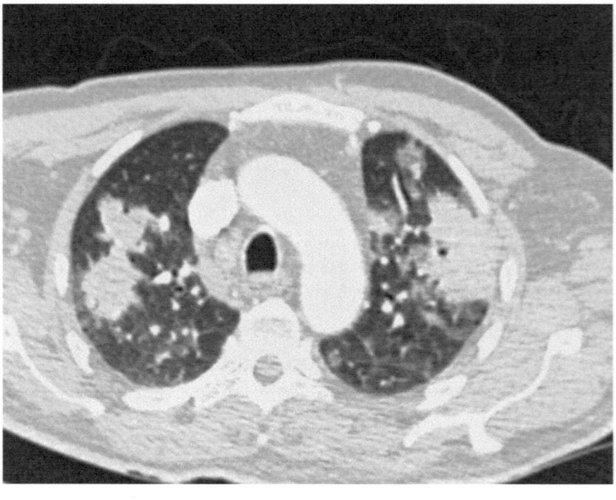

Fig. 16.1 Pulmonary involvement of pyoderma gangrenosum in a 57-year-old man. Chest CT scan shows bilateral asymmetric alveolar infiltrate (Courtesy Prof. M-S. Doutre MD, Bo1rdeaux, France)

Generalized pustular psoriasis (GPP) associated with aseptic pneumonitis is a rare, and perhaps underestimated complication of psoriasis, previously reported under the term "acute respiratory distress syndrome", "capillary leak syndrome" or "sterile pneumonitis". By 2017, ten cases had been described [7, 8]. The female/male ratio 1.5 and the average age 41 years old (range 14–62 years old). Time of psoriasis onset doesn't appear to be a risk factor for lung involvement. All patients develop rapid respiratory deterioration with dyspnea and arterial hypoxemia in a febrile context and an elevation of circulating neutrophils. Chest radiograph (X-ray or CT scan) shows bilateral interstitial infiltration with alveolar alterations (Fig. 16.2). Lung infection or drug-induced hypersensitivity reaction related to systemic treatment of psoriasis (methotrexate, acitretin, anti-tumor necrosis factor-alpha, ustekinumab) should be promptly considered in the

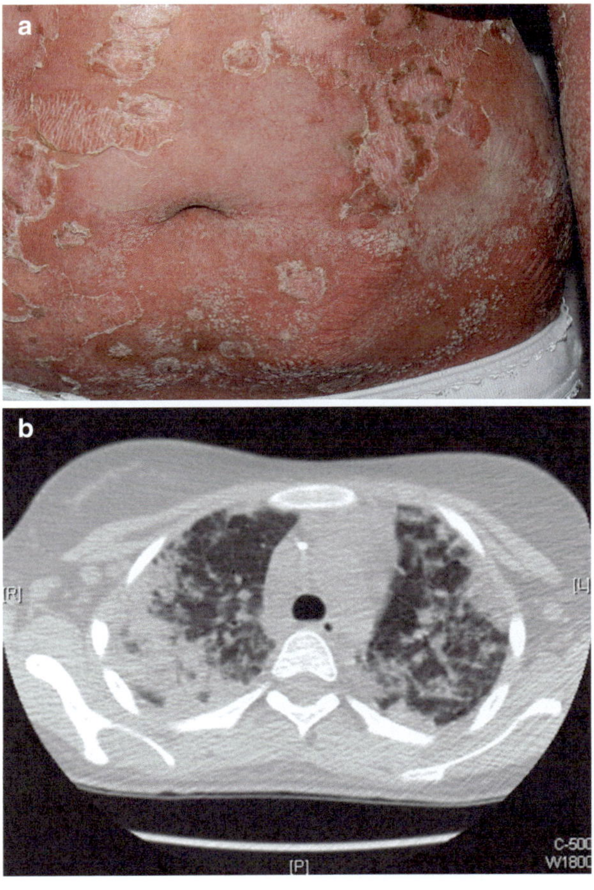

Fig. 16.2 Generalized pustular psoriasis associated with aseptic pneumonitis in a 14-year-old girl. (**a**) Pustular psoriasis of the abdomen. (**b** and **c**) Thoracic CT scan shows bilateral interstitial infiltrate and alveolar findings. Note the predominance of infiltrate in upper lobes and bilateral pleurisy

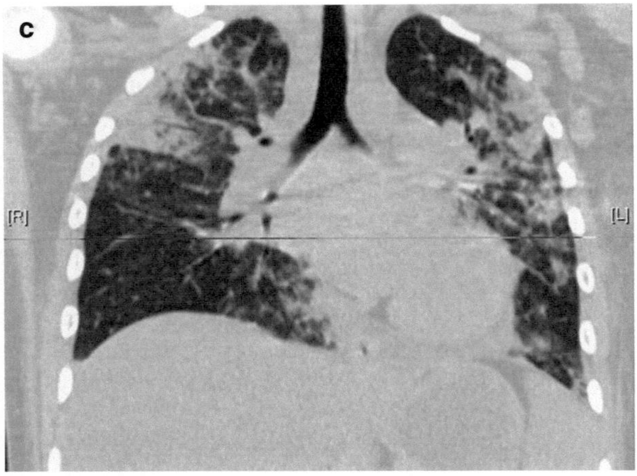

Fig. 16.2 (continued)

differential diagnosis. The outcome of GPP associated aseptic pneumonitis shows a high risk of death (three of the ten reported cases) and treatment requires transfer to an intensive care unit as mechanical ventilation and hemodynamic control is often necessary. It relies on systemic corticosteroid therapy at high doses in association with antibiotics, as ruling out primary or secondary pulmonary infection is usually impossible.

Bone

Chronic recurrent multifocal osteomyelitis (CRMO) belongs to the group of non-infectious osteomyelitis (NIO) and is characterized by recurrent, chronic and multifocal sterile bone lesions. Among the other specific entities within the group of NIO, including Majeed syndrome, deficiency of interleukin-1 receptor antagonist (DIRA) and synovitis, acne, pustulosis, hyperostosis and osteitis (SAPHO) syndrome, the latter is mostly considered as the adult form of CRMO due to clinical and radiological similarities [9]. Clinical features of CRMO are bone pain, usually with an insidious onset, associated with swelling and tenderness over the affected bones, predominantly the metaphyses and epiphyses of the long bones including femur, tibia or humerus, or more rarely clavicle, sternum, mandible or vertebrae. One to nearly 20 sites could be involved, with a median number of two bone lesions at onset of disease. Fever, arthralgias and myalgias are often present. In most cases, bone biopsies showed non-specific inflammatory changes in early stage combining osteolysis and infiltrate composed mainly of neutrophils and giant cells, followed by the presence of lymphocytes, plasma cells and monocytes and, in latter stage, sclerosis and hyperostosis. During flares, mild elevations in the leukocyte count, erythrocyte sedimentation rate and C-reactive protein are noted. Radiological signs (X-rays) are osteolysis (radiolucent areas), sclerosis and new bone formation, sometimes associated with periosteal reactions or soft tissue swelling. CRMO is strongly associated with ND including palmoplantar pustulosis (about 20%), mostly considered as a variant of pustular psoriasis, and nonpalmoplantar pustulosis. Direct temporal correlation between ND and bony lesions is not constant [10]. About ten cases of PG associated with CRMO have been described, some of them being associated with Crohn's disease [11, 12] and Takayasu arteritis [13, 14], these latter conditions being also possible etiologies of CRMO. Association of SwS and CRMO remains exceptional [15] and is mostly reported in pediatric patients during Majeed syndrome, an exceedingly rare autoinflammatory bone disease due to homozygous mutations in *LPIN2*, which encodes LIPIN2, a phosphatidase phosphatase acting in lipid metabolism [16]. Rare cases of focal aseptic osteitis underlying PG with contiguous osteolysis have been reported in PG of the scalp [17], ulna [18], tibia [19] and wrist [20]. Treatment of CRMO-associated ND relies on nonsteroidal anti-inflammatory drugs (indomethacin, naproxen) or systemic corticosteroid therapy (i.v. methylprednisolone, oral prednisolone).

Joints and Muscle

Articular manifestations are frequently mentioned during SwS and PG with an average frequency of 40%, varying from 31% to 62% in SwS [5, 21–23] and 19 to 56% in PG [24–26]. Articular involvement appears more rarely during EED, between 5 and 25% [27] and is anecdotal during subcorneal pustular dermatosis [28]. However, the origin of joint involvement in ND remains difficult to establish, taking in account various systemic associated diseases, in particular inflammatory bowel diseases and inflammatory rheumatic diseases (rheumatoid polyarthritis, ankylosing spondylitis). Three patterns of arthritis have been individualized in ND, mostly SwS and PG: chronic, progressive, seronegative destructive polyarthritis with axial or peripheral involvement mainly in PG and usually antedating the PG; seronegative, nondestructive, nondeforming polyarthritis that parallels the evolution of ND flares; and acute, seronegative monoarticular inflammation involving large joints [2, 29, 30]. They may precede ND but they are most often observed during the course of ND, occurring simultaneously with recurrences of skin lesions [31]. Favorable outcome is usually observed with systemic corticosteroid therapy.

Muscle involvement with myalgias is barely mentioned during ND, fewer than 10% in a large series of ND [31]. Specific neutrophilic myositis revealed by muscle weakness of the limbs and histologically characterized by intense neutrophilic infiltration throughout the muscle has been reported in one observation of PG associated with acute myelogenous leukemia [32].

Central Nervous System

Neuro-SwS disease was first defined in 1999 to design cases of encephalitis associated with SwS [33] and subsequently, in a large manner, for SwS with neurological involvement, including a wide range of symptoms and signs. Based on a large series of 42 patients with SwS disease and neurologic manifestations, diagnostic criteria of neuro-SwS have been proposed (Table 16.2) [34]. A review of the literature in 2017 compiles 69 cases of neuro-SwS disease [35]. The male/female ratio was 2, with a

Table 16.2 Criteria for neuro-Sweet disease

1. Neurologic features	
	Highly systemic glucocorticoid responsive or sometimes spontaneously remitting, but frequently recurrent encephalitis or meningitis, usually accompagnied with fever over 38 °C
2. Dermatologic features	
	Painful or tender, dull red erythematous plaques or nodules preferentially occuring on the face, neck, upper limbs, and upper part of the trunk
	Predominantly neutrophilic infiltration of the dermis, spared epidermis, and absence of leukocytoclastic vasculitis
3. Other features	
	Absence of cutaneous vasculitis and thrombosis, which are seen in Behçet disease
	Absence of typical uveitis, which is seen in Behçet disease
4. HLA association	
	HLA-Cw1 or B54 positive
	HLA-B51 negative

Probable neuro-Sweet disease: all of 1, 2 and 3
Possible neuro-Sweet disease: any neurologic manifestations, either 2 or 4 and one item or more of 3
Any other neurologic diseases that can explainthe neurologic symptoms and signs, except neuro-Behçet disease, should be excluded before the diagnosis of neuro-Sweet disease is made

greater predilection for Asian patients (81%) than Caucasian (19%), and the average age was 48.7 years old (range 7 weeks to 76 years old). The initial episodes of neurologic symptoms usually followed (44.9%) or occurred concurrently (27.5%) with cutaneous SwS. The neurological symptoms were varied, including disturbances of consciousness (confusion, somnolence, coma) in almost half of cases, followed by headache (42%) and memory disorders (27.5%). Many other additional signs/symptoms have been described with lower frequencies including generalized seizures, hemi/tetraparesis, dysarthria, ocular movement disorders, meningitis, disorientation, psychiatric symptoms, involuntary movements, ataxia, sensory disturbances and diplopia [35]. Brain magnetic resonance and/or computed tomography imaging findings are usually found (90%), non-specific, asymmetric and rather disseminated without site predilection: brainstem, cortex, basal ganglia, sub-cortex and thalamus, and less frequently subcortical white matter. Cerebrospinal fluid examination might show a mild increase in protein content and mild to moderate pleocytosis, with a predominance of lymphocytes. The main differential diagnosis of neuro-SwS remains neuro-Behçet disease, the latter sharing common clinical features including oral and genital aphthous, erythema nodosum-like lesions and inflammatory ocular symptoms. The arguments supporting the preferred diagnosis of neuro-Behçet disease are based on earlier age at neurological onset (20–30 years old), an elective location of basal ganglia and brainstem, the frequent and sometimes severe neurological sequelae and the typical lesions of Behçet's disease including vasculitis (frequent in skin lesions), thrombosis and uveitis (*versus* episcleritis and conjunctivitis in neuro-SwS). HLA typing could also be relevant insofar as frequency of HLA-B51 is increased in Behçet's disease while HLA-B54 and -Cw1 are mostly positive in case series of neuro-SwS of Japanese patients (usually not tested in Caucasian patients) [35]. The outcome of neuro-SwS is usually benign and transient, neurologic recurrences or sequelae being infrequent, respectively in 23.5% and 13.2% [35]. Treatment relies on systemic oral or intravenous corticosteroids at high doses, sometimes associated with dapsone or ciclosporine in initial management or as corticosteroid-sparing agents.

Intra-abdominal Viscera

Specific hepatic, splenic and/or pancreatic involvement has rarely been reported associated with ND [36–40]. Increased levels of alkaline phosphatase, when present, could be related to the inflammatory syndrome commonly observed during SwS. Mild liver enzymes abnormalities are rare and, in such cases, role of associated comorbidities directly associated or not with SwS or drug intake must be sought. One case of neutrophilic cholangitis associated with Sweet syndrome has been reported [41].

Three observations of PG with aseptic neutrophilic abscesses of the liver (Fig. 16.3), associated with pancreatic (2 cases) or spleen (1 case) or bone (1 case) involvement, have been described [37–39]. Cytological and bacteriological examination of abscesses after direct needle aspiration showed a purulent sterile fluid composed of neutrophils. Favorable and rapid response was consistently observed with corticosteroid therapy. Ten observations of PG with spleen involvement were compiled in 2016 [40]. Spleen involvement was always consistent with multiple spleen abscesses, mostly diagnosed after appearance of PG skin lesions (70%). Spleen lesions can occur at any age (mean age 45 years; range 8–82 years), more frequently in men and can be asymptomatic or revealed by fever, malaise, abdominal pain and splenomegaly. When histologic assessment was performed, it showed a non-specific neutrophil infiltration. Most patients respond well to corticosteroids associated or not with other suppressive agents. Similar observations of spleen neutrophilic abscesses, although much rarer, have also been described associated with SwS [42–44]. and subcorneal pustular dermatosis [45].

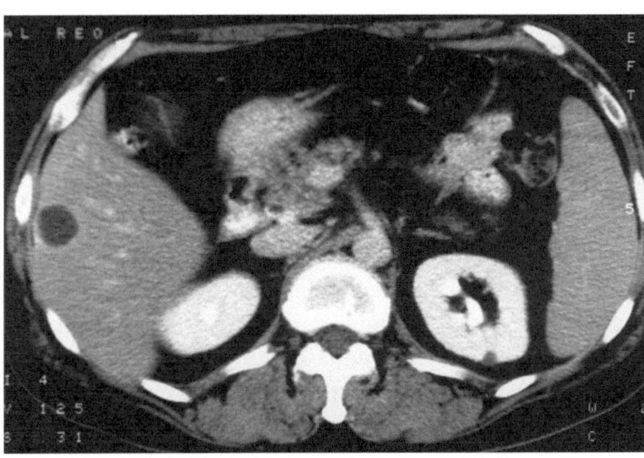

Fig. 16.3 Hepatic involvement of pyoderma gangrenosum in a 45-year-old woman. Abdominal CT scan shows hepatic abscess in the right lobe of liver

Abnormalities in liver enzymes with GPP are frequent and reported between 47% and 90% of cases [46, 47], evolving in parallel with cutaneous flares. Mostly asymptomatic, they can be associated with epigastric pain or jaundice reflecting specific neutrophilic involvement of the biliary tract due to neutrophilic cholangitis [47]. Rapid resolution of biological abnormalities and hepatobiliary clinical manifestations could be observed with anti-tumour necrosis factor agents (infliximab, etanercept) [48, 49].

Heart and Blood Vessels

Cardiac manifestations associated with neutrophilic dermatosis are very unusual, in less than ten cases, being reported almost exclusively with SwS. They include schematically two types of manifestations: (1) myopericarditis with histological neutrophilic infiltration of the myocardium [50–52], sometimes associated with acute valvulitis of aortic or mitral valve [50, 53]. The main suggestive symptoms are dyspnea, chest pain or heart failure and usually occurred simultaneously with the cutaneous lesions of SwS; (2) Acquired post-inflammatory cutis laxa (elastolysis) in children leading to multiple dilatations and aneurysms of the aorta, pulmonary, and coronary arteries or mitral valvulitis, observed months to years following the cutaneous SwS [54–56]. In these cases, asymptomatic cardiac and vascular arterial neutrophilic infiltrates parallel to the initial cutaneous eruption and complicated by scarring lesions seem probable although not proved [54]

Eye

Ocular inflammation occurs in about 20–30% of patients with SwS [5, 31, 57]. A review of the different manifestations of ocular involvement in SwS in 2008, based on 20 patients with SwS, included periorbital and orbital inflammation, dacryoadenitis, conjunctivitis, episcleritis, scleritis, limbal nodules, peripheral ulcerative keratitis, iritis, glaucoma and choroiditis [58]. The initial episodes of ophthalmologic symptoms usually occurred concurrently with the cutaneous lesions of SwS, or a few days later. In half of cases, ocular inflammation was unilateral. Biopsies of periocular or ocular tissue have been performed in 7 of the 20 cases and showed a similar histopathology to that of the cutaneous lesions, with dense neutrophilic infiltrates [58]. About ten cases of involvement of posterior structures in the eye (vitreous and retina) during SwS have been published, including bilateral retinal vasculitis and panuveitis, always complicated by a decrease in visual acuity [59–62]. In these cases, differential diagnosis may be difficult with ocular involvement of Behçet disease that shares common clinical features with SwS. Treatment of ocular inflammation of the anterior structures of the eye relies on oral corticosteroid therapy with a rapid response. In cases of retinal vasculitis or panuveitis, treatment is a medical emergency due to the risk of irreversible vision impairment induced by retinal ischemia. Systemic or intraocular steroids are the first line treatment, depending on the severity. Association with methotrexate, azathioprine or ciclosporine is also reported without definitive conclusion about their interest.

In a recent review of the literature, published in 2017, 34 cases of PG involving the eye and periorbital area have been recorded [63]. Most patients were older than 60 years (mean age 58; range 27–90 years old) with a slight predilection for females (male/female ratio 1:1.2). Ocular PG was most commonly due to cutaneous periocular PG (38%) and ocular diseases associated with PG (35%) including peripheral ulcerative keratitis, scleritis and scleromalacia. Ocular PG was mostly unilateral and often occurs at site of trauma, even minor. The most common cutaneous presenting sign was ulceration while the main ophthalmic signs were peripheral ulcerative keratitis, eye redness and decreased visual acuity. Close to 45% of ocular PG were associated with an underlying disease commonly described in classic PG cases, including inflammatory bowel disease, myeloproliferative disorders, rheumatoid arthritis and diabetes mellitus. Systemic corticosteroids are the first line treatment, usually paired with another systemic immunomodulatory agent including cyclosporine, azathioprine or dapsone due to the risk of corticosteroid-resistance. Surgical intervention is avoided in the initial phase of treatment because of the risk of pathergic reaction but could be considered after stabilization of the disease with medical treatment in order to improve wound healing and reduce morbidity [63].

Ocular involvement associated with EED has been reported in less than ten cases [64, 65], mostly peripheral keratitis, ranging from slowly progressive corneal thinning (Terrien marginal degeneration) to rapidly progressive keratolysis resulting in corneal perforation [64]. Treatment mostly relies on dapsone (except one case with cyclophosphamide and oral prednisone) with rapid therapeutic efficacy.

Ocular changes associated with GPP are rarely reported and included blepharitis, sterile purulent conjunctivitis, iridocyclitis, corneal ulceration, exfoliation of the cornea and uveitis particularly of the anterior uveal tract [66, 67]. The latter complication doesn't appear more frequent than in psoriasis vulgaris [68].

Kidney

Renal involvement in neutrophilic dermatoses is rarely reported, mostly during SwS, and usually manifesting as proteinuria, less often as hematuria, renal insufficiency, biopsy-diagnosed mesangiocapillary glomerulonephritis [2] and more rarely nodular kidney involvement [69]. Skin and renal involvement are usually simultaneous, with a parallel outcome, treatment by systemic corticosteroids restoring normal kidney function in most patients. Only few PG cases with renal involvement have been described [2], one of which with histopathologic findings of renal biopsy consistent with PG [70].

Fallopian Tube

A unique observation of aseptic pyosalpinx extending to ileocaecal junction, associated with PG during pregnancy has been reported [71]. Although about ten cases of cutaneous PG have already been reported during pregnancy [72], no other case of neutrophilic disease with Fallopian tube localization has been described since.

References

1. Vignon-Pennamen MD, Wallach D. Cutaneous manifestations of neutrophilic disease. A study of seven cases. Dermatologica. 1991;183(4):255–64.
2. Prat L, Bouaziz JD, Wallach D, Vignon-Pennamen MD, Bagot M. Neutrophilic dermatoses as systemic diseases. Clin Dermatol. 2014;32(3):376–88.
3. Astudillo L, Sailler L, Launay F, Josse AG, Lamant L, Couret B, Arlet-Suau E. Pulmonary involvement in Sweet's syndrome: a case report and review of the literature. Int J Dermatol. 2006;45(6):677–80.
4. Fernandez-Bussy S, Labarca G, Cabello F, Cabello H, Folch E, Majid A. Sweet's syndrome with pulmonary involvement: Case report and literature review. Respir Med Case Rep. 2012;6:16–9.
5. Fett DL, Gibson LE, Su WP. Sweet's syndrome: systemic signs and symptoms and associated disorders. Mayo Clin Proc. 1995;70(3):234–40.
6. Gade M, Studstrup F, Andersen AK, Hilberg O, Fogh C, Bendstrup E. Pulmonary manifestations of pyoderma gangrenosum: 2 cases and a review of the literature. Respir Med. 2015;109(4):443–50.
7. Kluger N, Bessis D, Guillot B, Girard C. Acute respiratory distress syndrome complicating generalized pustular psoriasis (psoriasis-associated aseptic pneumonitis). J Am Acad Dermatol. 2011;64(6):1154–8.
8. Maehara Lde S, Mariano MM, Góis AF, Padilha MH, Yamada S, Porro AM. Acute respiratory distress syndrome as a complication of generalized pustular psoriasis. An Bras Dermatol. 2011;86(3):579–81.
9. Costa-Reis P, Sullivan KE. Chronic recurrent multifocal osteomyelitis. J Clin Immunol. 2013;33(6):1043–56.
10. Tlougan BE, Podjasek JO, O'Haver J, Cordova KB, Nguyen XH, Tee R, Pinckard-Hansen KC, Hansen RC. Chronic recurrent multifocal osteomyelitis (CRMO) and synovitis, acne, pustulosis, hyperostosis, and osteitis (SAPHO) syndrome with associated neutrophilic dermatoses: a report of seven cases and review of the literature. Pediatr Dermatol. 2009;26(5):497–505.
11. Felton S, Al-Niaimi F, Lyon C. Severe back pain in a young patient with pyoderma gangrenosum and Crohn's disease controlled with anti-tumor necrosis factor therapy: sterile osteomyelitis. Dermatol Ther (Heidelb). 2014;4(1):137–40.
12. Omidi CJ, Siegfried EC. Chronic recurrent multifocal osteomyelitis preceding pyoderma gangrenosum and occult ulcerative colitis in a pediatric patient. Pediatr Dermatol. 1998;15(6):435–8.
13. Dagan O, Barak Y, Metzker A. Pyoderma gangrenosum and sterile multifocal osteomyelitis preceding the appearance of Takayasu arteritis. Pediatr Dermatol. 1995;12(1):39–42.
14. Vettiyil G, Punnen A, Kumar S. An unusual association of chronic recurrent multifocal osteomyelitis, pyoderma gangrenosum, and Takayasu arteritis. J Rheumatol. 2017;44(1):127–8.
15. Hospach T, von den Driesch P, Dannecker GE. Acute febrile neutrophilic dermatosis (Sweet's syndrome) in childhood and adolescence: two new patients and review of the literature on associated diseases. Eur J Pediatr. 2009;168(1):1–9.
16. Ferguson PJ, Chen S, Tayeh MK, Ochoa L, Leal SM, Pelet A, Munnich A, Lyonnet S, Majeed HA, El-Shanti H. Homozygous mutations in LPIN2 are responsible for the syndrome of

chronic recurrent multifocal osteomyelitis and congenital dyserythropoietic anaemia (Majeed syndrome). J Med Genet. 2005;42(7):551–7.
17. Samlaska CP, Smith RA, Myers JB, Bottini AG, Person DA. Pyoderma gangrenosum and cranial osteolysis: case report and review of the paediatric literature. Br J Dermatol. 1995;133(6):972–7.
18. Hayes RC, Curtis A. Pyoderma gangrenosum with a contiguous erosion of the distal ulna. J Cutan Med Surg. 2004;8(3):162–5.
19. Marie I, Boyer A, Heron F, Joly P, Levesque H, Thomine E, Courtois H. Focal aseptic osteitis underlying neutrophilic dermatosis. Br J Dermatol. 1998;139(4):744–5.
20. Choe H, Sakano H, Takigami H, Inaba Y, Matsuo K, Saito T. Pyoderma gangrenosum with wrist joint destruction: case report. J Hand Surg Am. 2013;38(2):357–61.
21. Kemmett D, Hunter JA. Sweet's syndrome: a clinicopathologic review of twenty-nine cases. J Am Acad Dermatol. 1990;23(3 Pt 1):503–7.
22. Sitjas D, Puig L, Cuatrecasas M, De Moragas JM. Acute febrile neutrophilic dermatosis (Sweet's syndrome). Int J Dermatol. 1993;32(4):261–8.
23. Cohen PR, Kurzrock R. Sweet's syndrome and cancer. Clin Dermatol. 1993;11(1):149–57.
24. Vidal D, Puig L, Gilaberte M, Alomar A. Review of 26 cases of classical pyoderma gangrenosum: clinical and therapeutic features. J Dermatolog Treat. 2004;15(3):146–52.
25. Mlika RB, Riahi I, Fenniche S, Mokni M, Dhaoui MR, Dess N, Dhahri AB, Mokhtar I. Pyoderma gangrenosum: a report of 21 cases. Int J Dermatol. 2002;41(2):65–8.
26. Binus AM, Qureshi AA, Li VW, Winterfield LS. Pyoderma gangrenosum: a retrospective review of patient characteristics, comorbidities and therapy in 103 patients. Br J Dermatol. 2011;165(6):1244–50.
27. Momen SE, Jorizzo J, Al-Niaimi F. Erythema elevatum diutinum: a review of presentation and treatment. J Eur Acad Dermatol Venereol. 2014;28(12):1594–602.
28. Cheng S, Edmonds E, Ben-Gashir M, Yu RC. Subcorneal pustular dermatosis: 50 years on. Clin Exp Dermatol. 2008;33(3):229–33.
29. Wallach D, Vignon-Pennamen MD. From acute febrile neutrophilic dermatosis to neutrophilic disease: forty years of clinical research. J Am Acad Dermatol. 2006;55(6):1066–71.
30. Powell FC, WP S, Perry HO. Pyoderma gangrenosum: classification and management. J Am Acad Dermatol. 1996;34(3):395–409.
31. Moreland LW, Brick JE, Kovach RE, DiBartolomeo AG, Mullins MC. Acute febrile neutrophilic dermatosis (Sweet syndrome): a review of the literature with emphasis on musculoskeletal manifestations. Semin Arthritis Rheum. 1988;17(3):143–53.
32. Marie I, Levesque H, Joly P, Reumont G, Courville P, Baudrimont M, Baubion D, Cailleux N, Courtois H. Neutrophilic myositis as an extracutaneous manifestation of neutrophilic dermatosis. J Am Acad Dermatol. 2001;44(1):137–9.
33. Hisanaga K, Hosokawa M, Sato N, Mochizuki H, Itoyama Y, Iwasaki Y. "Neuro-sweet disease": benign recurrent encephalitis with neutrophilic dermatosis. Arch Neurol. 1999;56(8):1010–3.
34. Hisanaga K, Iwasaki Y, Itoyama Y, Neuro-Sweet Disease Study Group. Neuro-Sweet disease: clinical manifestations and criteria for diagnosis. Neurology. 2005;64(10):1756–61.
35. Drago F, Ciccarese G, Agnoletti AF, Sarocchi F, Parodi A. Neuro sweet syndrome: a systematic review. A rare complication of Sweet syndrome. Acta Neurol Belg. 2017;117(1):33–42.
36. Petit A, Dupuy A, Pépin È, Gardies A, Gaulier A, Sigal M. Sweet's syndrome associated with pancreatitis. A chance association? Eur J Dermatol. 1994;4:453–5.
37. Hastier P, Caroli-Bosc FX, Bartel HR, Harris AG, Maes B, Arpurt JP, Taillan B, Bodock I, Dumas R, Delmont JP. Pyoderma gangrenosum with hepatopancreatic manifestations in a patient with rheumatoid arthritis. Dig Dis Sci. 1996;41(3):594–7.
38. Vadillo M, Jucgla A, Podzamczer D, Rufi G, Domingo A. Pyoderma gangrenosum with liver, spleen and bone involvement in a patient with chronic myelomonocytic leukaemia. Br J Dermatol. 1999;141(3):541–3.
39. Ferrazzi V, Rivière S, Sany J. Association of pyoderma gangrenosum with hepato-pancreatic involvement in rheumatoid polyarthritis. Rev Med Interne. 1996;17(3):266–7.

40. Cosgarea R, Senilă SC, Badea R, Ungureanu L. Pyoderma gangrenosum with spleen involvement. Review of the literature and case report. J Dermatol Case Rep. 2016;10(2):26–31.
41. Matta M, Malak J, Tabet E, et al. Sweet's syndrome: systemic associations. Cutis. 1973;12:561–5.
42. Quilichini R, Mazzerbo F, Baume D, Carsuzaa F, Burtey S. Sweet's syndrome and aseptic abscess of the spleen. Rev Med Interne. 1996;17(12):1029–31.
43. Klinger S, Mathis N, Jackson S. Bullous Sweet syndrome associated with an aseptic splenic abscess. Cutis. 2009;84(5):255–8.
44. Fortna RR, Toporcer M, Elder DE, Junkins-Hopkins JM. A case of sweet syndrome with spleen and lymph node involvement preceded by parvovirus B19 infection, and a review of the literature on extracutaneous sweet syndrome. Am J Dermatopathol. 2010;32(6):621–7.
45. Dallot A, Decazes JM, Drouault Y, Rybojad M, Verola O, Morel P, Modai J, Puissant A. Subcorneal pustular dermatosis (Sneddon-Wilkinson disease) with amicrobial lymph node suppuration and aseptic spleen abscesses. Br J Dermatol. 1988;119(6):803–7.
46. Borges-Costa J, Silva R, Gonçalves L, Filipe P, Soares de Almeida L, Marques Gomes M. Clinical and laboratory features in acute generalized pustular psoriasis: a retrospective study of 34 patients. Am J Clin Dermatol. 2011;12(4):271–6.
47. Viguier M, Allez M, Zagdanski AM, Bertheau P, de Kerviler E, Rybojad M, Morel P, Dubertret L, Lémann M, Bachelez H. High frequency of cholestasis in generalized pustular psoriasis: evidence for neutrophilic involvement of the biliary tract. Hepatology. 2004;40(2):452–8.
48. Chandran NS, Chong WS. A dramatic response to a single dose of infliximab as rescue therapy in acute generalized pustularpsoriasis of von Zumbusch associated with a neutrophilic cholangitis. Australas J Dermatol. 2010;51(1):29–31.
49. Rodríguez-Lomba E, Baniandrés O, Cano N, Suárez-Fernández R. Generalised pustular psoriasis and neutrophilic cholangitis: an infrequently reported association with excellent response to tumour necrosis factor inhibitors. Australas J Dermatol. 2017;58(1):70–1.
50. Dorenkamp M, Weikert U, Meyer R, Schwimmbeck PL, Morguet AJ. Heart failure in acute febrile neutrophilic dermatosis. Lancet. 2003;362(9393):1374.
51. Shimizu K. Neutrophilic infiltration of the myocardium in a patient with myelodysplastic syndrome. Am J Hematol. 1998;58(4):337–8.
52. WY Y, Manrriquez E, Bhutani T, Chaganti RK, Ruben BS, Schwartz BS, Fox LP. Sweet heart: a case of pregnancy-associated acute febrile neutrophilic dermatosis with myopericarditis. JAAD Case Rep. 2014;1(1):12–4.
53. Hayashi I, Hosoda Y, Kawasaki S, Yamamoto T, Dohi S, Kawai S. Aortic and mitral valve replacement in a patient with acute febrile neutrophilic dermatosis (Sweet's syndrome): report of a case. Surg Today. 2001;31(9):810–3.
54. Guia JM, Frias J, Castro FJ, Gracián M. Cardiovascular involvement in a boy with Sweet's syndrome. Pediatr Cardiol. 1999;20(4):295–7.
55. Stos B, Hatchuel Y, Bonnet D. Mitral valvar regurgitation in a child with Sweet's syndrome. Cardiol Young. 2007;17(2):218–9.
56. Muster AJ, Bharati S, Herman JJ, Esterly NB, Gonzales-Crussi F, Holbrook KA. Fatal cardiovascular disease and cutis laxa following acute febrile neutrophilic dermatosis. J Pediatr. 1983;102(2):243–8.
57. von den Driesch P. Sweet's syndrome (acute febrile neutrophilic dermatosis). J Am Acad Dermatol. 1994;31(4):535–56.
58. Gottlieb CC, Mishra A, Belliveau D, Green P, Heathcote JG. Ocular involvement in acute febrile neutrophilic dermatosis (Sweet syndrome): new cases and review of the literature. Surv Ophthalmol. 2008;53(3):219–26.
59. Baartman B, Kosari P, Warren CC, Ali S, Jorizzo JL, Sato M, Kurup SK. Sight-threatening ocular manifestations of acute febrile neutrophilic dermatosis (Sweet's syndrome). Dermatology. 2014;228(3):193–7.
60. Sato M, Kawamura T, Hase S, Katsumata S, Oshika T. A case of bilateral retinal vasculitis associated with Sweet syndrome. Retina. 2005;25(6):800–2.

61. Matsumiya W, Kusuhara S, Yamada Y, Azumi A, Negi A. Sweet's syndrome with panuveitis resembling Behçet's disease. Jpn J Ophthalmol. 2012;56(3):268–72.
62. Song WK, Bang D, Choi YJ, Lee SC, Oh SH. Sudden visual loss due to occlusive venous vasculitis associated with Sweet syndrome. Arch Dermatol. 2009;145(2):216–8.
63. Gupta AS, Ortega-Loayza AG. Ocular pyoderma gangrenosum: a systematic review. J Am Acad Dermatol. 2017;76(3):512–8.
64. Aldave AJ, Shih JL, Jovkar S, McLeod SD. Peripheral keratitis associated with erythema elevatum diutinum. Am J Ophthalmol. 2003;135(3):389–90.
65. Lekhanont K, Patarakittam T, Mantachote K, Waiyawatjamai P, Vongthongsri A. Progressive keratolysis with pseudopterygium associated with erythema elevatum diutinum. Ophthalmology. 2011;118(5):927–33.
66. Yamamoto T, Yokozeki H, Katayama I, Nushioka K. Uveitis in patients with generalized pustular psoriasis. Br J Dermatol. 1995;132(6):1023–4.
67. Hatchome N, Tagami H. Hypopyon-iridocyclitis as a complication of pustular psoriasis. J Am Acad Dermatol. 1985;13(5 Pt 1):828–9.
68. Rehal B, Modjtahedi BS, Morse LS, Schwab IR, Maibach HI. Ocular psoriasis. J Am Acad Dermatol. 2011;65(6):1202–12.
69. Daloul R, Gupta S, Marin M. Nodular kidney involvement in a patient with idiopathic Sweet's syndrome. BMJ Case Rep. 2013;11:2013.
70. Carvalho LR, Zanuncio VV, Gontijo B. Pyoderma gangrenosum with renal and splenic impairment--case report. An Bras Dermatol. 2013;88(6 Suppl 1):150–3.
71. Dinulescu M, Vigy P, Droitcourt C, Adamski H, Rioux N, Bretagne JF, Chevrant-Breton J. Pyoderma gangrenosum and aseptic pyosalpinx in a pregnant patient. Ann Dermatol Venereol. 2007;134(2):179–80.
72. Takeshita N, Takashima A, Ishida H, Manrai M, Kinoshita T. Pyoderma gangrenosum in a pregnant patient: a case report and literature review. J Obstet Gynaecol Res. 2017;43(4):775–8.

Neutrophilic Dermatoses in Blood Disorders

17

Maxime Battistella

Introduction

Neutrophilic dermatoses have long been associated with neoplastic blood disorders. As early as 1955, a 16-year-old patient with acute myeloid leukemia and recurrent cutaneous lesions including mature neutrophilic infiltrate was reported [1]. In 1973, 9 years after the seminal paper by Dr. Robert Douglas Sweet describing "acute febrile neutrophilic dermatosis", proper Sweet syndrome was reported in two women as the presenting manifestation of their previously unsuspected acute myeloid leukemia [2].

Since then, most types of neutrophilic dermatoses have been reported in association with blood disorders: Sweet syndrome (SS) and its histiocytoid variant (H-SS), pyoderma gangrenosum (PG), erythema elevatum diutinum (EED), subcorneal pustular dermatosis (SPD), neutrophilic eccrine hidradenitis (NEH), and less frequently aseptic abscesses or neutrophilic panniculitis.

In this chapter will be discussed the relations between neutrophilic dermatoses and neoplastic or non-neoplastic hematologic diseases. First, the type of hematologic diseases associated with neutrophilic diseases will be presented. Second, the data on the pathophysiology of hemopathy-associated neutrophilic dermatoses will be reviewed. Finally, the clinical, histopathological and therapeutical particularities of hemopathy-associated neutrophilic dermatoses will be described.

M. Battistella
Pathology Department, APHP Hôpital Saint Louis, INSERM UMR_S1165, Université Paris Diderot, Paris, France
e-mail: maxime.battistella@aphp.fr

D. Wallach et al. (eds.), *Neutrophilic Dermatoses*,
https://doi.org/10.1007/978-3-319-72649-6_17

Blood Disorders Associated with Neutrophilic Dermatoses

A bunch of blood disorders have been reported in association with neutrophilic dermatoses. Most of them comprise neoplastic hematologic diseases, either acute or chronic. The neutrophilic dermatosis can precede, follow or appear concurrent with the diagnosis of the patient's blood disorder. Drugs used to treat hematologic disorders have also been reported to induce neutrophilic dermatoses.

Neoplastic Blood Disorders

Neutrophilic dermatosis is most often associated with **myeloid neoplasms**. In one study, myeloid neoplasms represented 62% of the neoplastic blood disorders associated with Sweet syndrome [3]. In a review of 448 Sweet syndrome patients in 15 studies, Cohen *et al.* showed that more than 70% of neoplastic blood disorders were myeloid neoplasms. However, in this study, monoclonal gammopathy of unknown significance (MGUS) was not considered in the neoplastic blood disorders, which may have overrepresented myeloid diseases [4].

Myeloid neoplasms associated with neutrophilic dermatosis include acute myeloid leukemia (AML), chronic myeloproliferative neoplasms (MPN) (chronic myeloid leukemia, polycythemia vera, essential thrombocytemia, primary myelofibrosis), chronic or juvenile myelomonocytic leukemia (CMML/JMML), and myelodysplastic syndromes (MDS) [5].

Neutrophilic dermatosis also occurs, but less frequently, in **chronic or acute lymphoid neoplasms**, i.e. chronic lymphocytic lymphoma/leukemia (CLL), non-Hodgkin B-cell or T-cell lymphoma, hairy cell leukemia, Hodgkin lymphoma, or lymphoblastic lymphoma/leukemia [4, 5].

Paraproteinemia has also been associated with neutrophilic dermatoses, at all stages of plasma cell dyscrasia, i.e. monoclonal gammopathy of unknown significance (MGUS), monoclonal cryoglobulinemia, plasmocytoma, smoldering multiple myeloma, or multiple myeloma. Neutrophilic dermatosis is most often associated with the IgA subtype of paraproteinemia in this context [6, 7].

Overall, in myeloid, lymphoid or paraproteinemia-associated hematologic proliferations, neutrophilic dermatoses are considered of the malignancy-associated type. For the majority of patients, the onset of the neutrophilic dermatosis is prior or concurrent with the diagnosis of their hematologic neoplastic disease. It may also be the harbinger of a disease recurrence after a period of remission [8]. Few data exist regarding the prognostic value of the occurrence of a neutrophilic dermatosis in patients with neoplastic blood disorders. In 2178 AML patients, 21 patients with SS did not have worse or better survival than those without SS [9], suggesting no prognostic effect.

Drug-Induced Neutrophilic Dermatosis in Blood Disorders

Hematologic diseases may also be treated by drugs responsible for drug-associated neutrophilic dermatosis. Granulocyte-colony stimulating factor (G-CSF), granulocyte-macrophage-colony stimulating factor (GM-CSF), bortezomib, imatinib mesylate, 5-azacitidine, decitabine, all-*trans*-retinoic acid or lenalidomide have been reported to induce SS or other forms of neutrophilic dermatoses [8–10].

Drug-induced PG is scarce but recently there have been more reported cases, including cases implicating imatinib, G-CSF, and azacitidine [11].

Most NEH cases in the context of AML patients occur shortly after cytotoxic chemotherapy initiation. The main drugs responsible for NEH are cytarabine and anthracyclins, but other cytotoxic regimen, G-CSF, or antibiotics/antiviral drugs may also be implicated [12].

It is sometimes difficult to assess in a patient with a neoplastic blood disorder if the underlying disease, the treatment or both are causative of the neutrophilic dermatosis. In this context, the chronology is of paramount importance, as drug-induced neutrophilic dermatosis will occur shortly after initiation of the responsible drug, after neoplastic blood disorder diagnosis.

Other Associations Between Blood Disorders and Neutrophilic Dermatosis

Anecdotically, neutrophilic dermatoses have been reported to occur in patients with aplastic anemia or hemophilia [13–17]. In the patient with acquired aplastic anemia, neutrophilic dermatosis was due to G-CSF treatment [13]. In the patient with hemophilia, the link between the underlying blood disorder and the neutrophilic dermatosis is difficult to assess [14]. Their co-occurrence may be coincidental. Patients with Fanconi anemia and SS seem prone to extracutaneous involvement by the neutrophilic infiltrate [15–17].

Neutrophilic dermatosis (amicrobial pustulosis of the skin folds) has been reported in one patient with auto-immune erythroblastopenia [18]. Neutrophilic dermatosis has not been reported in association with sickle cell disease, thalassemia, von Willebrand disease, idiopathic thrombopenic purpura or thrombotic thrombocytopenic purpura.

Pathophysiology of Neutrophilic Dermatoses Associated with Blood Disorders

The pathogenesis of neutrophilic dermatoses remains uncompletely deciphered as only few mechanistic biological studies have been done to date.

Increased rates of circulating and *in situ* proinflammatory cytokines and chemokines have been reported in SS and PG. Interleukin (IL)-1β and its receptor, IL-8, IL-17, tumor necrosis factor (TNF)-α, G-CSF, and the chemokines CXCL1/2/3 and CXCL16 are particularly involved [19]. All of these overexpressed cytokines amplify the inflammatory response and neutrophil recruitment. Abnormal neutrophil functions have also been found in PG [20]. In addition, the recent discovery of neutrophilic dermatosis associated with monogenic autoinflammatory diseases paved the way for progress in understanding the pathogenesis of neutrophilic dermatoses [21]. Indeed, many monogenic inherited autoinflammatory diseases feature neutrophilic dermatosis with various phenotypes. These genetic diseases often involve mutations in the IL-1 pathway, emphasizing the importance of this pathway in the pathophysiology of neutrophilic dermatosis. However, the specific homing mechanisms of neutrophils in the skin are not yet elucidated, in idiopathic neutrophilic dermatoses or in monogenic autoinflammatory disease-associated neutrophilic dermatoses.

Neutrophilic dermatoses associated with a neoplastic hemopathy are considered as paraneoplastic, which is a general non-mechanistic term. They may rely on different pathogenetic mechanisms according to the underlying blood disorder. The neutrophilic skin lesions in patients with monoclonal gammopathies and in patients with myeloid neoplastic disease have been the subject of specific studies, and constitute pseudo-experimental models to study the mechanisms of neutrophilic dermatoses.

Neutrophilic Dermatoses Associated with Monoclonal Gammopathies

The clinical association of neutrophilic dermatoses with monoclonal gammopathy is well described. In this context, the monoclonal immunoglobulin is mostly of the IgA isotype (64% in a literature review), with the exception of Sweet syndrome that is more often associated to IgG isotype [7]. Among IgA receptors, FcαRI is expressed in cells of the myeloid lineage including neutrophils. Specific cytokinic environment is known to up-regulate FcαRI expression (IL-8, TNF-α). In case of neutrophilic dermatoses associated with clonal IgA, a ligation between IgA and its receptor may occur with high IgA affinity, high IgA receptor avidity, or both [7]. The skin deposition of the clonal Ig has been hypothesized as an initial factor for the development of some neutrophilic dermatoses (namely SPD, IgA pemphigus, EED). In EED, it has been suggested that immune complexes are primary deposited in post-capillary venules, initiating the vasculitic process [22]. In SPD, IgA has been found within vesicles, together with IL-8 and TNF-α [23]. In IgA pemphigus, sometimes clinically similar to SPD, intraepidermal IgA deposits initiate the disease.

In patients with neutrophilic dermatosis and monoclonal gammopathy, the systemic inflammation involves a particular cytokinic pattern with increased rated of IL-6, vascular endothelial growth factor, EGF, intercellular adhesion molecule-1, G-CSF, and MCP-1, but not GM-CSF [7]. This profile may be the cause or the consequence of the neutrophilic dermatosis. An inappropriate secretion of cytokine by the clonal plasma cells may be hypothesized, because EGF and MCP-1 are known to be produced by myeloma cells.

Neutrophilic Dermatoses in Myeloid Malignancies

In myeloid malignancy-associated neutrophilic dermatosis, the hypothesis that neutrophils in the cutaneous infiltrate are related to the underlying myeloid malignancy has been investigated in the past few years. Initially, in two case reports, fluorescent in situ hybridization identified the same 20q deletion in mucosal or skin infiltrating cells as well as in the marrow cells in two patient with SS and MDS/AML [24, 25]. Since then, various studies using fluorescent in situ hybridization have been able to identify common cytogenetic alterations in skin-infiltrating cells and in the underlying myeloid malignancy [26–28]. The cytogenetic alteration-bearing cells in the skin can be mature neutrophils, but also immature non blastic myeloid cells in the context of MDS. In addition, common FLT3 mutational status has been found in skin samples and bone marrow samples in some patients with AML and SS [9]. All these findings indicate that the mature neutrophils or immature myeloid cells in myeloid malignancy-associated neutrophilic dermatosis are clonally related to the underlying hemopathy. In the context of AML-associated neutrophilic dermatosis, this also indicates that blastic tumor cells may differentiate to neutrophils, either before entering the skin or in the skin. This clonal differentiation process is consistent with the similarities between SS and the differentiation syndrome observed in patients with acute promyelocytic leukemia treated with all-trans retinoic acid, i.e. the association of fever, multiorgan infiltration by neutrophils and the marked response to corticosteroids [26].

The chemotactic or homing factors eliciting the recruitment of clonal myeloid cells in the skin, and the factors involved in clonal cell maturation remain to be identified.

Particularities of Hemopathy-Associated Neutrophilic Dermatoses

Neutrophilic dermatoses associated with hematologic disorders, and especially with hematologic malignancies, may have particular clinical features. Prototypical SS, PG, EED, SPD, or NEH is encountered, but the neutrophilic dermatosis may present some clinical particularities, or may be composed of clinical lesions of more than one prototypical neutrophilic dermatosis. Overlap of SS and PG, or transitional forms with the less frequent entities EED, SPD or NEH, have all been described, frequently in association with an underlying myeloid neoplasm [29]. Extracutaneous neutrophilic involvement may also occur, mainly in SS and PG, a feature that has led to the proposition of the concept of systemic neutrophilic disease [29].

Sweet Syndrome

Sweet syndrome (SS) is a skin condition classically characterized by tender erythematous plaques, nodules, or papules; prodromal symptoms such as fever, malaise, or arthralgia; and diffuse infiltrate of neutrophils in the papillary dermis. Less common lesions include vesicles, bullae, and pustules.

SS is associated with underlying neoplastic hemopathy in 15–27% of cases according to published series [3, 4]. Acute myeloid leukemia (AML) is the most common hemopathy associated with SS, although most myeloid and lymphoid neoplastic diseases may be associated with SS. In a series of 2178 AML patients, SS frequency was of 1% [9]. Hemopathy-associated SS may precede the neoplastic disease, occurring months to years before diagnosis, or co-occur with the hemopathy. SS may also sign the recurrence of the disease in a patient considered in remission. Less frequently SS occur during the course of the hematologic disease. In this case, it may be drug-associated. The main responsible drugs are G-CSF, GM-CSF, bortezomib, all-*trans*-retinoic acid, and hypomethylating agents with or without histone deacetylase inhibitors [8–10].

When comparing clinical and biological features of hemopathy-associated SS to those of classic idiopathic SS, few significant differences appear. In a cohort study, hemopathy-associated SS patients were older (mean aged 68), but did not show significant clinical difference with classic SS (Fig. 17.1) [3]. Indeed, bullous or ulcerated lesions may occur both in hemopathy-associated SS and in classic SS (Fig. 17.2) [30, 31]. Biologically, patients with hemopathy-associated SS have lower hemoglobin level than in classic SS [3]. Anemia is present in most patients with hemopathy-associated SS, even before the hemopathy diagnosis. Of note, hemopathy-associated SS may occur in neutropenic patients. Sometimes, SS and PG lesions exist on a continuum in patients with hematologic neoplasm. Definitive differential diagnosis may be difficult to make between SS and PG in this context. Subcutaneous involvement in SS is possible, and is sometimes named neutrophilic panniculitis in the literature.

Recurrent skin lesions are not more frequent in hemopathy-associated SS than in classic SS [3]. However, when looking closely at the associated hemopathy, it

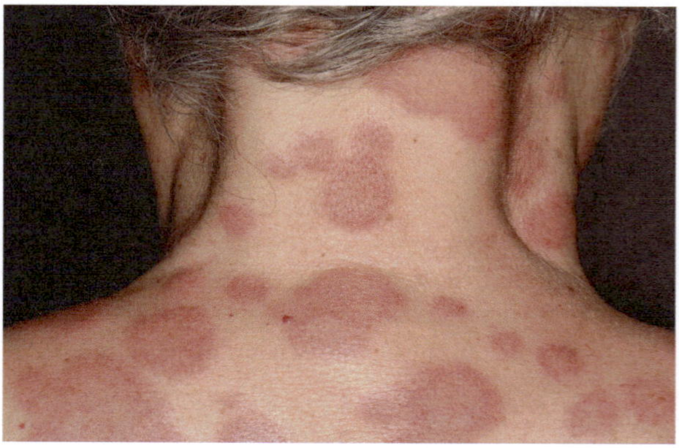

Fig. 17.1 Sweet syndrome in a patient with IgA multiple myeloma, with classical erythematous edematous plaque on the trunk and the neck

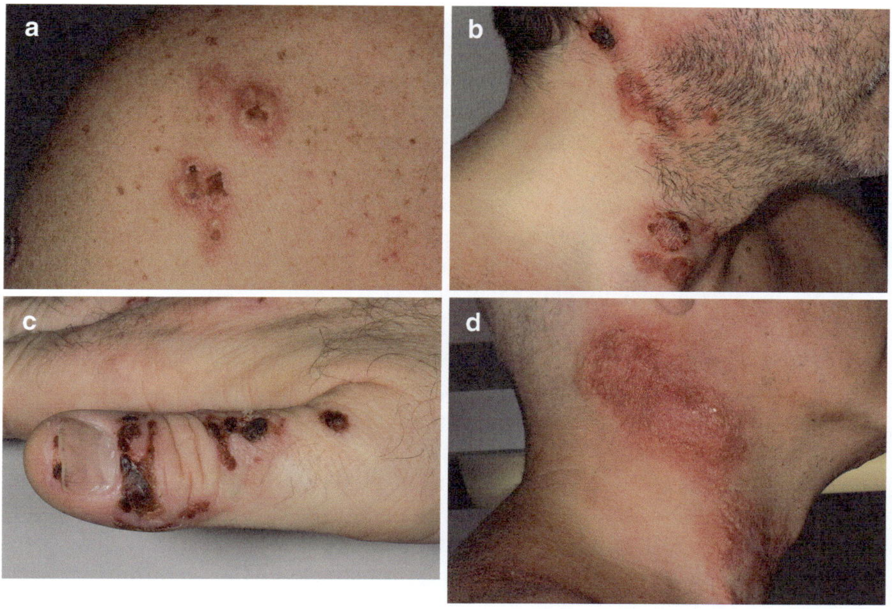

Fig. 17.2 Sweet syndrome with ulcerated lesions in a patient with AML. (**a–c**) Erythematous edematous plaques with ulceration and acral involvement occurring some months before AML diagnosis; (**d**) Recurring erythemato-vesicular plaque after initial AML treatment, heralding AML relapse

appears that chronic recurrent SS is associated with MDS, and often of the histiocytoid type [3, 27, 32, 33].

Histopathologically, hemopathy-associated SS often shows classical features. In some patients with MDS, the skin infiltrate may initially be lymphocyte-rich or display immature non-blastic myeloid cells (histiocytoid Sweet syndrome) [33, 34]. Rarely, mature neutrophils may be associated with blastic leukemia cells infiltrating the skin, [35].

The treatment of hemopathy-associated SS includes hemopathy-directed drugs and SS directed drugs. Among the latter, systemic corticosteroids are the most often employed, followed by topical corticosteroids [3, 9]. Complete response is very often reached, mostly with steroids, sometimes without specific SS treatment. SS may relapse, requiring multiple courses of glucocorticoids, especially if the underlying hemopathy is not in complete remission or recur. There is no indication that SS associated with a hemopathy is a factor of poor prognosis for the hemopathy [3].

Histiocytoid Sweet Syndrome

Histiocytoid Sweet syndrome (H-SS) is a histopathological variant of SS where cellular components of the infiltrate include lymphocytes and mononuclear cells resembling histiocytes and expressing myeloperoxidase, in addition to mature neutrophils

(Fig. 17.3) [33, 36, 37]. These mononuclear cells also express CD163, a feature that led to their interpretation as M2-like macrophages [38]. However, more recent works argue more in favor of immature myelomonocytic cells with histiocytoid morphology [39].

Clinically, the tender erythematous plaques and nodules of H-SS are more often relapsing remitting than in SS [37]. Most studies report a male predominance. As in SS, neutrophilic panniculitides and episcleritis are possible; fever and arthralgia are frequent. In some patients, the erythematous plaques are annular, purpuric or may involve the face, ears and extremities (Fig. 17.4).

H-SS is particularly associated with hematological malignancies (as frequently as 55.5% in [37]), especially with MDS [32, 33, 37, 39]. The eruption may precede MDS diagnosis by months to years [28, 32, 33]. As cells in the infiltrate of H-SS sometimes portend the clonal molecular alteration of underlying MDS, the concept of *myelodysplasis cutis* has been proposed to describe such condition [28]. H-SS in MDS patients does not have the poor prognosis of blastic leukemia cutis, and does not modify the survival of MDS patients [28].

The treatment of H-SS relies on systemic and high potent topical corticosteroids, and on the treatment of the underlying hematological disorder. Corticosteroids alone may have to be maintained on a higher dose of prednisolone (>15–20 mg/day) to prevent recurrent episodes in patients with untreated MDS, as in this context H-SS may be recalcitrant to treatment [32, 37].

Pyoderma Gangrenosum

Although more than 50% of pyoderma gangrenosum (PG) have an associated systemic disease, hematologic disorders are less frequent in association with PG than inflammatory bowel diseases [11]. In a review of four case series including 138 PG patients, 7.2% had associated malignancy [40]. More recent monocentric series on

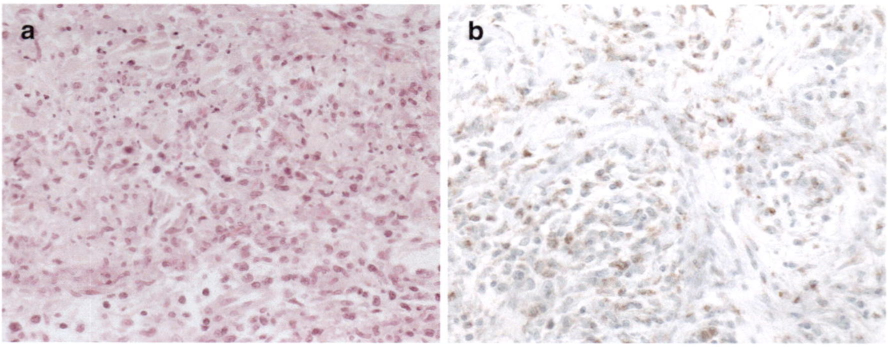

Fig. 17.3 Histiocytoid Sweet syndrome—histopathology. (**a**) Polymorphic infiltrate containing nuclear debris, lymphocytes, some mature neutrophils and histiocytoid cells corresponding to immature non-blastic myeloid cells (hematoxylin and eosin, ×400 magnification); (**b**) Myeloperoxydase expression by mononucleated cells in the infiltrate (×400 magnification)

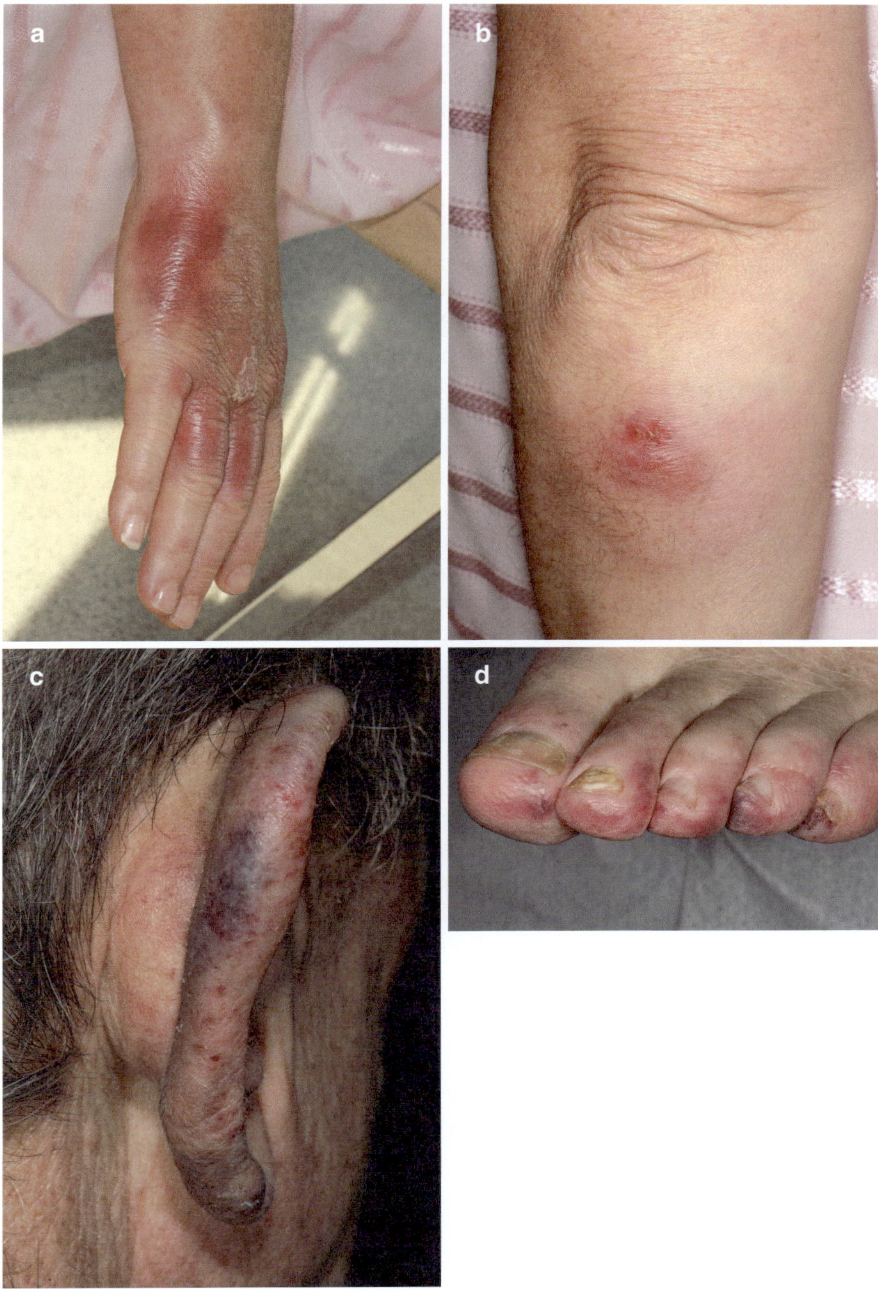

Fig. 17.4 Histiocytoid Sweet syndrome in two patients with MDS. (**a**, **b**) Erythematous plaques on the hand and nodule on the forearm; (**c**, **d**) Erythematho-violaceous purpuric plaques on the ear and the toes

103 and 31 patients report around 20% of associated hematological disorders (including MGUS in about 10% of PG patients and hematological malignancies in about 10% of PG patients) [41, 42]. Hematological malignancies in PG patients include AML, MDS, MPN, malignant myeloma and lymphomas. The paraprotein in MGUS and myeloma associated with PG is mostly of the IgA isotype [7, 43].

The specific clinical features of hemopathy-associated PG have not been studied comparatively to idiopathic PG or inflammatory bowel disease-associated PG. Among the currently recognized clinical variants of PG, i.e. classic ulcerative, bullous, pustular, vegetative, and peristomal, it is repeatedly said in the literature that ulcerative and bullous types are associated with hematological malignancy (Fig. 17.5) [11, 40, 44]. In a study of 86 patients with PG, hematologic disease or malignancy was more common in patients with bullous PG (also known as atypical PG) than in patients with typical ulcerative PG [45]. Bullous PG is characterized by tense, often hemorrhagic bullae which break down to form large painful superficial ulcers, on the face, the limbs or trunk at sites of trauma (Fig. 17.6). It has a predilection for the upper extremity, particularly the dorsal aspect of the hands. Histopathologically, bullous PG shows epidermal necrosis, spongiosis, intraepidermal vesiculation and pustulation, intraepidermal bullae, or subcorneal abscess formation [40].

Hemopathy-associated PG may involve extracutaneous sites (eyes, lung, spleen, musculoskeletal system). Pulmonary involvement is rare in PG, more commonly reported in patients with underlying disease [46].

The choice of treatment depends on the location of lesion(s), number, size, extracutaneous involvement and the type of associated hemopathy. Systemic therapy with corticosteroids or topical high potent corticosteroids in case of limited skin involvement is the first-line therapy [11]. In patients with malignant hemopathy, immunosuppressive or immunomodulatory drugs as cyclosporine or TNF-alpha inhibitors are usually not recommended, and treatment of the underlying hemopathy is mandatory. Therapy of PG associated with malignant hemopathy can be difficult. Cytotoxic chemotherapy administered to treat the hemopathy may sometimes interfere with the healing of skin lesions; in addition, the loss of epidermal integrity can also be a source of sepsis in these

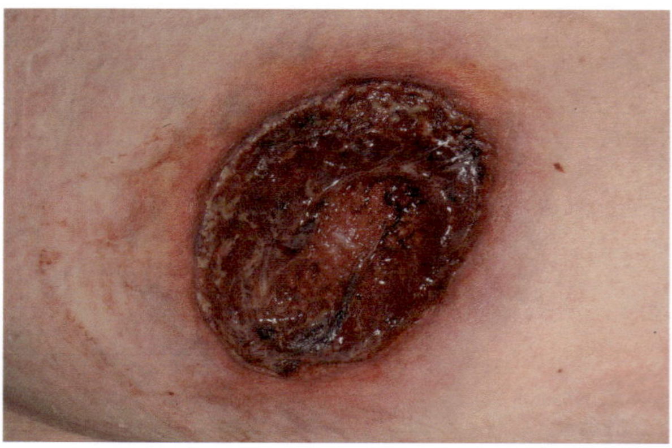

Fig. 17.5 Pyoderma gangrenosum of the ulcerative type, in a patient with IgA monoclonal gammopathy of unknown significance

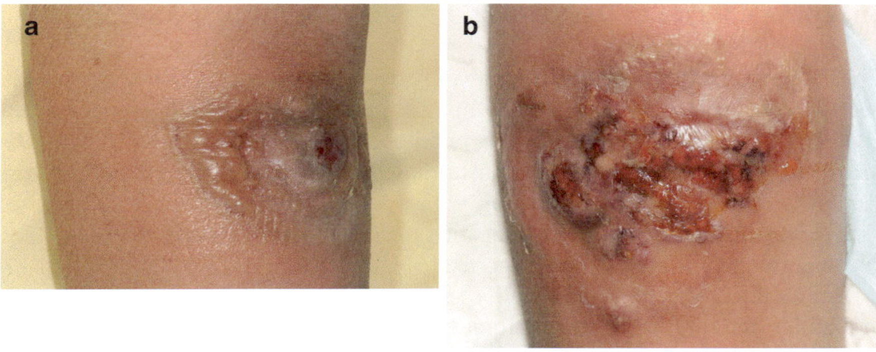

Fig. 17.6 Bullous (atypical) pyoderma gangrenosum in a patient with chronic myeloid leukemia. (**a**) Bullous plaque initially; (**b**) Evolution to an ulcerated vegetative plaque

immunosuppressed patients [47]. In patients with MGUS-associated PG, many treatments have been reported, sometimes in association with corticosteroids, i.e. dapsone, colchicine, thalidomide, cyclosporine, or intravenous immunoglobulins [7].

Erythema Elevatum Diutinum

Erythema elevatum diutinum (EED) is a rare chronic inflammatory dermatosis characterized by brownish, red, elevated lesions occurring symmetrically over extensor surfaces. It is considered to be a chronic localized variant of leukocytoclastic vasculitis [47]. The brown to purple papules are persistent and may coalesce to form larger nodules or plaques [48]. The lesions are located near joints, and may also be palmo-plantar, truncal, or retroauricular. Their resolution may give a yellowish or brown hue, resembling xanthomata. Late-stage nodular pseudotumoral EED may be histopathologically challenging, as the lesion contains less neutrophils and more sclerosis and fibroblastic proliferation [49].

EED is sometimes associated with hematologic disorder. In a series of 13 patients, 6 had hematologic abnormalities, including IgA MGUS, multiple myeloma, MDS and MPN [50]. The EED preceded the hematologic disease by 7.8 years. Other hematologic diseases reported in EED include hairy cell leukemia, Waldenström's macroglobulinemia, and non-Hodgkin lymphoma [49]. Overall, EED is particularly associated with IgA paraproteinemia (MGUS or myeloma) [7, 49].

The disease is very responsive to oral dapsone (complete resolution in around 80% of cases in the literature) [49]. Maintenance therapy may be required to suppress recurrences as dapsone is suppressive rather than curative [47, 49]. In late-stage lesions with fibrosis, dapsone may have less effect. Dapsone in association with corticosteroids, colchicine, sulphonamide or surgical excision are options [49]. Systemic, topical or intralesional corticosteroids alone seem less effective than in other neutrophilic dermatoses.

Subcorneal Pustular Dermatosis

This rare chronic relapsing condition mainly occurs in middle-aged women but has been reported in all age groups. Asymptomatic pustules, typically grouped in an annular pattern, are mainly located around the axillary and inguinal folds, symmetrically. They are sterile, flaccid pustules, which can appear with hypopyon formation (Fig. 17.7). Cases presenting with systemic symptoms such as malaise, fever, arthralgias, anormalities of hepatic enzymes, aseptic neutrophilic abscesses or glomerulonephritis have been reported [51].

Hematologic disorders reportedly seen with SPD include monoclonal gammopathies (MGUS, multiple myeloma), aplastic anemia, IgG cryoglobulinemia, lymphomas, chronic lymphocytic leukemia and chronic myeloid leukemia [51]. The most frequent associated hemopathy in the literature is by far monoclonal gammopathy, most often of the IgA isotype [7, 52]. It is difficult to determine the true incidence of paraproteinemia in SPD because of the low incidence of the disease. The latency between SPD presentation and myeloma has been inconsistently reported. SPD may appear years before detection of the gammopathy.

SPD usually responds well to oral dapsone therapy, in 1–4 weeks [51]. Relapses are common with discontinuation of the treatment. Other treatments include topical corticosteroids, oral corticosteroids, oral retinoids such as acitretin and etretinate. Light therapy (psoralen plus ultraviolet A) alone or with dapsone or retinoid has been used with good results [53]. The skin lesions of SPD may improve with the treatment of an underlying IgA myeloma.

IgA pemphigus may be regarded as a variant of SPD. IgA intercellular deposits are directed against interkeratinocyte adhesion molecules, and detectable by direct immunofluorescence, which is mandatory in case of SPD.

Neutrophilic Eccrine Hidradenitis

This rare neutrophilic dermatosis has a slight male predominance, and a particular association to adult AML patients receiving chemotherapy. The cutaneous lesions

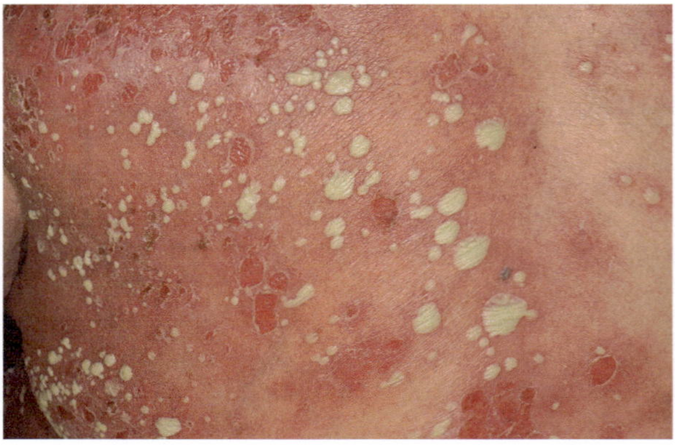

Fig. 17.7 Subcorneal pustular dermatosis in a patient with IgA multiple myeloma

of NEH are featured by the rapid development of infiltrated or edematous papules or plaques, asymptomatic or painful, close to SS. The lesions may be purpuric. They involve the trunk, limbs and face, particularly the periorbital areas, mimicking orbital cellulitis, or develop in a distal disposition affecting the extremities [12]. Fever is frequently observed, but may be due to other cause than NEH, as patients are often neutropenic when NEH occurs.

The diagnosis relies on the histological examination showing a degeneration of eccrine gland and a neutrophilic infiltrate.

In a review of 51 patients with NEH, 67% had AML treated with chemotherapy. Other associated hematological malignancies included chronic lymphocytic leukemia, chronic myelomonocytic leukemia, Hodgkin's disease or non-Hodgkin lymphoma [12, 47]. Eighty-four percent of patients had received anti-cancer chemotherapy before the onset of NEH, the two main administered drug being cytarabine or anthracyclins.

Spontaneous resolution of NEH is the rule, within a few days or weeks. No specific treatment is administered in most patients, but they usually receive antibiotics in the context of fever and neutropenia. Topical or systemic corticosteroids may shorten the disease evolution in cases with pain or ocular occlusion, but should be used with caution in neutropenic patients [54]. Occasionally, NEH may constitute a clinical marker for the relapse of the hematologic malignancy.

Other Forms of Neutrophilic Dermatosis

Deep neutrophilic dermatoses that are clinically different from PG may occur in association with hematologic disorders [29]. They consist in neutrophilic infiltrates in the subcutaneous fat. According to the density of the neutrophilic infiltrate and to the presence of pus formation, neutrophilic panniculitis or aseptic abscesses have been reported. Such neutrophilic subcutaneous lesions may also occur in the context of more typical SS or PG lesions in a patient with hematologic disorder.

References

1. Costello MJ, Canizares O, Montague M III, Buncke CM. Cutaneous manifestations of myelogenous leukemia. Arch Dermatol. 1955;71:605–14.
2. Matta M, Lurban AK. Sweet's syndrome: systemic association. Cutis. 1973;12:561–5.
3. Rochet NM, Chavan RN, Cappel MA, Wada DA, Gibson LE. Sweet syndrome: clinical presentation, association and response to treatment in 77 patients. J Am Acad Dermatol. 2013;69:557–64.
4. Cohen PR, Talpaz M, Kurzrock R. Malignancy-associated Sweet's syndrome: review of the world literature. J Clin Oncol. 1988;6:1887–97.
5. Cohen PR, Kurzrock R. Sweet's syndrome and cancer. Clin Dermatol. 1993;11:149–57.
6. Chevrant-Breton J, Logeais B, Pibouin M. Pyoderma gangrenosum (pyodermite phagédénique). Ann Dermatol Venereol. 1989;116:577–89.
7. Szalat R, Monsel G, Le Goff W, Battistella M, Bengouffa D, Schlageter MH, et al. The spectrum of neutrophilic dermatoses associated with monoclonal gammopathy: association with IgA isotype and inflammatory profile. J Am Acad Dermatol. 2015;73:809–20.

8. Cohen PR. Sweet's syndrome – a comprehensive review of an acute febrile neutrophilic dermatosis. Orphanet J Rare Dis. 2007;2:34.
9. Kazmi SM, Pemmaraju N, Patel KP, Cohen PR, Daver N, Tran KM, et al. Characteristics of Sweet syndrome in patients with acute myeloid leukemia. Clin Lymphoma Myeloma Leuk. 2015;15:358–63.
10. Alencar C, Abramowtiz M, Parekh S, Braunschweig I, Jacobson M, Silverman L, et al. Atypical presentations of Sweet's syndrome in patients with MDS/AML receiving combinations of hypomethylating agents with histone deacetylase inhibitors. Am J Hematol. 2009;84: 688–9.
11. Alavi A, French LE, Davis MD, Brassard A, Kirsner RS. Pyoderma gangrenosum: an update on pathophysiology, diagnosis and treatment. Am J Clin Dermatol. 2017;18:355–72.
12. Bachmeyer C, Aractingi S. Neutrophilic eccrine hidradenitis. Clin Dermatol. 2000;18:319–30.
13. Fukutoku M, Shimizu S, Ogawa Y, Takeshita S, Masaki Y, Arai T, et al. Sweet's syndrome during therapy with granulocyte colony-stimulating factor in a patient with aplastic anemia. Br J Haematol. 1994;84:645–8.
14. Deasy AM, Walker B, Layton AM, Lacey CJ. Sweet's syndrome in a patient with haemophilia, HIV, and hepatitis C infection. Int J STD AIDS. 2012;23:e11–3.
15. Mc Dermott MB, Corbally MT, O'Marcaigh AS. Extracutaneous Sweet syndrome involving the gastrointestinal tract in a patient with Fanconi anemia. J Pediatr Hematol Oncol. 2001;23:59–62.
16. Chatham-Stephens K, Devere T, Guzman-Cottrill J, Kurre P. Metachronous manifestations of Sweet's syndrome in a neutropenic patient with Fanconi anemia. Pediatr Blood Cancer. 2008;51:128–30.
17. Baron F, Sybert VP, Andrews RG. Cutaneous and extracutaneous neutrophilic infiltrates (Sweet syndrome) in three patients with Fanconi anemia. J Pediatr. 1989;115:726–9.
18. Saint-Jean M, Gagey-Caron V, Jossic F, Barbarot S, Hamidou M, Stalder JF. Amicrobial pustulosis of the skin folds and autoimmune erythroblastopenia. Ann Dermatol Venereol. 2011;138:399–404.
19. Marzano AV, Fanoni D, Antiga E, Quaglino P, Caproni M, Crosti C, et al. Expression of cytokines, chemokines and other effector molecules in two prototypic autoinflammatory skin diseases, pyoderma gangrenosum and Sweet's syndrome. Clin Exp Immunol. 2014;178:48–56.
20. Adachi Y, Kindzelskii AL, Cookingham G, Shaya S, Moore EC, Todd RF III, et al. Aberrant neutrophil trafficking and metabolic oscillations in severe pyoderma gangrenosum. J Invest Dermatol. 1998;111:259–68.
21. Maalouf D, Battistella M, Bouaziz JD. Neutrophilic dermatosis: disease mechanism and treatment. Curr Opin Hematol. 2015;22:23–9.
22. Porneuf M, Duterque M, Sotto A, Jourdan J. Unusual erythema elevatum diutinum with fibrohistiocytic proliferation. Br J Dermatol. 1996;143:1131–4.
23. Grob JJ, Mege JL, Capo C, Jancovicci E, Fournerie JR, Bongrand P, et al. Role of tumor necrosis factor-alpha in Sneddon-Wilkinson subcorneal pustular dermatosis. A model of neutrophil priming in vivo. J Am Acad Dermatol. 1991;25:944–7.
24. Van Loon K, Gill RM, McMahon P, Chigurupati R, Siddiqi I, Fox L, et al. 20q-clonality in a case of oral sweet syndrome and myelodysplasia. Am J Clin Pathol. 2012;137:310–5.
25. Van Kamp H, van den Berg E, Timens W, Kraaijenbrink RA, Halie MR, Daenen SM. Sweet's syndrome in myeloid malignancy: a report of two cases. Br J Haematol. 1994;86:415–7.
26. Sujobert P, Cuccuini W, Vignon-Pennamen MD, Martin-Garcia N, Albertini AF, Uzunov M, et al. Evidence of differentiation in myeloid malignancies associated neutrophilic dermatosis: a fluorescent in situ hybridization study of 14 patients. J Invest Dermatol. 2013;133(4):1111.
27. Chavan RN, Cappel MA, Ketterling RP, Wada DA, Rochet NM, Knudson R, et al. Histiocytoid Sweet syndrome may indicate leukemia cutis : a novel application of fluorescence in situ hybridization. J Am Acad Dermatol. 2014;70:1021–7.
28. Osio A, Battistella M, Feugeas JP, Cuccuini W, Noguera ME, Petrella T, et al. Myelodysplasis cutis versus leukemia cutis. J Invest Dermatol. 2015;135:2321–4.

29. Wallach D, Vignon-Pennamen MD. From acute febrile neutrophilic dermatosis to neutrophilic disease: forty years of clinical research. J Am Acad Dermatol. 2006;55:1066–71.
30. Bielsa S, Baradad M, Marti RM, Casanova JM. Sweet's syndrome with bullous lesions. Actas Dermosifiliogr. 2005;96:315–6.
31. Voelter-Mahlknecht S, Bauer J, Metzler G, Fierlbeck G, Rassner G. Bullous variant of Sweet's syndrome. Int J Dermatol. 2005;44:946–7.
32. Kulasekararaj AG, Kordasti S, Basu T, Salisbury JR, Mufti GJ, du Vivier AWP. Chronic relapsing remitting Sweet syndrome – harbinger of myelodysplastic syndrome. Br J Haematol. 2015;170:649–56.
33. Vignon-Pennamen MD, Juillard C, Rybojad M, Wallach D, Daniel MT, Morel P, et al. Chronic recurrent lymphocytic Sweet syndrome as a predictive marker of myelodysplasia: a report of 9 cases. Arch Dermatol. 2006;142:1170–6.
34. Tomasini C, Aloi F, Osella-Abate S, Dapavo P, Pippione M. Immature myeloid precursors in chronic neutrophilic dermatosis associated with myelodysplastic syndrome. Am J Dermatopathol. 2000;22:429–33.
35. Deguchi M, Tsunoda T, Yuda F, Tagami H. Sweet's syndrome in acute myelogenous leukemia showing dermal infiltration of leukemic cells. Dermatology. 1997;194:182–4.
36. Requena L, Kutzner H, Palmedo G, Pascual M, Fernandez-Herrera J, Fraga J, et al. Histiocytoid Sweet syndrome: a dermal infiltration of immature neutrophilic granulocytes. Arch Dermatol. 2005;141:834–42.
37. Ghoufi L, Ortonne N, Ingen-Housz-Oro S, Barhoumi W, Begon E, Haioun C, et al. Histiocytoid Sweet syndrome is more frequently associated with myelodysplastic syndromes than the classical neutrophilic variant. Medicine. 2016;95:e3033.
38. Peroni A, Colato C, Schena D, Rongioletti F, Girolomoni G. Histiocytoid Sweet syndrome is infiltrated predominantly by M2-like macrophages. J Am Acad Dermatol. 2015;72:131–9.
39. Alegria-Landa V, Rodriguez-Pinilla SM, Santos-Briz A, Rodriguez-Peralto JL, Alegre V, Cerroni L, et al. Clinicopathologic, immunohistochemical, and molecular features of histiocytoid Sweet syndrome. JAMA Dermatol. 2017;153(7):651–9.
40. Duguid CM, Powell FC. Pyoderma gangrenosum. Clin Dermatol. 1993;11:129–33.
41. Binus AM, Qureshi AA, Li VW, Winterfield LS. Pyoderma gangrenosum: a retrospective review of patients characteristics, comorbidities and therapy in 103 patients. Br J Dermatol. 2011;165:1244–50.
42. Vacas A, Torre AC, Bollea-Garlatti ML, Warley F, Galimberti RL. Pyoderma gangrenosum: clinical characteristics, associated diseases, and responses to treatment in a retrospective cohort study of 31 patients. Int J Dermatol. 2017;56:386–91.
43. Powell FC, Schroeter AL, Su WP, Perry HO. Pyoderma gangrenosum and monoclonal gammopathy. Arch Dermatol. 1983;119:468–72.
44. DeFilippis EM, Feldman SR, Huang WW. The genetics of pyoderma gangrenosum and implications for treatment: a systematic review. Br J Dermatol. 2015;172:1487–97.
45. Bennett ML, Jackson JM, Jorizzo JL, Fleischer AB Jr, White WL, Callen JP. Pyoderma gangrenosum. A comparison of typical and atypical forms with an emphasis on time to remission. Case review of 86 patients from 2 institutions. Medicine (Baltimore). 2000;79:37–46.
46. Gade M, Studstrup F, Andersen AK, Hilberg O, Fogh C, Bendstrup E. Pulmonary manifestations of pyoderma gangrenosum: 2 cases and a review of the literature. Respir Med. 2015;109:443–50.
47. Hensley CD, Caughman SW. Neutrophilic dermatoses associated with hematologic disorders. Clin Dermatol. 2000;18:355–67.
48. Gibson LE, El-Azhari RA. Erythema elevatum diutinum. Clin Dermatol. 2000;18:295–9.
49. Momen SE, Jorizzo J, Al-Niaimi F. Erythema elevatum diutinum: a review of presentation and treatment. J Eur Acad Dermatol Venereol. 2014;28:1594–602.
50. Yiannias JA, El-Azhari RA, Gibson LE. Erythema elevatum diutinum: a clinical and histopathologic study of 13 patients. J Am Acad Dermatol. 1992;26:38–44.
51. Watts PJ, Khachemoune A. Subcorneal pustular dermatosis: a review of 30 years of progress. Am J Clin Dermatol. 2016;17:653–71.

52. Lutz ME, Daoud MS, MT ME, Gibson LE. Subcorneal pustular dermatosis: a clinical study of ten patients. Cutis. 1998;61:203–8.
53. Bauwens M, De Coninck A, Roseeuw D. Subcorneal pustular dermatosis treated with PUVA therapy: a case report and review of the literature. Dermatology. 1999;198:203–5.
54. Copaescu AM, Castilloux JF, Chababi-Atallah M, Sinave C, Bertrand J. A classic clinical case: neutrophilic eccrine hidradenitis. Case Rep Dermatol. 2013;5:340–6.

18 Neutrophilic Dermatoses in Digestive Disorders

Sébastien Buche and Emmanuel Delaporte

Inflammatory Bowel Disease (IBD) is a group of chronic immune-mediated, polygenic disorders that relapse and remit, affecting predominantly adolescents and young adults. The pediatric population, however, accounts for 10–15% of cases, most often in those older than 10 years of age. Patients under the age of 20 account for 25% of newly diagnosed cases with IBD. IBD affects more than one in every 1000 individuals in Western countries and is becoming more common in the rest of the world. It arises when an inappropriate immune response of the intestine is mounted against the components of the bacterial flora occurring in genetically predisposed individuals [1]. The instability and reduction of microbiota biodiversity (dysbiosis) are currently the most studied etiopathogenic factors in Crohn's disease [2].

IBD encompass two major forms, known as Ulcerative Colitis (UC) and Crohn's disease (CD). In certain atypical forms limited to the colon with little evocative histology, the distinction between the two may be impossible. It is important to note that there is often a clinico-anatomical dissociation with delayed clinical signs contrasting with endoscopic and histological findings. It is no longer required for IBD to be clinically active for an individual to be treated. Digestive exploration must be done in the case of the slightest doubt to avoid tissue destruction, especially in young affected individuals (with CD) who are as well smokers. This notion is particularly important for the dermatologist who is likely to encounter preceding manifestations. Indeed, mucocutaneous lesions are, together with the musculoskeletal involvement, the most prevalent extra-intestinal manifestations (EIM) of IBD [3]. Neutrophilic dermatoses classified amongst reactional diseases, represent a major group of these EIM [4].

S. Buche • E. Delaporte (✉)
Service de Dermatologie, Hôpital Nord, Marseille, France
e-mail: emmanuel.delaporte@ap-hm.fr

D. Wallach et al. (eds.), *Neutrophilic Dermatoses*,
https://doi.org/10.1007/978-3-319-72649-6_18

Pyoderma gangrenosum (PG) is a cutaneous complication noted in 1–3% of IBD, more frequently in individuals with CD with colonic involvement or in individuals with UC with extensive colitis [5]. Pyoderma gangrenosum is, however, not correlated with the severity of IBD. Inversely, IBD represents the most common cause of pyoderma gangrenosum (accounting for 20–30% of cases). IBD gene loci associated with PG have been identified, including IL8RA, MUC 17 and MMP24 [5]. PG lesions may be single or multiple. They characteristically predominate on the lower extremities, relapse in one-third of the cases and are sometimes accompanied by mucosal lesions. PG appears approximately 10 years after the onset of IBD, most often during periods of regression (66% vs. 34% during periods of remission). PG can appear in patients under systemic steroids and needs to be distinguished from infectious complications, especially in cases with systemic (pulmonary, hepatosplenic…) involvement [6]. An ophthalmological attack (uveitis) is also frequently associated. It may, nonetheless, precede intestinal symptomatology. Then, in the absence of a hematological or rheumatological cause, a systematic endoscopic exploration is warranted if it is a recurrent form or if there are digestive signs and a positive family history of IBD.

The peristomal area is affected in about 10% of cases, essentially seen in patients affected with CD that had undergone abdominal surgery with placement of an ileostomy. This peristomal location of PG lesions is favored by the various irritations in which the peristomal skin is subjected to. They appear on average 2 months after stoma's appliance. However, longer periods of up to 3 years have also been observed. Iodine antiseptics should be avoided due to a pathergy phenomenon (activation of polynuclear neutrophils).

PG lesions do not always respond to the treatment of IBD. This resistance has been found in up to 80% of cases that received treatment for IBD. Corticosteroids have long been the treatment of choice. Their intra-lesional use makes it possible to achieve approximately 40% complete response and 40% partial response. Immunosuppressants especially anti-TNF agents, represent remarkable therapeutic alternatives. Anti-TNF therapy as a first-line agent for PG should be considered, as it appears to be highly effective [7–9].

Smoking cessation should be considered as an essential associated preventative measure, given the stimulating effect of tobacco on neutrophils. Arguelles-Arias et al. stated that active smoking was noted in 28% of patients during PG surveillance [10].

Sweet syndrome (SS) also known as acute febrile neutrophilic dermatosis has been knowingly associated with UC since its description. The association with CD, however, is of more recent knowledge; several cases have been reported in the last few years. However, the association of SS with IBD is much rarer than that of PG [11]. Cutaneous eruption is usually typical, both concerning lesion topography and appearance, which are mostly pustular but rarely bullous or necrotic, as in SS associated with haemopathies. When SS appears, IBD is not always known, but it is most often targeted, prompting , as for erythema nodosum, to carry out a systematic digestive exploration after having eliminated an infectious cause (particularly Yersinia, Salmonellosis). Several observations of SS revealing the diagnosis of IBD have been reported. Hypersensitivity to azathioprine may mimic clinically and histologically a neutrophilic dermatosis, especially a SS. As azathioprine is still widely used, clinicians should be aware of this adverse reaction. In severe forms of SS, systemic steroid therapy is the treatment of choice. NSAIDs (indometacin) and colchicine may also be used after obtaining the gastroenterologist's professional advice.

Bowel-Associated Dermatosis-Arthritis Syndrome (BADAS) has also been reportedly associated with IBD. It was only until during the 1970s that attention was drawn to the possible cutaneous and joint complications of bariatric surgery. BADAS also known as "Bowel-Bypass Syndrome" is associated with patients who underwent bowel bypass surgery but also patients with IBD. It is caused by bacterial multiplication in a blind loop of the bowel and the formation of circulating immune complexes. This rare but not unusual syndrome is typically observed in the course of UC and has been mentioned in the literature under other names: vesicular eruption of UC or Pustular Vasculitis [12].

BADAS often occurs and evolves in parallel with the IBD. Cutaneous eruptions consist of non-follicular pustules, resting on an erythematous base (Fig. 18.1). Their sizes vary between 2 and 8 mm in diameter, and they mainly appear on the external surface of the upper limbs, the extensor surface of the lower limbs, but also the trunk and the scalp. Erythema nodosum-like lesions could also be associated. This eruption is always accompanied by systemic manifestations including fever, myalgia, polyarthralgia, peripheral arthritis, and conjunctivitis. The histological image reveals signs of subcorneal pustulosis and SS with vasculitis but no fibrinoid necrosis.

The main differential diagnoses are cutaneous manifestations of septicemia, Behcet's disease, SS and PG on which the issue is mainly nosological. Indeed, in some cases, pustular lesions and elements of larger size coexist suggestive of SS or PG, reinforcing the notion of neutrophilic disease that may indeed represent overlapping and co-occurrence of the neutrophilic dermatoses (Fig. 18.2).

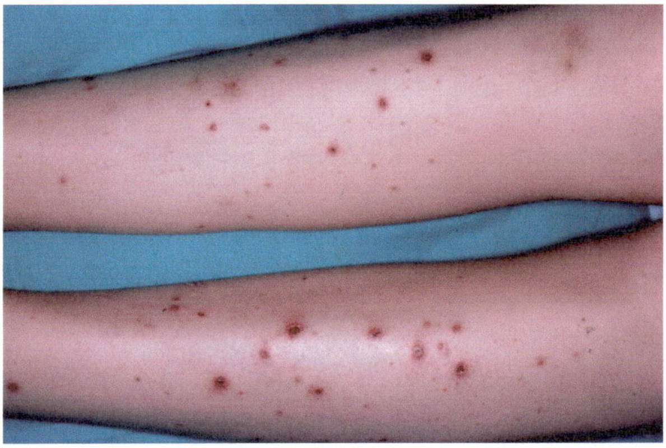

Fig. 18.1 BADAS. Non-follicular pustules, resting on an erythematous base

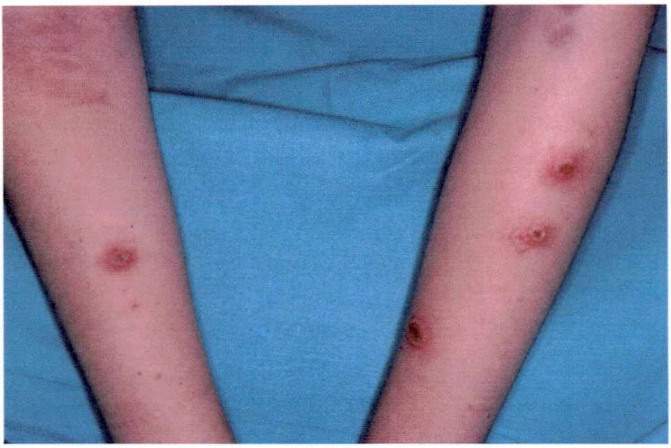

Fig. 18.2 BADAS. Same patient. Note largest pustular lesions evocative for borderline form of PG

In acute phase, the treatment of the underlying disease is required, more often based on systemic steroid therapy rather than on sulfasalazine or mesalazine. Antibiotics (quinolones or metronidazole) that are active against intestinal bacterial multiplication are often added when treatment is started.

Pyodermatitis-Pyostomatitis Vegetans (PPV) is a rare condition of which approximately 60 cases have only been reported. It is strongly associated with IBD (about 75% of the reported cases).This condition is more commonly found in individuals with UC than CD. Hallopeau initially described PD-PSV. The positive results of direct immunofluorescence (DIF) found in some cases, explain the confusion that is often made with pemphigus vegetans, another condition that has also been described by the same author. PPV is a condition that must be integrated into the spectrum of neutrophilic dermatoses. Observations in which PPV is contemporaneous with PG reinforce this nosological concept [13].

Clinically, PPV manifests as pustules on the buccal mucosa giving a very characteristic appearance that is known as "snail-tracks". It affects mainly the gums, the internal side of the cheeks, the palate and the lips (Figs. 18.3 and 18.4). The tongue and buccal floor are spared. These painless lesions break easily and give way to erosions with a tendency to vegetate. Genital mucosal sites are possible but are considered an exception. In half of the cases, they are pustular lesions and cutaneous vegetations, localized preferentially to the scalp and the large folds, justifying the name "pyodermatitis-pyostomatitis vegetans". Cutaneous lesions generally appear at the same time as mucosal lesions, but can also appear secondary facilitating their diagnosis.

Histologically, the pustules are intra- and/or subepithelial, and contain many neutrophils associated with few eosinophils. Acantholysis is present in some cases but remains only focal. A low positivity of DIF that is non-specific can be observed. Other cases with epidermal pattern of DIF probably correspond to pemphigus

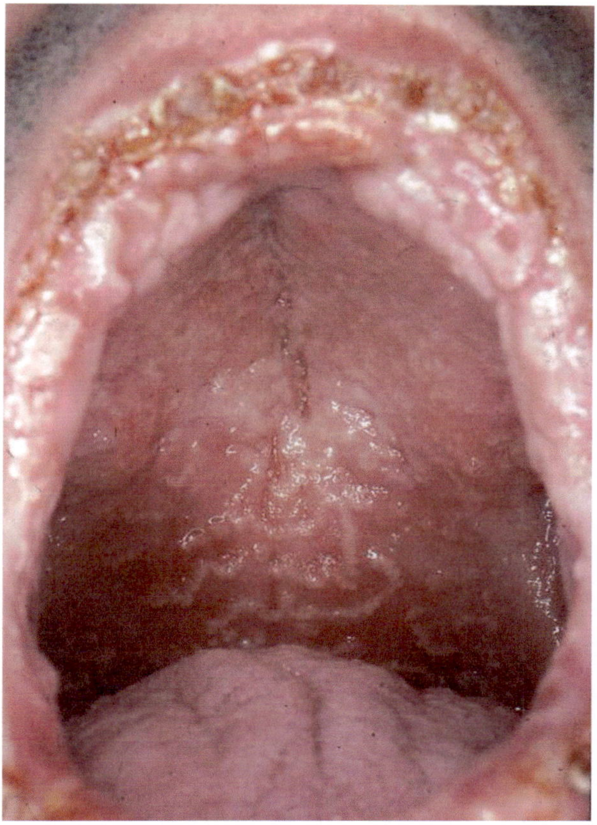

Fig. 18.3 PPV. Pustules of the palate giving the typical aspect of snail tracks

vegetans [14]. Systemic steroid therapy is the treatment of choice for PPV but is not always effective. Dapsone and anti-TNF agents are interesting therapeutic alternatives.

Aseptic abscesses. Subcutaneous aseptic abscesses corresponding probably to deep forms of SS have been reported in CD and more rarely in UC. Moreover, visceral abscesses can also be observed in CD. They may precede the bowel disease by several months [15]. Such abscesses may involve the spleen, the liver, the lymph nodes. TNF antagonists have been used successfully in some steroid-resistant or dependent patients.

Other neutrophilic dermatoses including Sneddon-Wilkinson's subcorneal pustulosis, erythema elevatum diutinum, and intraepidermal IgA pustulosis have also been observed during both forms of IBD. Parallel evolutions between cutaneous and digestive manifestations have not always been observed. These associations are extremely rare but certainly not fortuitous [16].

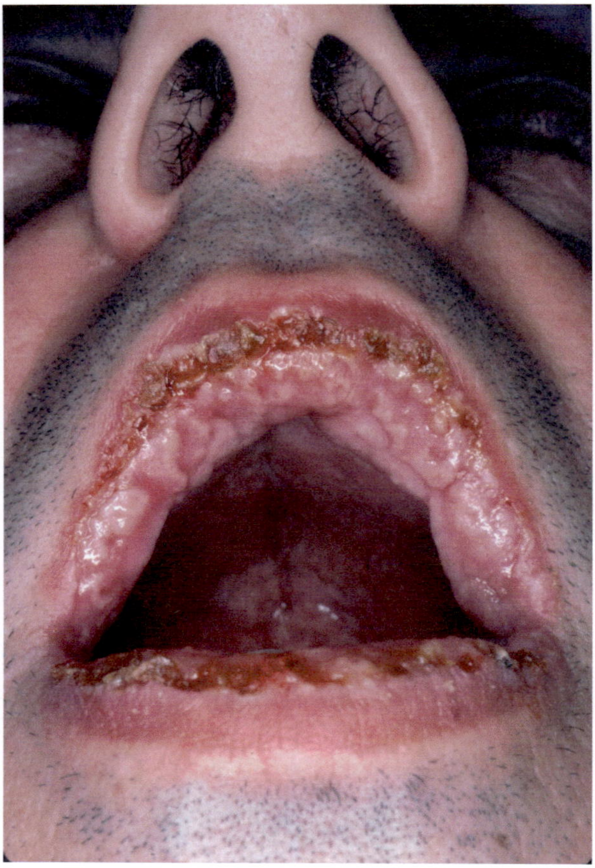

Fig. 18.4 PPV. Pustules of the lips with the same typical aspect

References

1. Van Limbergen J, Radford-Smith G, Satsangi J. Advances in IBD genetics. Nat Rev Gastroenterol Hepatol. 2014;11:372–85.
2. Knights D, Lassen KG, Xavier RJ. Advances in inflammatory bowel disease pathogenesis: linking host genetics and the microbiome. Gut. 2013;62:1505–10.
3. Gerson LB. Use and misuse of small bowel video capsule endoscopy in clinical practice. Clin Gastroenterol Hepatol. 2013;11:1224–31.
4. Delaporte E, Piette F. Peau et affections du tube digestif. EMC – Dermatologie. 2015;10:1–12. [Article 98-876-A-10].
5. Thrash B, Patel M, Shah KR, Boland R, Menter A. Cutaneous manifestations of gastrointestinal disease. Part II. J Am Acad Dermatol. 2013;68:211.e1–33.
6. Weizman AV, Huang B, Targan S, et al. Pyoderma gangrenosum among patients with inflammatory bowel disease: a descriptive cohort study. J Cut Med Surg. 2015;19:125–31.
7. DeFilippis EM, Feldman SR, Huang WW. The genetics of pyoderma gangrenosum and implications for treatment: a systematic review. Br J Dermatol. 2015;172:1487–97.

8. Deregnaucourt D, Buche S, Coopman S, Basraoui D, Turck D, Delaporte E. Pyoderma gangrenosum avec localisations pulmonaires traité par infliximab. Ann Dermatol Vénéréol. 2013;140:363–6.
9. Peyrin-Biroulet L, Van Assche G, Gómez-Ulloa D, et al. Systematic review of tumor necrosis factor antagonists in extraintestinal manifestations in inflammatory bowel disease. Clin Gastroenterol Hepatol. 2017;15:25–36.
10. Argüelles-Arias F, Castro-Laria L, Lobaton T, et al. Characteristics and treatment of pyoderma gangrenosum in inflammatory bowel disease. Dig Dis Sci. 2013;58:2949–54.
11. Marzano AV, Ishak RS, Saibeni S, Crosti C, Meroni PL, Cugno M. Autoinflammatory skin disorders in inflammatory bowel diseases, pyoderma gangrenosum and Sweet's syndrome: a comprehensive review and disease classification criteria. Clinic Rev Allergol Immunol. 2013;45:202–10.
12. DeFilippis EM, Magro C, Jorizzo JL. Bowel-associated dermatosis – arthritis syndrome in a patient with ulcerative colitis: an extraintestinal manifestation of inflammatory bowel disease. Clin J Gastroenterol. 2014;7:410–3.
13. Clark LG, Tolkachjov SN, Bridges AG, Camilleri MJ. Pyostomatitis vegetans (PSV)-pyodermatitis vegetans (PDV): a clinicopathologic study of 7 cases at a tertiary referral center. J Am Acad Dermatol. 2016;75:578–84.
14. Nico MMS, Hussein TP, Aoki V, Lourenço SV. Pyostomatitis vegetans and its relation to inflammatory bowel disease, pyoderma gangreosum, pyodermatitis vegetans, and pemphigus. J Oral Pathol Med. 2012;41:584–8.
15. André M, Aumaître O. Le syndrome des abcès aseptiques. Rev Med Int. 2010;32:678–88.
16. Shipman AR, Reddy H, Wojnarowska F. Association between the subepidermal autoimmune blistering diseases linear IgA disease and the pemphigoid group and inflammatory bowel disease: two case reports and literature review. Clin Exp Dermatol. 2012;37:461–8.

Neutrophilic Dermatoses and Joint Disorders

19

Roberta Gualtierotti, Angelo Valerio Marzano, and Massimo Cugno

Introduction

Inflammatory joint disorders such as rheumatoid arthritis and spondyloarthritis are chronic systemic diseases with an immune-mediated pathogenesis. They may be associated with neutrophilic dermatoses, particularly pyoderma gangrenosum, Sweet's syndrome and hidradenitis suppurativa [1–3].

Both inflammatory joint disorders and neutrophilic dermatoses share a number of pathophysiological features related to the pro-inflammatory cytokine expression profile [4, 5]. Furthermore, it is well recognized that in neutrophilic dermatoses any organ system can be potentially involved, giving rise to the concept of "neutrophilic disease" [6, 7]. Among the extracutaneous manifestations of neutrophilic dermatoses, joint involvement is regarded as the most frequent [6, 7].

In this chapter, we focus on the main rheumatic diseases associated with neutrophilic dermatoses as well as on the articular involvement of "neutrophilic disease", providing a simple approach for the recognition of these associations.

R. Gualtierotti
Divisione e Cattedra di Reumatologia, Dipartimento di Scienze Cliniche e di Comunità, Università degli Studi di Milano, Milan, Italy

A. V. Marzano
Dipartimento di Fisiopatologia Medico-Chirurgica e dei Trapianti, Università degli Studi di Milano, Unità Operativa di Dermatologia, IRCCS Fondazione Ca' Granda, Ospedale Maggiore Policlinico, Milan, Italy
e-mail: angelo.marzano@unimi.it

M. Cugno (✉)
Dipartimento di Fisiopatologia Medico-Chirurgica e dei Trapianti, Università degli Studi di Milano, Medicina Interna, IRCCS Fondazione Ca' Granda, Ospedale Maggiore Policlinico, Milan, Italy
e-mail: massimo.cugno@unimi.it

D. Wallach et al. (eds.), *Neutrophilic Dermatoses*,
https://doi.org/10.1007/978-3-319-72649-6_19

Rheumatoid Arthritis (RA)

Rheumatoid arthritis (RA) is a chronic systemic autoimmune disease characterized not only by inflammation of the joints (synovitis), but also by a systemic inflammation that may lead, if untreated, to severe extra-articular manifestations [8]. RA may be seropositive, in the presence of rheumatoid factors (RF) and/or anti-citrullinated peptide autoantibodies (ACPA), or seronegative, in their absence. Seropositive RA seems to have a worse prognosis in terms of bone erosions and disability [9]. The diagnosis of RA is straightforward in the presence of tender and swollen joints, morning joint stiffness with duration >1 h, abnormal laboratory tests such as elevated concentrations of C reactive protein or erythrocyte sedimentation rate and if RF or ACPA positivity are present. Bone erosions of the small joints of the hands or feet are typical of the disease [8, 10]. However, radiographic signs of erosions usually are not present in the early phase of the disease and antibodies may be absent. Therefore, classification criteria for RA have been recently revised in order to help achieving a definite diagnosis also in early arthritis (Table 19.1) [11]. Both seropositive and seronegative RA may present various cutaneous manifestations, among which there are neutrophilic dermatoses [12]. A possible common pathway may be represented by the involvement of autoinflammatory mechanisms related to the overproduction of IL-1beta,

Table 19.1 The 2010 classification criteria for rheumatoid arthritis (RA) of the American College of Rheumatology/European League Against Rheumatism

	Score
A. Joint involvement	
1 large joint	0
2–10 large joints	1
1–3 small joints (with or without involvement of large joints)	2
4–10 small joints (with or without involvement of large joints)	3
>10 joints (at least 1 small joint)	5
B. Serology (at least 1 test result is needed for classification)	
Negative RF *and* negative ACPA	0
Low-positive RF *or* low-positive ACPA	2
High-positive RF *or* high-positive ACPA	3
C. Acute-phase reactants (at least 1 test result is needed for classification)	
Normal CRP *and* normal ESR 0	0
Abnormal CRP *or* abnormal ESR	1
D. Duration of symptoms	
<6 weeks	0
≥6 weeks	1

A total score higher than 6/10 is needed for classification of a patient as having definite RA
ACPA anticitrullinated protein antibody, *CRP* C reactive protein, *ESR* erythrocyte sedimentation rate, *RF* rheumatoid factor

a pivotal pro-inflammatory cytokine in both RA and neutrophilic dermatoses [5, 13, 14]. Furthermore, IL-8, a pro-inflammatory chemokine, which is able to attract neutrophils and lymphocytes, is elevated in the joints and serum of patients with RA and may play a role in the development of neutrophilic dermatoses in these patients [4, 5, 15].

Although neutrophilic dermatoses are not commonly reported in RA, possibly due to misdiagnosis, their early recognition is important to avoid potentially severe complications. In RA, the most frequent neutrophilic dermatosis is pyoderma gangrenosum, followed by Sweet's syndrome and rheumatoid neutrophilic dermatosis.

Pyoderma Gangrenosum

Pyoderma gangrenosum in RA usually presents with single or multiple painful skin ulcers with undermined erythematous-violaceous borders on the lower extremities. Other rare atypical variants are recognized, mainly including the pustular, bullous and vegetative forms [16]. It is still controversial whether pyoderma gangrenosum is a true skin manifestation of RA, since pyoderma gangrenosum often occurs in other systemic disorders and has no relation with the course of RA. Furthermore, pyoderma gangrenosum associated with RA has no specific histologic presentation but early lesions demonstrate a predominant neutrophilic infiltrate in the dermis and subcutaneous tissue [17, 18].

In a classic retrospective study of 86 patients with pyoderma gangrenosum from the Mayo Clinic, RA was the second most common disease association (14%) after inflammatory bowel diseases [18]. These findings have been more recently confirmed in a larger series of patients with pyoderma gangrenosum, by Langan et al., who observed a similar prevalence of RA (12% of cases) [1].

Sweet's Syndrome

Sweet's syndrome can be associated with RA, although uncommonly. Lesions present as single or multiple erythematous papules, nodules or raised plaques, associated with fever, malaise, arthralgia and myalgia. Localisation is prominent at the face, neck and upper extremities, however, any site could be potentially targeted. The lesions are usually tender and sharply demarcated with a characteristic superficial vesiculation on their surface [19, 20]. Histopathology reveals a dense neutrophilic infiltrate in the superficial derma with massive oedema. Leukocytoclastic vasculitis is usually absent [21].

Neutrophilic dermatosis of the hands can be regarded as a localised variant of Sweet's syndrome [22]. The cutaneous picture is similar to that of Sweet's syndrome, with lesions located exclusively on the hands, especially at their dorsal aspect, and is usually not associated with systemic symptoms [22].

Rheumatoid Neutrophilic Dermatosis

Rheumatoid neutrophilic dermatosis is a rare cutaneous manifestation in patients with severe RA. It was described in 1978 by Ackerman [23]. It mainly affects patients with severe seropositive RA, predominantly women (ratio 2:1), but it has been observed also in seronegative RA [24].

Clinically, it presents with symmetric asymptomatic erythematous papulo-nodular lesions and/or plaques, which may persist and sometimes ulcerate. They are usually distributed on the extensor surfaces of forearms and hands as well as the neck, the shoulders and the trunk. Rheumatoid neutrophilic dermatosis lesions may resemble those of Sweet's syndrome. Histopathological examination reveals a dense neutrophilic infiltrate without vasculitis. The course of rheumatoid neutrophilic dermatosis seems to follow RA disease course [25]. Resolution may occur spontaneously or in association with improvement of RA, without scarring.

Spondyloarthritis

With the term spondyloarthritis we refer to the spectrum of diseases comprising several related but clinically distinct diseases: psoriatic arthritis, arthritis related to inflammatory bowel disease, reactive arthritis, a subgroup of juvenile idiopathic arthritis, and ankylosing spondylitis [26]. The various clinical forms include spinal (axial) features with inflammatory back pain, peripheral arthritis predominantly of the lower limbs, dactylitis ('sausage'-like fingers or toes), enthesopathy, and extra-articular features such as uveitis, psoriasis, and inflammatory bowel diseases.

All these diseases are associated with the major histocompatibility complex HLA-B27. The presence of a common genetic basis is demonstrated by the observation of a familial clustering of different forms of spondyloarthritis [26].

The members of the Assessment of SpondyloArthritis international Society (ASAS) (Table 19.2) have recently reviewed previous criteria of the European Spondylarthropathy Study Group (ESSG) [27] and those of Amor [28].

Although spondyloarthritis has been traditionally regarded as a condition depending on an altered adaptive immunity, recently, a contributing role of autoinflammatory mechanisms has been proposed based on the observation of a genetic polymorphism in genes related to IL-1 pathway [29].

Although psoriasis is by far the most common skin manifestation in spondyloarthritis, also neutrophilic dermatoses have been reported [30]. In particular, hidradenitis suppurativa and bowel-associated dermatosis-arthritis syndrome (BADAS) are the most frequently reported in spondyloarthritis patients.

Table 19.2 Classification criteria for axial spondyloarthritis (SpA) according to the Assessment of SpondyloArthritis International Society (ASAS)

Sacroiliitis on imaging[a] *plus*	HLA-B27 *plus*
≥ 1 SpA feature[b]	≥ 2 other SpA feature[b]

The criteria encompass both patients with and without definite radiographic sacroiliitis in patients with chronic back pain (>3 months) and age at onset <45 years

[a]Active (acute) inflammation on MRI highly suggestive of sacroiliitis associated with SpA *or* definite radiographic sacroiliitis according to modified New York criteria

[b]Inflammatory back pain; arthritis; enthesitis (heel); uveitis; dactylitis; psoriasis; Crohn's disease/ulcerative colitis; good response to non-steroidal anti-inflammatory drugs; family history for SpA; HLA-B27; elevated C reactive protein

Hidradenitis Suppurativa

Hidradenitis suppurativa, also called acne inversa, is a chronic, frequently debilitating inflammatory disease manifesting as nodules, abscesses and fistulae involving skin folds, predominantly in the axillary and inguinal regions, as well as the anogenital areas [31]. It may present in association with other neutrophilic dermatoses, also in the context of syndromic forms, or in combination with inflammatory diseases, particularly psoriasis [32]. Hidradenitis suppurativa is also often associated with extracutaneous diseases, such as inflammatory bowel diseases [33] and spondyloarthritis [3]. Strong evidence for a non-fortuitous association of spondyloarthritis and hidradenitis suppurativa is supported by the study by Richette et al., demonstrating that spondyloarthritis had a prevalence of 3.7% in their large cohort, a much higher value than the prevalence of spondyloarthritis in the general population [3].

A dysregulation of the innate immune system has been demonstrated in both hidradenitis suppurativa [34] and spondyloarthritis [26, 35]. The enhanced presence or expression in tissue lesions of neutrophils and macrophages as well as cytokines, such as IL-1beta, TNF-alpha, and IL-6 further supports this view [34, 36]. Interestingly, all these pro-inflammatory cytokines are upregulated and play a pivotal role also in the pathogenesis of spondyloarthritis [26, 37].

Bowel-Associated Dermatosis-Arthritis Syndrome (BADAS)

BADAS is characterised by fever, flu-like symptoms, arthritis and inflammatory skin involvement. The latter is characterised by lesions recalling different neutrophilic dermatoses such as papules and plaques (Sweet's syndrome), pustules and ulcers (pyoderma gangrenosum) or nodules, abscesses or fistulae (hidradenitis suppurativa) [38]. In addition, acne and neutrophilic panniculitis can be associated [38, 39]. Patients usually experience a symmetrical, non-erosive polyarthritis that predominantly involves small joints [40].

This syndrome has been initially described in patients undergoing jejunoileal bypass for bariatric surgery and named "bowel-bypass syndrome" [41, 42]. Later, the term BADAS was introduced, based on the observation that a similar presentation could occur also in patients undergoing surgery such as Billroth II for peptic ulcer disease, biliopancreatic diversion [43] and in patients with chronic inflammatory bowel diseases such as Crohn's disease and ulcerative colitis [44]. More recently, it has been described also in patients with diverticulosis and appendicitis [45].

The pathogenesis of BADAS is still poorly understood. Evidence suggests that gut microbiota could play a pivotal role in its pathogenesis [46]. In particular, BADAS could be caused by small intestine bacterial overgrowth [39]. This condition may predispose to the release of pro-inflammatory cytokines and chemokines and effector molecules eventually leading to neutrophil-mediated inflammation.

Joint Involvement in the "Neutrophilic Disease" and Syndromic Forms

Since the first reports of neutrophilic disorders, the observation of a possible multisystem involvement has led researchers to coin the term "neutrophilic disease" [6, 7]. During the course of neutrophilic dermatoses almost any organ can be involved, particularly lungs, with parenchymal infiltrates, or kidneys, usually with a nephrotic syndrome. However, joints are the most frequent extracutaneous site with arthralgia in more than in 50% or overt arthritis in 10–37% of patients [6]. Joint manifestations may precede by years the onset of dermatosis [47].

It is not always easy to distinguish chronic inflammatory arthritis such as RA or spondyloarthritis and neutrophilic dermatosis-related arthritis. Nevertheless, the clinical presentation, the distribution and the localisation together with laboratory findings may help in the differential diagnosis.

For example, RA and spondyloarthritis are chronic, characterised by recurrent flares and may progress with erosions and deformity if untreated [48]. By contrast, arthritis associated with neutrophilic dermatoses seems to follow the course of skin involvement with remission after treatment and usually no flare-up [6]. When a flare-up of arthritis occurs, a chronic inflammatory rheumatic disorder should be suspected. Nolla et al. reported in patients with Sweet's syndrome an asymmetric non-erosive arthritis with predominant neutrophilic and mildly inflammatory infiltrate usually involving large joints [49]. These characteristics can be found also in RA and therefore are not useful in differential diagnosis. Radiographs are often normal in arthritis related to neutrophilic dermatoses [49]. However, in the early phase of the disease also RA and spondyloarthritis may not show erosions or other signs. In this case, ultrasound with power-Doppler assessment or magnetic resonance imaging are more sensitive than plain radiographs [50]. It is possible that the pattern of arthritis mainly described by Holt et al., namely a chronic, progressive, symmetric, seronegative destructive polyarthritis with axial and peripheral involvement or both, could actually be a seronegative arthritis or a spondyloarthritis [47]. Furthermore, this kind of arthritis could also be associated with hidradenitis suppurativa or acne conglobata and in some patients, “the arthritis of ulcerative colitis” was hypothesised [47]. Finally, undifferentiated spondyloarthritis in association with pyoderma gangrenosum has been reported [51].

No data regarding the prevalence of ACPA is available in patients with neutrophilic dermatoses. Although not very sensitive, ACPA are very specific for RA and may help in the differential diagnosis. The specificity of RF depends on its titre: low titres are not specific, whereas high titres are more specific for RA, particularly when associated with ACPA [52].

Therefore, it is advisable that patients with articular symptoms are referred as soon as possible to a rheumatologist in order to make a correct diagnosis, to decide the optimal treatment and to perform regular follow-up of the patients.

Joint involvement also typically occurs in the context of several syndromic forms of neutrophilic dermatoses, namely SAPHO (synovitis, acne, pustulosis, hyperostosis and osteitis), PAPA (pyogenic arthritis, pyoderma gangrenosum and acne) and PAPASH (pyogenic arthritis, pyoderma gangrenosum, acne and suppurative hidradenitis) syndromes.

SAPHO Syndrome

Synovitis, acne, pustulosis, hyperostosis, and osteitis (SAPHO) syndrome was initially described in 1987 [53]. SAPHO syndrome is a rare condition, also possibly due to misdiagnosis [54].

Although its pathogenesis is still elusive, there is increasing understanding that SAPHO shares similarities with other autoinflammatory diseases [55]. The proline-serine-threonine phosphatase interacting protein 2 (PSTPIP2), which is involved in macrophage activation, neutrophil motility and osteoclast differentiation, has recently been supposed to play a role in innate immunity and development of autoinflammatory bone disorders, including SAPHO syndrome [56]. Proinflammatory cytokines, such as IL-1beta and TNF-alpha, as well as the chemokine IL-8, seem to be important in the pathogenesis of SAPHO [57, 58]. It has been suggested that *Propionibacterium acnes*, the main pathogenic responsible for acne, may trigger autoinflammation via inflammasome activation [59, 60]. Furthermore, Th17 cells were recently found to be increased in the peripheral blood of patients with SAPHO [61].

The diagnosis of SAPHO syndrome is based upon typical clinical findings. A set of criteria has been proposed for SAPHO in 1994: (i) multifocal osteitis with or without skin symptoms; (ii) sterile acute/chronic joint inflammation with either pustules or psoriasis of the palms/soles, or acne or hidradenitis suppurativa; and (iii) sterile osteitis and any one of the above skin manifestations, with any one of the criteria being sufficient for the diagnosis [62].

Actually, the term SAPHO refers to a group of diseases in which pustular skin involvement—manifesting as acne fulminans or acne conglobata, psoriasis and palmoplantar pustulosis,—is associated with bone and joint involvement presenting as hyperostosis and osteitis—chronic inflammatory reactions involving the cortical and medullary bone—and arthritis (synovitis) [63]. Other cutaneous manifestations of SAPHO syndrome include pyoderma gangrenosum, Sweet's syndrome and Sneddon–Wilkinson disease [55]. The sternoclavicular joints are often involved, followed by the spine and sacroiliac joints [64]. Total body bone scintigraphic imaging may show the "bullhead sign", a pattern of bone inflammation localised at the sternum and sternocostoclavicular joints, which is regarded as characteristic of this syndrome [65]. Although arthritis (synovitis) in SAPHO presents with a pattern that resembles spondyloarthritis, HLA-B27 is not characteristic of this syndrome [54]. Arthritis is erosive and usually involves axial joints, less frequently peripheral joints, with a reported association with inflammatory bowel diseases [66]. SAPHO syndrome is usually self-limiting, but may also have a chronic course, particularly if inflammatory indices, anterior chest wall involvement, peripheral synovitis and skin involvement are present at the onset and are associated with female sex [67]. It is important to consider that skin and joint/bone involvement may not be present at the same time [63].

PAPA and PAPASH Syndromes

PAPA and PAPASH belong to a group of autoinflammatory syndromes characterised by the association of pyoderma gangrenosum and sterile pyogenic arthritis. Also in these forms an over-activation of the innate immune system may lead to increased production of IL-1beta. From a genetic point of view, a number of mutations affecting the proteins of the inflammasome complex or the proteins that regulate its function have been described in these disorders [68–70]. In particular, mutations of the PSTPIP1 gene are the genetic hallmark of PAPA, which is nowadays regarded as a monogenic autoinflammatory syndrome [55, 69].

Pyogenic arthritis in these cases presents as a painful, recurrent, monoarticular arthritis mainly involving large joints such as elbows, knees and ankles. Synovial fluid appears as a seropurulent or purulent, cloudy, yellow and sterile liquid due to the prominent neutrophilic infiltrate [68]. The first episodes usually occur in childhood and may be the presenting sign of the disease. The episodes may occur spontaneously, but traumatic events may precipitate episodes of arthritis, similarly to what is observed in a "Koebner's phenomenon" in the skin [71]. Erosions and joint destruction are reported in persistent (untreated) disease, even though in young adults joint symptoms tend to decrease, whereas cutaneous symptoms become more prominent [72].

Drug-Induced Neutrophilic Dermatoses in Rheumatic Diseases

The treatment of neutrophilic dermatoses is mainly based on corticosteroids, which in most cases are effective in controlling the disease. Targeted therapies including TNF blocking agents seem to be another effective option [73]. However, treatment with anti-TNF alpha may also be responsible for a number of cutaneous adverse reactions, the most frequent of which are pustular eruptions [74]. Indeed, neutrophilic dermatoses have been reported during the course of anti-TNF therapy with infliximab [75] adalimumab [76, 77] or etanercept [78]. The causal mechanism is still a matter of debate, but may implicate an imbalance of cytokines toward interferons, chemokines and probably IL-17 [79]. Cases of pyoderma gangrenosum have been reported also during treatment with abatacept [80, 81]. CTLA-4-Ig therapy diminishes the frequency but enhances the function of Treg cells in patients with RA and a possible explanation could be a paradoxical inhibition of T-cell function in response to CTLA-4 blockade [82, 83].

References

1. Langan SM, Groves RW, Card TR, Gulliford MC. Incidence, mortality, and disease associations of pyoderma gangrenosum in the United Kingdom: a retrospective cohort study. J Invest Dermatol. 2012;132(9):2166–70.
2. Levin J, Werth VP. Skin disorders with arthritis. Best Pract Res Clin Rheumatol. 2006;20(4):809–26.
3. Richette P, Molto A, Viguier M, Dawidowicz K, Hayem G, Nassif A, et al. Hidradenitis suppurativa associated with spondyloarthritis—results from a multicenter national prospective study. J Rheumatol. 2014;41(3):490–4.
4. Firestein GS, McInnes IB. Immunopathogenesis of rheumatoid arthritis. Immunity. 2017;46(2):183–96.
5. Marzano AV, Fanoni D, Antiga E, Quaglino P, Caproni M, Crosti C, et al. Expression of cytokines, chemokines and other effector molecules in two prototypic autoinflammatory skin diseases, pyoderma gangrenosum and Sweet's syndrome. Clin Exp Immunol. 2014;178(1):48–56.
6. Prat L, Bouaziz JD, Wallach D, Vignon-Pennamen MD, Bagot M. Neutrophilic dermatoses as systemic diseases. Clin Dermatol. 2014;32(3):376–88.
7. Wallach D, Vignon-Pennamen MD. From acute febrile neutrophilic dermatosis to neutrophilic disease: forty years of clinical research. J Am Acad Dermatol. 2006;55(6):1066–71.
8. Smolen JS, Aletaha D, McInnes IB. Rheumatoid arthritis. Lancet. 2016;388(10055):2023–38.
9. Malmstrom V, Catrina AI, Klareskog L. The immunopathogenesis of seropositive rheumatoid arthritis: from triggering to targeting. Nat Rev Immunol. 2017;17(1):60–75.
10. Arnett FC, Edworthy SM, Bloch DA, McShane DJ, Fries JF, Cooper NS, et al. The American Rheumatism Association 1987 revised criteria for the classification of rheumatoid arthritis. Arthritis Rheum. 1988;31(3):315–24.
11. Aletaha D, Neogi T, Silman AJ, Funovits J, Felson DT, Bingham CO III, et al. 2010 Rheumatoid arthritis classification criteria: an American College of Rheumatology/European League Against Rheumatism collaborative initiative. Arthritis Rheum. 2010;62(9):2569–81.
12. Sayah A, English JC III. Rheumatoid arthritis: a review of the cutaneous manifestations. J Am Acad Dermatol. 2005;53(2):191–209; quiz 10–2.
13. Stehlik C. Multiple interleukin-1beta-converting enzymes contribute to inflammatory arthritis. Arthritis Rheum. 2009;60(12):3524–30.
14. Dinarello CA. Immunological and inflammatory functions of the interleukin-1 family. Annu Rev Immunol. 2009;27:519–50.
15. Catrina AI, Svensson CI, Malmstrom V, Schett G, Klareskog L. Mechanisms leading from systemic autoimmunity to joint-specific disease in rheumatoid arthritis. Nat Rev Rheumatol. 2017;13(2):79–86.
16. Ahmadi S, Powell FC. Pyoderma gangrenosum: uncommon presentations. Clin Dermatol. 2005;23(6):612–20.
17. von den Driesch P. Pyoderma gangrenosum: a report of 44 cases with follow-up. Br J Dermatol. 1997;137(6):1000–5.

18. Powell FC, Schroeter AL, Su WP, Perry HO. Pyoderma gangrenosum: a review of 86 patients. Q J Med. 1985;55(217):173–86.
19. Gay-Crosier F, Dayer JM, Chavaz P, Hauser C. Rheumatoid neutrophilic dermatitis/Sweet's syndrome in a patient with seronegative rheumatoid arthritis. Dermatology. 2000;201(2):185–7.
20. Yamauchi PS, Turner L, Lowe NJ, Gindi V, Jackson JM. Treatment of recurrent Sweet's syndrome with coexisting rheumatoid arthritis with the tumor necrosis factor antagonist etanercept. J Am Acad Dermatol. 2006;54(3 Suppl 2):S122–6.
21. Cohen PR, Kurzrock R. Sweet's syndrome: a neutrophilic dermatosis classically associated with acute onset and fever. Clin Dermatol. 2000;18(3):265–82.
22. Wolf R, Tuzun Y. Acral manifestations of Sweet syndrome (neutrophilic dermatosis of the hands). Clin Dermatol. 2017;35(1):81–4.
23. Ackerman AB. Histologic diagnosis of inflammatory skin diseases: a method by pattern analysis. Philadelphia: Lea & Febiger; 1978.
24. Brown TS, Fearneyhough PK, Burruss JB, Callen JP. Rheumatoid neutrophilic dermatitis in a woman with seronegative rheumatoid arthritis. J Am Acad Dermatol. 2001;45(4):596–600.
25. Mashek HA, Pham CT, Helm TN, Klaus M. Rheumatoid neutrophilic dermatitis. Arch Dermatol. 1997;133(6):757–60.
26. Dougados M, Baeten D. Spondyloarthritis. Lancet. 2011;377(9783):2127–37.
27. Dougados M, van der Linden S, Juhlin R, Huitfeldt B, Amor B, Calin A, et al. The European Spondylarthropathy Study Group preliminary criteria for the classification of spondylarthropathy. Arthritis Rheum. 1991;34(10):1218–27.
28. Amor B, Dougados M, Mijiyawa M. Criteria of the classification of spondylarthropathies. Rev Rhum Mal Osteoartic. 1990;57(2):85–9.
29. Sims AM, Timms AE, Bruges-Armas J, Burgos-Vargas R, Chou CT, Doan T, et al. Prospective meta-analysis of interleukin 1 gene complex polymorphisms confirms associations with ankylosing spondylitis. Ann Rheum Dis. 2008;67(9):1305–9.
30. El Maghraoui A. Extra-articular manifestations of ankylosing spondylitis: prevalence, characteristics and therapeutic implications. Eur J Intern Med. 2011;22(6):554–60.
31. Jemec GB. Clinical practice. Hidradenitis suppurativa. N Engl J Med. 2012;366(2):158–64.
32. Marzano AV, Trevisan V, Gattorno M, Ceccherini I, De Simone C, Crosti C. Pyogenic arthritis, pyoderma gangrenosum, acne, and hidradenitis suppurativa (PAPASH): a new autoinflammatory syndrome associated with a novel mutation of the PSTPIP1 gene. JAMA Dermatol. 2013;149(6):762–4.
33. van der Zee HH, van der Woude CJ, Florencia EF, Prens EP. Hidradenitis suppurativa and inflammatory bowel disease: are they associated? Results of a pilot study. Br J Dermatol. 2010;162(1):195–7.
34. van der Zee HH, de Ruiter L, van den Broecke DG, Dik WA, Laman JD, Prens EP. Elevated levels of tumour necrosis factor (TNF)-alpha, interleukin (IL)-1beta and IL-10 in hidradenitis suppurativa skin: a rationale for targeting TNF-alpha and IL-1beta. Br J Dermatol. 2011;164(6):1292–8.
35. Monnet D, Kadi A, Izac B, Lebrun N, Letourneur F, Zinovieva E, et al. Association between the IL-1 family gene cluster and spondyloarthritis. Ann Rheum Dis. 2012;71(6):885–90.
36. Lima AL, Karl I, Giner T, Poppe H, Schmidt M, Presser D, et al. Keratinocytes and neutrophils are important sources of proinflammatory molecules in hidradenitis suppurativa. Br J Dermatol. 2016;174(3):514–21.
37. Ambarus C, Yeremenko N, Tak PP, Baeten D. Pathogenesis of spondyloarthritis: autoimmune or autoinflammatory? Curr Opin Rheumatol. 2012;24(4):351–8.
38. Delaney TA, Clay CD, Randell PL. The bowel-associated dermatosis—arthritis syndrome. Australas J Dermatol. 1989;30(1):23–7.
39. Brouard MC, Chavaz P, Borradori L. Acute pustulosis of the legs in diverticulitis with sigmoid stenosis: an overlap between bowel-associated dermatosis-arthritis syndrome and pustular pyoderma gangrenosum. J Eur Acad Dermatol Venereol. 2004;18(1):89–92.
40. Callen JP. Neutrophilic dermatoses. Dermatol Clin. 2002;20(3):409–19.

41. Shagrin JW, Frame B, Duncan H. Polyarthritis in obese patients with intestinal bypass. Ann Intern Med. 1971;75(3):377–80.
42. Kennedy C. The spectrum of inflammatory skin disease following jejuno-ileal bypass for morbid obesity. Br J Dermatol. 1981;105(4):425–35.
43. Slater GH, Kerlin P, Georghiou PR, Fielding GA. Bowel-associated dermatosis-arthritis syndrome after biliopancreatic diversion. Obes Surg. 2004;14(1):133–5.
44. Dicken CH. Bowel-associated dermatosis-arthritis syndrome: bowel bypass syndrome without bowel bypass. J Am Acad Dermatol. 1986;14(5 Pt 1):792–6.
45. Prpic-Massari L, Kastelan M, Brajac I, Cabrijan L, Zamolo G, Massari D. Bowel-associated dermatosis-arthritis syndrome in a patient with appendicitis. Med Sci Monit. 2007;13(8):CS97–100.
46. Marzano AV, Ishak RS, Saibeni S, Crosti C, Meroni PL, Cugno M. Autoinflammatory skin disorders in inflammatory bowel diseases, pyoderma gangrenosum and Sweet's syndrome: a comprehensive review and disease classification criteria. Clin Rev Allergy Immunol. 2013;45(2):202–10.
47. Holt PJ, Davies MG, Saunders KC, Nuki G. Pyoderma gangrenosum: clinical and laboratory findings in 15 patients with special reference to polyarthritis. Medicine. 1980;59(2):114–33.
48. Aletaha D, Funovits J, Breedveld FC, Sharp J, Segurado O, Smolen JS. Rheumatoid arthritis joint progression in sustained remission is determined by disease activity levels preceding the period of radiographic assessment. Arthritis Rheum. 2009;60(5):1242–9.
49. Nolla JM, Juanola X, Valverde J, Roig-Escofet D, Pagerols X, Servitge O. Arthritis in acute febrile neutrophilic dermatosis (Sweet's syndrome). Ann Rheum Dis. 1990;49(2):135.
50. McQueen FM. Imaging in early rheumatoid arthritis. Best Pract Res Clin Rheumatol. 2013;27(4):499–522.
51. Olivieri I, Costa AM, Cantini F, Niccoli L, Marini R, Ferri S. Pyoderma gangrenosum in association with undifferentiated seronegative spondylarthropathy. Arthritis Rheum. 1996;39(6):1062–5.
52. Ingegnoli F, Castelli R, Gualtierotti R. Rheumatoid factors: clinical applications. Dis Markers. 2013;35(6):727–34.
53. Chamot AM, Benhamou CL, Kahn MF, Beraneck L, Kaplan G, Prost A. Acne-pustulosis-hyperostosis-osteitis syndrome. Results of a national survey. 85 cases. Rev Rhum Mal Osteoartic. 1987;54(3):187–96.
54. Van Doornum S, Barraclough D, McColl G, Wicks I. SAPHO: rare or just not recognized? Semin Arthritis Rheum. 2000;30(1):70–7.
55. Marzano AV, Borghi A, Meroni PL, Cugno M. Pyoderma gangrenosum and its syndromic forms: evidence for a link with autoinflammation. Br J Dermatol. 2016;175(5):882–91.
56. Liao HJ, Chyuan IT, Wu CS, Lin SW, Chen KH, Tsai HF, et al. Increased neutrophil infiltration, IL-1 production and a SAPHO syndrome-like phenotype in PSTPIP2-deficient mice. Rheumatology. 2015;54(7):1317–26.
57. Rukavina I. SAPHO syndrome: a review. J Child Orthop. 2015;9(1):19–27.
58. Hurtado-Nedelec M, Chollet-Martin S, Nicaise-Roland P, Grootenboer-Mignot S, Ruimy R, Meyer O, et al. Characterization of the immune response in the synovitis, acne, pustulosis, hyperostosis, osteitis (SAPHO) syndrome. Rheumatology. 2008;47(8):1160–7.
59. Qin M, Pirouz A, Kim MH, Krutzik SR, Garban HJ, Kim J. Propionibacterium acnes Induces IL-1beta secretion via the NLRP3 inflammasome in human monocytes. J Invest Dermatol. 2014;134(2):381–8.
60. Sahdo B, Sarndahl E, Elgh F, Soderquist B. Propionibacterium acnes activates caspase-1 in human neutrophils. APMIS. 2013;121(7):652–63.
61. Firinu D, Barca MP, Lorrai MM, Perra S, Cabras S, Muggianu E, et al. TH17 cells are increased in the peripheral blood of patients with SAPHO syndrome. Autoimmunity. 2014;47(6):389–94.
62. Kahn MF, Khan MA. The SAPHO syndrome. Baillieres Clin Rheumatol. 1994;8(2):333–62.
63. Nguyen MT, Borchers A, Selmi C, Naguwa SM, Cheema G, Gershwin ME. The SAPHO syndrome. Semin Arthritis Rheum. 2012;42(3):254–65.

64. Hayem G, Bouchaud-Chabot A, Benali K, Roux S, Palazzo E, Silbermann-Hoffman O, et al. SAPHO syndrome: a long-term follow-up study of 120 cases. Semin Arthritis Rheum. 1999;29(3):159–71.
65. Freyschmidt J, Sternberg A. The bullhead sign: scintigraphic pattern of sternocostoclavicular hyperostosis and pustulotic arthroosteitis. Eur Radiol. 1998;8(5):807–12.
66. Naves JE, Cabre E, Manosa M, Grados D, Olive A, Domenech E. A systematic review of SAPHO syndrome and inflammatory bowel disease association. Dig Dis Sci. 2013;58(8):2138–47.
67. Kundu BK, Naik AK, Bhargava S, Srivastava D. Diagnosing the SAPHO syndrome: a report of three cases and review of literature. Clin Rheumatol. 2013;32(8):1237–43.
68. Lindor NM, Arsenault TM, Solomon H, Seidman CE, McEvoy MT. A new autosomal dominant disorder of pyogenic sterile arthritis, pyoderma gangrenosum, and acne: PAPA syndrome. Mayo Clin Proc. 1997;72(7):611–5.
69. Wise CA, Gillum JD, Seidman CE, Lindor NM, Veile R, Bashiardes S, et al. Mutations in CD2BP1 disrupt binding to PTP PEST and are responsible for PAPA syndrome, an autoinflammatory disorder. Hum Mol Genet. 2002;11(8):961–9.
70. Yeon HB, Lindor NM, Seidman JG, Seidman CE. Pyogenic arthritis, pyoderma gangrenosum, and acne syndrome maps to chromosome 15q. Am J Hum Genet. 2000;66(4):1443–8.
71. Hsieh J, Kadavath S, Efthimiou P. Can traumatic injury trigger psoriatic arthritis? A review of the literature. Clin Rheumatol. 2014;33(5):601–8.
72. Cugno M, Borghi A, Marzano AV. PAPA, PASH and PAPASH syndromes: pathophysiology, presentation and treatment. Am J Clin Dermatol. 2017;18(4):555–62.
73. Donmez S, Pamuk ON, Gedik M, KR A, Bulut G. A case of granulomatosis with polyangiitis and pyoderma gangrenosum successfully treated with infliximab and rituximab. Int J Rheum Dis. 2014;17(4):471–5.
74. Marzano AV, Borghi A, Meroni PL, Crosti C, Cugno M. Immune-mediated inflammatory reactions and tumors as skin side effects of inflammatory bowel disease therapy. Autoimmunity. 2014;47(3):146–53.
75. Vandevyvere K, Luyten FP, Verschueren P, Lories R, Segaert S, Westhovens R. Pyoderma gangrenosum developing during therapy with TNF-alpha antagonists in a patient with rheumatoid arthritis. Clin Rheumatol. 2007;26(12):2205–6.
76. Stichenwirth M, Riedl E, Pehamberger H, Tappeiner G. Pyoderma gangrenosum in a patient with seronegative rheumatoid arthritis during therapy with adalimumab: toxic effects of adalimumab or failure of adalimumab to prevent the onset of this phenomenon? Arch Dermatol. 2008;144(6):817–8.
77. Kikuchi N, Hiraiwa T, Ohashi T, Hanami Y, Satoh M, Takenoshita H, et al. Pyoderma gangrenosum possibly triggered by adalimumab. Eur J Dermatol. 2012;22(6):804–5.
78. Kowalzick L, Bertolini J, Baumann C, Walther B, Truhm B, Eickenscheidt L. Paradoxical reaction to etanercept: development of pyoderma gangraenosum during therapy of psoriasis arthritis. J Dtsch Dermatol Ges. 2013;11(5):447–9.
79. Wendling D, Prati C. Paradoxical effects of anti-TNF-alpha agents in inflammatory diseases. Expert Rev Clin Immunol. 2014;10(1):159–69.
80. Akahoshi-Ikeda M, Yoshizawa S, Motoshita J, Furue M, Takeuchi S. A case of pyoderma gangrenosum in a patient with rheumatoid arthritis treated with abatacept. Acta Derm Venereol. 2016;96(6):822–3.
81. Tiwari SM, Wood BA, Skender-Kalnenas T, Cook N. A case of abatacept associated neutrophilic dermatosis and a review of the literature. Australas J Dermatol. 2014;55(3):214–7.
82. Alvarez-Quiroga C, Abud-Mendoza C, Doniz-Padilla L, Juarez-Reyes A, Monsivais-Urenda A, Baranda L, et al. CTLA-4-Ig therapy diminishes the frequency but enhances the function of Treg cells in patients with rheumatoid arthritis. J Clin Immunol. 2011;31(4):588–95.
83. Anderson DE, Bieganowska KD, Bar-Or A, Oliveira EM, Carreno B, Collins M, et al. Paradoxical inhibition of T-cell function in response to CTLA-4 blockade; heterogeneity within the human T-cell population. Nat Med. 2000;6(2):211–4.

Drug-Induced Neutrophilic Dermatoses 20

Lauryn M. Falcone, Rivka C. Stone, and Robert A. Schwartz

Introduction

Medications are substantial underlying contributors to the development of neutrophilic dermatoses. Many different classes of drugs have been shown to induce a variety of neutrophilic dermatoses, with the histopathologic presence of a dermal neutrophilic infiltrate remaining the unifying feature. Identifying a drug-induced neutrophilic dermatosis with certainty can be difficult, as many patients have underlying conditions that may independently contribute to the development of similar cutaneous findings. Diagnosis is therefore based upon the observation of a temporal relationship between drug initiation and appearance of the characteristic dermatosis, coupled with resolution of symptoms upon discontinuation of the drug. Drugs that have been reported to trigger five classic neutrophilic dermatoses are summarized in Table 20.1 and discussed in more detail below.

L. M. Falcone
West Virginia University School of Medicine, Morgantown, WV, USA
e-mail: lmfalcone@mix.wvu.edu

R. C. Stone
Dermatology, Rutgers-New Jersey Medical School, Newark, NJ, USA

R. A. Schwartz (✉)
Dermatology, Rutgers-New Jersey Medical School, Newark, NJ, USA

Rutgers School of Public Affairs and Administration, Newark, NJ, USA

D. Wallach et al. (eds.), *Neutrophilic Dermatoses*,
https://doi.org/10.1007/978-3-319-72649-6_20

Table 20.1 Drug triggers of neutrophilic dermatoses

Category	Drug	SS	PNGD	PG	AGEP	NEH
Infectious disease						
Anti-bacterial	Amoxicillin				[a]	
	Ampicillin				[b]	
	Cefepime				[b]	
	Cefotaxime				[b]	
	Ciprofloxacin				[b]	
	Clindamycin	[b]			[a]	
	Dapsone				[b]	
	Daptomycin				[b]	
	Doripenem				[b]	
	Flucloxacillin				[b]	
	Nitrofurantoin	[b]				
	Piperacillin/tazobactam				[b]	
	Quinolones	[b]				
	Quinupristin/dalfopristin	[b]				
	Televancin				[b]	
	Tetracyclines	[a]				
	Trimethoprim-sulfamethoxazole	[b]			[b]	
	Vancomycin				[b]	
Anti-viral	Abacavir	[b]				
	Zidovudine					[b]
Anti-fungal	Ketoconazole	[b]				
	Terbinafine				[b]	
Anti-parasitic	Hydroxychloroquine				[b]	
Cardiovascular						
	Diltiazem				[b]	
	Furosemide	[b]				
	Hydralazine	[a]				
	Midodrine				[b]	
	Ticagrelor	[b]				
Hematology/Oncology						
Chemotherapeutic	ATRA	[a]				
	Azacitidine	[b]		[b]		
	Bleomycin					[b]
	Bortezomib	[a]				
	BRAF inhibitor	[a]				[b]
	Cetuximab					[b]
	Cytarabine			[b]		[a]
	Decitabine					[b]
	Enzalutamide				[b]	
	Gefitinib			[b]		
	Imatinib	[b]		[b]	[b]	
	Ipilimumab	[a]		[b]		
	Lenalidomide	[b]				
	Rituximab			[b]		
	Sunitinib			[a]		
	Thalidomide	[b]				
	Topotecan	[b]				[b]

Table 20.1 (continued)

Category	Drug	SS	PNGD	PG	AGEP	NEH
Colony stimulating factor	G-CSF	[a]		[a]		[b]
	Pegfilgrastim	[b]		[b]		
Psychiatry						
	Carbamazepine					[b]
	Clozapine	[b]				
	Diazepam	[b]				
	Lormetazepam	[b]				
Endocrinology						
	Oral contraceptives	[a]				
	Propylthiouracil	[b]		[a]		
Rheumatology						
	Allopurinol		[b]			
	Azathioprine	[a]				
	Sulfasalazine	[b]				
Non-steroidal anti-inflammatory drugs	Acetominophen					[b]
	Celecoxib	[b]				
	Diclofenac	[b]				
	Piroxicam				[b]	
	Valdecoxib				[b]	
Immunology						
	Abatacept			[b]		
	Adalimumab		[b]	[b]		
	Etanercept		[b]	[b]		
	Interferon-alpha			[b]		
	Ranibizumab				[b]	
Other						
	Iodine			[b]		
	Iodixanol				[b]	
	Isotretinoin	[b]		[a]		
	Proton pump inhibitors	[b]				

SS Sweet's syndrome, *PNGD* palisaded neutrophilic and granulomatous dermatitis, *PG* pyoderma gangrenosum, *AGEP* acute generalized exanthematous pustulosis, *NEH* neutrophilic eccrine hidradenitis, *G-CSF* granulocyte colony stimulating factor, *ATRA* all-trans retinoic acid

[a]many case reports

[b]few case reports

Sweet's Syndrome

Sweet's syndrome (SS), also known as acute febrile neutrophilic dermatosis, is the prototypic neutrophilic dermatosis. It is characterized clinically by fever, neutrophilia, and painful erythematous papules, nodules or plaques most commonly on the extremities, head, neck, trunk and occasionally visceral mucosa such as gut [1, 2] (Fig. 20.1). While nearly 50% of diagnosed cases of SS are idiopathic [1, 3], a growing list of drugs has been reported to trigger Sweet's Syndrome. The precise etiology of drug-induced SS is unknown, but it is thought to be a hypersensitivity reaction to different stimuli and/or cytokine dysregulation [4]. Proposed diagnostic criteria for

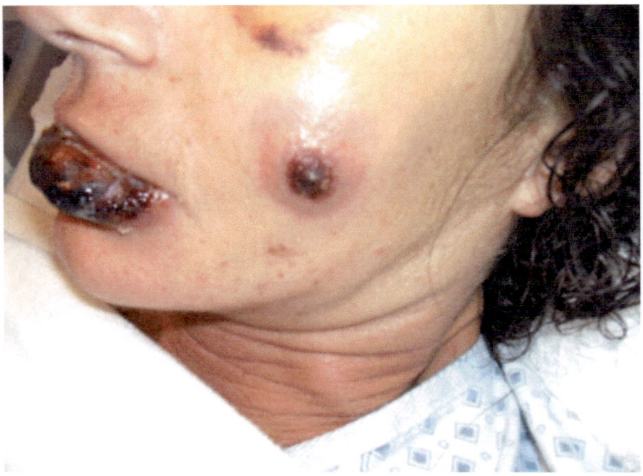

Fig. 20.1 Sweet's Syndrome. From: Buck T, González LM, Schwartz RA, Lambert WC: Acute neutrophilic dermatosis (Sweet's syndrome) with hematologic disorders: a review and reappraisal. Int J Dermatol 47: 775–782, 2008

drug-induced Sweet's syndrome include features of classic SS (i.e., characteristic clinical lesions and histopathologic findings; presence of constitutional symptoms; excellent response to corticosteroids), but with symptom onset following medication use, recurring with re-challenge, and resolving with drug withdrawal [3, 5].

The association of granulocyte colony stimulating factor (G-CSF) therapy with the development of SS has been particularly well-documented [6–11]. G-CSF induces neutrophil differentiation, survival and chemotaxis [4] and its use in healthy peripheral blood stem cell donors as well as in patients with hematologic malignancies has triggered SS [7, 9]. Serum levels of G-CSF are elevated in patients with SS [12]. It has been suggested that a common neoplastic clone gives rise to clonal neutrophil precursors which undergo maturation in the dermis (Magro et al. 2001). The G-CSF effect does not appear to be dose-dependent, as SS has been reported in patients after single and multiple courses of treatment [6]. Pegfilgrastim, a pegylated analog of G-CSF, may induce SS [13, 14]. Pegfilgrastim possesses a polyethylene glycol moiety which is cleared by neutrophils; it is hypothesized that this triggers additional neutrophil proliferation and may also contribute to the development of SS [14].

Anticancer therapies are among the most common triggers of drug-induced Sweet's Syndrome [4]. SS has been reported to develop in patients with acute myelogenous leukemia (AML) after all-trans retinoic acid (ATRA) treatment, which increases G-CSF as well as interleukin-1β expression [15]. ATRA may also alter neutrophil function and migratory abilities thereby contributing to SS [4]. However, AML itself has been associated with SS, which may complicate the diagnosis of ATRA-induced SS [16]. The temporal relationship of AML diagnosis versus commencement of ATRA treatment with the onset of symptoms may aid in differentiating ATRA-induced versus AML-induced SS. Imatinib and bortezomib, classically used in the treatment of chronic myelogenous leukemia and multiple myeloma, respectively, may induce SS [17], perhaps due to an imbalance of pro-inflammatory cytokines that stimulate neutrophil chemotaxis [18]. Similarly, SS has been described in melanoma patients after treatment with ipilimumab, a CTLA-4 receptor blocker that modulates T cell activity and may thus promote cytokine release leading to neutrophil stimulation [19].

Other medications associated with SS include azathioprine, which may induce SS in patients being treated for inflammatory bowel disease [20–23]. Trimethoprim sulfamethoxazole and celecoxib both contain a sulfonamide moiety that can trigger a neutrophil-associated allergic response manifesting clinically as SS [24]. Ketoconazole, a broad-spectrum antifungal medication, is associated with the development of SS, perhaps by increasing neutrophil chemotaxis [25]. Benzodiazepines may also produce SS [26, 27], postulated to occur through a type III (antibody-mediated) hypersensitivity reaction, as diazepam-associated SS usually appears after a latency period of several days during which antibodies may be synthesized [26]. A few cases of oral contraceptive induced SS have been noted, suggesting that sex hormones may be triggers of SS as well [28–30].

Palisaded Neutrophilic and Granulomatous Dermatitis

Palisaded neutrophilic and granulomatous dermatitis (PNGD) is a rare neutrophilic dermatosis that develops primarily in patients with autoimmune and/or connective tissue disorders, commonly systemic lupus erythematosus and rheumatoid arthritis [31]. It may be first evident as skin-colored or erythematous papules or plaques of the extremities. As a consequence, cases of drug-induced PNGD are invariably evident in patients undergoing treatment for these underlying diseases, making it difficult to differentiate the disorder itself from its treatments as the true trigger for PNGD. As with other drug-induced neutrophilic dermatoses, resolution of PNGD after discontinuation of the suspected drug supports the treatment rather than the disease as the etiology. Several cases of drug-induced PNGD have been delineated following treatment with TNF-alpha inhibitors, including infliximab [32] and adalimumab [33] in patients with rheumatoid arthritis. It has been proposed that TNF-α inhibitors may act as allergens and stimulate a type III hypersensitivity reaction to induce an immune complex-mediated leukocytoclastic vasculitis and ischemic damage or may disrupt self-tolerance leading to an autoimmune reaction, culminating in granulomatous inflammation and the appearance of PNGD [33]. To this end, Immunoglobulin M and C3 have been identified in the walls of small vessels of patients with PNGD [31]. A case of allopurinol-induced PNGD was also reported in a patient with impaired drug clearance due to underlying renal disease [34]; the mechanism was similarly attributed to type III-mediated immune complex deposition that led to neutrophil recruitment, complement activation, and dermal collagen damage.

Pyoderma Gangrenosum

Pyoderma gangrenosum (PG) is a rare neutrophilic dermatosis often first evident as an exquisitely painful ulcer with a mucopurulent base and a violaceous undermined border surrounded by a peripheral zone of erythema [35, 36]. PG usually develops in association with underlying systemic diseases such as inflammatory bowel disease, hematologic disorders, and rheumatoid arthritis, suggesting a potential role of inflammation in inducing PG [36–38], Immunohistochemical studies have also demonstrated increased levels of proinflammatory cytokines in the ulcers of PG [38]. However, many cases of drug-induced PG have also been reported, both in response to systemic medications as well as at sites of local injection. One of the first reported cases was in a patient being treated with G-CSF for small cell lung cancer who subsequently developed bullous PG [39]. There have also been reports of patients developing PG on combination chemotherapy which included G-CSF [40]. G-CSF is believed to stimulate neutrophil activity by increasing superoxide release and enhancing the presence of effector molecules on neutrophils [40].

Chemotherapeutic agents such as CTLA-4 inhibitor ipilimumab and tyrosine kinase inhibitor sunitinib may also rarely induce PG [41, 42]. Although the mechanisms are not fully understood, ipilimumab may deplete T regulatory cells and trigger effector T cells to release cytokines which activate neutrophils [42], while sunitinib may trigger PG through inhibition of growth factor receptors such as vascular endothelial growth factor receptor, stem cell factor receptor KIT, and platelet-derived growth factor receptor [41].

The association of isotretinoin therapy with PG is incompletely understood, as several case reports support isotretinoin as a trigger of PG [43–46] while others support its use in the treatment of PG [47]. Isotretinoin modulates keratinocyte desmosomes, thus perhaps increasing the risk of ulcerative toxicities such as PG [44]; it may also alter adhesion molecules to induce pathologic neutrophil migration present in PG [43]. However, studies have suggested that low dose isotretinoin inhibits neutrophil function, which may explain its use as a therapy for PG [47].

Finally, PG has been reported to develop locally at sites of interferon alpha injection in a dose-dependent fashion [48, 49]. It has been proposed that interferons induce interleukin-1 which attracts neutrophils and increases chemotactic acute phase proteins.

Acute Generalized Exanthematous Pustulosis

Unlike most neutrophilic dermatoses, acute generalized exanthematous pustulosis (AGEP) is characterized by the acute onset of generalized, nonfollicular, pustules with fever and most often develops in response to drugs rather than to underlying systemic disease [50–52] (Fig. 20.2). Over 50 medications have been reported to trigger AGEP, with antibiotics serving as the most common culprits. The temporal relationship between drug administration and onset of AGEP differs by medication, as antibiotics usually trigger symptoms within 24 h while non-antibiotics induce AGEP with a median lag of 11 days [53].

The mechanism of drug-induced AGEP may also differ by medication. Drug-induced T cells in AGEP produce significantly more interleukin-8, a neutrophil-attracting cytokine, as compared with drug-induced T cells in non-AGEP disorders [54]. Antibiotics may induce AGEP via delayed T cell response to the beta-lactam ring, a mechanism that is supported by reports of patch testing positive for beta-lactams in patients with AGEP [55]. Additionally, β-lactam specific T_H17 cells have

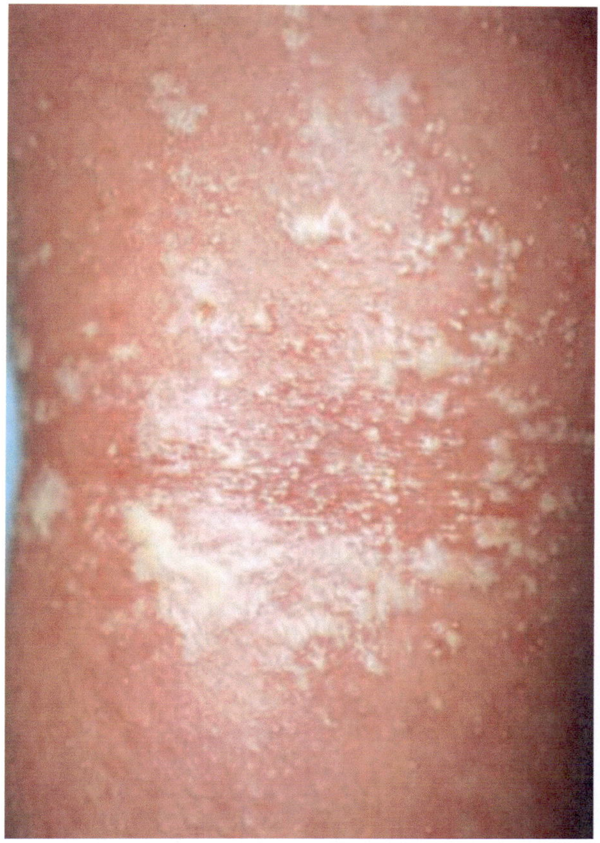

Fig. 20.2 Acute generalized exanthematous pustulosis. In this patient, AGEP was induced by oral ketoconazole. From: Miteva L, Kadurina M, Schwartz R: Childhood acute generalized exanthematous pustulosis induced by oral ketoconazole. Acta Derm Venerol Croatica 18: 267–270, 2010

been identified in antibiotic-triggered AGEP; these cells produce cytokines that recruit neutrophils and eosinophils and account for drug-specific circulating IgE that has been reported [56]. Certain non-antibiotic medications such as the α_1-adrenergic receptor agonist midodrine contain aromatic rings that provoke an immune response manifesting clinically as AGEP [57, 58].

It may be important to differentiate AGEP from other drug-induced cutaneous reactions including pustular psoriasis, Stevens Johnson Syndrome (SJS) and toxic epidermal necrolysis (TEN), due to differences in management. Both AGEP and pustular psoriasis feature non-follicular, generalized pustules, though AGEP has a greater predilection for body folds and more rapidly desquamates [59, 60]. An associated personal or family history of psoriasis as well as arthritis is usually absent in patients with AGEP [53, 59]. The drugs which induce AGEP and pustular psoriasis also typically differ, with drugs such as lithium and beta-blockers more likely to induce pustular psoriasis [61, 62]. Similarly, while pustules in AGEP can sometimes converge and give a false Nikolsky's sign [63], common causes of SJS/TEN including allopurinol and anti-epileptic drugs do not typically trigger AGEP [53].

Neutrophilic Eccrine Hidradenitis (NEH)

Neutrophilic eccrine hidradenitis (NEH), a neutrophilic dermatosis characterized by erythematous, edematous or purpuric papules, nodules or plaques and neutrophils surrounding eccrine glands, is often associated with underlying malignancies. They are often hyperpigmented and may be tender to touch, most often involving the trunk or limbs. They may involve the face, resembling cellulitis too. Drug triggers of NEH encompass many anti-cancer medications including cytarabine, bleomycin, topotecan, cetuximab, vemurafenib, and mitoxantrone, either as single agents or in combination [64–71]. A variety of mechanisms for chemotherapy-induced NEH have been proposed. One hypothesis suggests that anti-cancer therapies may induce myeloblasts to differentiate into neutrophils and accumulate in eccrine glands [72]. Chemotherapy drugs are also secreted from eccrine glands, where they may also act as local irritants to provoke necrosis and degeneration followed by inflammatory damage and neutrophil influx around the ducts [73]. Cetuximab, which targets the epidermal growth factor receptor (EGFR), may also uniquely induce NEH by inhibiting EGF receptors that are present in sweat duct epithelia, promoting inflammation [64]. G-CSF, which as mentioned can trigger Sweet syndrome and PG, may also induce NEH [74]. NEH has also been reported following treatment with carbamazepine, zidovudine and acetaminophen [72, 75, 76]. Like chemotherapeutics, zidovudine and other human immunodeficiency virus (HIV) medications are secreted from eccrine glands. The resulting local inflammatory response may thus represent a shared mechanism for the development of drug-induced NEH [76].

Management of Drug-Induced Neutrophilic Dermatoses

Treatment of drug-induced neutrophilic dermatoses is similar to non-medication-induced disease and is often guided by the severity of clinical presentation. Systemic steroids are first-line therapies [77, 78]. Dapsone, which inhibits the recruitment and adhesion of neutrophils [79], also plays a prominent role in the management of neutrophilic dermatoses. Adjunctive treatments may include topical and intralesional corticosteroids, cyclosporine, colchicine, and retinoids [77].

References

1. Yi S, Bhate C, Schwartz RA. Sweet's syndrome: an update and review. G Ital Dermatol Venereol. 2009;144(5):603–12.
2. Buck T, Gonzalez LM, Lambert WC, Schwartz RA. Sweet's syndrome with hematologic disorders: a review and reappraisal. Int J Dermatol. 2008;47(8):775–82.
3. Alavi A, Sajic D, Cerci FB, Ghazarian D, Rosenbach M, Jorizzo J. Neutrophilic dermatoses: an update. Am J Clin Dermatol. 2014;15(5):413–23.
4. Raza S, Kirkland RS, Patel AA, Shortridge JR, Freter C. Insight into Sweet's syndrome and associated-malignancy: a review of the current literature. Int J Oncol. 2013;42(5):1516–22.

5. Cohen PR. Sweet's syndrome—a comprehensive review of an acute febrile neutrophilic dermatosis. Orphanet J Rare Dis. 2007;2:34.
6. Thompson DF, Montarella KE. Drug-induced Sweet's syndrome. Ann Pharmacother. 2007;41(5):802–11.
7. Garty BZ, Levy I, Nitzan M, Barak Y. Sweet syndrome associated with G-CSF treatment in a child with glycogen storage disease type Ib. Pediatrics. 1996;97(3):401–3.
8. Kim MJ, Choe YH. EPONYM Sweet syndrome. Eur J Pediatr. 2010;169(12):1439–44.
9. Magro CM, De Moraes E, Burns F. Sweet's syndrome in the setting of CD34-positive acute myelogenous leukemia treated with granulocyte colony stimulating factor: evidence for a clonal neutrophilic dermatosis. J Cutan Pathol. 2001;28(2):90–6.
10. Oiso N, Watanabe K, Kawada A. Granulocyte colony-stimulating factor-induced Sweet syndrome in a healthy donor. B J Haematol. 2006;135(2):148.
11. Paydas S, Sahin B, Seyrek E, Soylu M, Gonlusen G, Acar A, et al. Sweet's syndrome associated with G-CSF. B J Haematol. 1993;85(1):191–2.
12. Reuss-Borst MA, Muller CA, Waller HD. The possible role of G-CSF in the pathogenesis of Sweet's syndrome. Leuk Lymphoma. 1994;15(3–4):261–4.
13. Llamas-Velasco M, Garcia-Martin P, Sanchez-Perez J, Fraga J, Garcia-Diez A. Sweet's syndrome with subcutaneous involvement associated with pegfilgrastim treatment: first reported case. J Cutan Pathol. 2013;40(1):46–9.
14. Draper BK, Robbins JB, Stricklin GP. Bullous Sweet's syndrome in congenital neutropenia: association with pegfilgrastim. J Am Acad Dermatol. 2005;52(5):901–5.
15. Park CJ, Bae YD, Choi JY, Heo PS, Lee KS, Park YS, et al. Sweet's syndrome during the treatment of acute promyelocytic leukemia with all-trans retinoic acid. Korean J Intern Med. 2001;16(3):218–21.
16. Christ E, Linka A, Jacky E, Speich R, Marincek B, Schaffner A. Sweet's syndrome involoving the musculoskeletal system during treatment of promyelocytic leukemia with all-trans retinoic acid. Leukemia. 1996;10(4):731–4.
17. Ayirookuzhi SJ, Ma L, Ramshesh P, Mills G. Imatinib-induced sweet syndrome in a patient with chronic myeloid leukemia. Arch Dermatol. 2005;141(3):368–70.
18. Kolb-Maurer A, Kneitz H, Goebeler M. Sweet-like syndrome induced by bortezomib. J Dtsch Dermatol Ges. 2013;11(12):1200–2.
19. Pintova S, Sidhu H, Friedlander PA, Holcombe RF. Sweet's syndrome in a patient with metastatic melanoma after ipilimumab therapy. Melanoma Res. 2013;23(6):498–501.
20. Cyrus N, Stavert R, Mason AR, Ko CJ, Choi JN. Neutrophilic dermatosis after azathioprine exposure. JAMA Dermatol. 2013;149(5):592–7.
21. Treton X, Joly F, Alves A, Panis Y, Bouhnik Y. Azathioprine-induced Sweet's syndrome in Crohn's disease. Inflamm Bowel Dis. 2008;14(12):1757–8.
22. Imhof L, Meier B, Frei P, Kamarachev J, Rogler G, Kolios A, et al. Severe Sweet's syndrome with elevated cutaneous interleukin-1beta after azathioprine exposure: case report and review of the literature. Dermatology. 2015;230(4):293–8.
23. Biswas SN, Chakraborty PP, Gantait K, Bar C. Azathioprine-induced bullous Sweet's syndrome: a rare association. BMJ Case Rep. 2016;2016. https://doi.org/10.1136/bcr-2016-215192.
24. Fye KH, Crowley E, Berger TG, LeBoit PE, Connolly MK. Celecoxib-induced Sweet's syndrome. J Am Acad Dermatol. 2001;45(2):300–2.
25. Baquerizo Nole KL, Lee E, Villada G, Romanelli P. Ketoconazole-induced Sweet syndrome: a new association. Am J Dermatopathol. 2015;37(5):419–22.
26. Guimera FJ, Garcia-Bustinduy M, Noda A, Saez M, Dorta S, Sanchez R, et al. Diazepam-associated Sweet's syndrome. Int J Dermatol. 2000;39(10):795–8.
27. Stenzel W, Frosch PJ, Schwarz M. Sweet's syndrome associated with acute benign encephalitis. A drug induced aetiology. J Neurol. 2003;250(6):770–1.
28. Kazlouskaya V, Junkins-Hopkins JM, KN W, Itenberg SJ. Sweet syndrome caused by oral contraceptives. Int J Dermatol. 2015;54(5):e189–91.
29. Saez M, Garcia-Bustinduy M, Noda A, Guimera F, Dorta S, Escoda M, et al. Sweet's syndrome induced by oral contraceptive. Dermatology. 2002;204(1):84.

30. Tefany FJ, Georgouras K. A neutrophilic reaction of Sweet's syndrome type associated with the oral contraceptive. Australas J Dermatol. 1991;32(1):55–9.
31. Chu P, Connolly MK, LeBoit PE. The histopathologic spectrum of palisaded neutrophilic and granulomatous dermatitis in patients with collagen vascular disease. Arch Dermatol. 1994;130(10):1278–83.
32. Collaris EJ, van Marion AM, Frank J, Poblete-Gutierrez P. Cutaneous granulomas in rheumatoid arthritis. Int J Dermatol. 2007;46(Suppl 3):33–5.
33. Stephenson SR, Campbell SM, Drew GS, Magro CM. Palisaded neutrophilic and granulomatous dermatitis presenting in a patient with rheumatoid arthritis on adalimumab. J Cutan Pathol. 2011;38(8):644–8.
34. Gordon K, Miteva M, Torchia D, Romanelli P. Allopurinol-induced palisaded neutrophilic and granulomatous dermatitis. Cutan Ocul Toxicol. 2012;31(4):338–40.
35. Birnkrant MJ, Papadopoulos AJ, Schwartz RA, Lambert WC. Pyoderma gangrenosum, acne conglobata, and IgA gammopathy. Int J Dermatol. 2003;42(3):213–6.
36. Romanska-Gocka K, Ciescinska C, Zegarska B, Schwartz RA, Ciescinski J, Olszewska-Slonina D, et al. Pyoderma gangrenosum with monoclonal IgA gammopathy and pulmonary tuberculosis. Illustrative case and review. Postepy Dermatol Alergol. 2015;32(2):137–41.
37. Powell FC, Su WP, Perry HO. Pyoderma gangrenosum: classification and management. J Am Acad Dermatol. 1996;34(3):395–409; quiz 10–2.
38. Wu BC, Patel ED, Ortega-Loayza AG. Drug-induced pyoderma gangrenosum: a model to understand the pathogenesis of pyoderma gangrenosum. Br J Dermatol. 2017;177(1):72–83.
39. Ross HJ, Moy LA, Kaplan R, Figlin RA. Bullous pyoderma gangrenosum after granulocyte colony-stimulating factor treatment. Cancer. 1991;68(2):441–3.
40. Takagi S, Ohsaka A, Taguchi H, Kusama H, Matsuoka T. Pyoderma gangrenosum following cytosine arabinoside, aclarubicin and granulocyte colony-stimulating factor combination therapy in myelodysplastic syndrome. Intern Med. 1998;37(3):316–9.
41. ten Freyhaus K, Homey B, Bieber T, Wilsmann-Theis D. Pyoderma gangrenosum: another cutaneous side-effect of sunitinib? Br J Dermatol. 2008;159(1):242–3.
42. Rudolph BM, Staib F, Von Stebut E, Hainz M, Grabbe S, Loquai C. Neutrophilic disease of the skin and intestines after ipilimumab treatment for malignant melanoma—simultaneous occurrence of pyoderma gangrenosum and colitis. Eur J Dermatol. 2014;24(2):268–9.
43. Tinoco MP, Tamler C, Maciel G, Soares D, Avelleira JC, Azulay D. Pyoderma gangrenosum following isotretinoin therapy for acne nodulocystic. Int J Dermatol. 2008;47(9):953–6.
44. Gangaram HB, Tan LP, Gan AT, Suraiya HH, Ganesapillai T. Pyoderma gangrenosum following treatment with isotretinoin. Br J Dermatol. 1997;136(4):636–7.
45. Freiman A, Brassard A. Pyoderma gangrenosum associated with isotretinoin therapy. J Am Acad Dermatol. 2006;55(5 Suppl):S107–8.
46. Exner JH, Dahod S, Pochi PE. Pyogenic granuloma-like acne lesions during isotretinoin therapy. Arch Dermatol. 1983;119(10):808–11.
47. Proudfoot LE, Singh S, Staughton RC. Superficial pyoderma gangrenosum responding to treatment with isotretinoin. Br J Dermatol. 2008;159(6):1377–8.
48. Sanders S, Busam K, Tahan SR, Johnson RA, Sachs D. Granulomatous and suppurative dermatitis at interferon alfa injection sites: report of 2 cases. J Am Acad Dermatol. 2002;46(4):611–6.
49. Montoto S, Bosch F, Estrach T, Blade J, Nomdedeu B, Nontserrat E. Pyoderma gangrenosum triggered by alpha2b-interferon in a patient with chronic granulocytic leukemia. Leuk Lymphoma. 1998;30(1–2):199–202.
50. Mysore V, Ghuloom A. A case of recurrent acute generalized exanthematous pustulosis due to beta-lactam antibiotics: a case report. J Dermatol Treat. 2003;14(1):54–6.
51. Miteva L, Kadurina M, Schwartz RA. Childhood acute generalized exanthematous pustulosis induced by oral ketoconazole. Acta Dermatovenerol Croat. 2010;18(4):267–70.

52. Szatkowski J, Schwartz RA. Acute generalized exanthematous pustulosis (AGEP): a review and update. J Am Acad Dermatol. 2015;73(5):843–8.
53. Sidoroff A, Dunant A, Viboud C, Halevy S, Bavinck JN, Naldi L, et al. Risk factors for acute generalized exanthematous pustulosis (AGEP)-results of a multinational case-control study (EuroSCAR). Br J Dermatol. 2007;157(5):989–96.
54. Britschgi M, Steiner UC, Schmid S, Depta JP, Senti G, Bircher A, et al. T-cell involvement in drug-induced acute generalized exanthematous pustulosis. J Clin Invest. 2001;107(11):1433–41.
55. Bomarrito L, Zisa G, Delrosso G, Farinelli P, Galimberti M. A case of acute generalized exanthematous pustulosis due to amoxicillin-clavulanate with multiple positivity to beta-lactam patch testing. Eur Ann Allergy Clin Immunol. 2013;45(5):178–80.
56. Fili L, Cardilicchia E, Severino MG, Testi S, Matucci A, Vultaggio A, et al. Hapten-specific TH17 cells in the peripheral blood of beta-lactam-induced AGEP. Allergol Int. 2014;63(1):129–31.
57. Sadeghpour M, Bunick CG, Robinson DM, Galan A, Tigelaar RE, Imaeda S. Midodrine-induced acute generalized exanthematous pustulosis. Cutis. 2014;93(5):E17–20.
58. Handoko KB, van Puijenbroek EP, Bijl AH, Hermens WA, Zwart-van Rijkom JE, Hekster YA, et al. Influence of chemical structure on hypersensitivity reactions induced by antiepileptic drugs: the role of the aromatic ring. Drug Saf. 2008;31(8):695–702.
59. Byerly FL, Nelson KC, Granko RP, Morrell DS, Cairns BA. Valdecoxib-associated acute generalized exanthematous pustulosis. Burns. 2005;31(3):383–7.
60. Sidoroff A, Halevy S, Bavinck JN, Vaillant L, Roujeau JC. Acute generalized exanthematous pustulosis (AGEP)—a clinical reaction pattern. J Cutan Pathol. 2001;28(3):113–9.
61. Roujeau JC, Bioulac-Sage P, Bourseau C, Guillaume JC, Bernard P, Lok C, et al. Acute generalized exanthematous pustulosis. Analysis of 63 cases. Arch Dermatol. 1991;127(9):1333–8.
62. Sulewski RJ Jr, Blyumin M, Kerdel FA. Acute generalized exanthematous pustulosis due to clindamycin. Dermatol Online J. 2008;14(7):14.
63. Chaabane A, Aouam K, Gassab L, Njim L, Boughattas NA. Acute generalized exanthematous pustulosis (AGEP) induced by cefotaxime. Fundam Clin Pharmacol. 2010;24(4):429–32.
64. Turan H, Kaya E, Gurlevik Z, Erdem H, Oktay M. Neutrophilic eccrine hidradenitis induced by cetuximab. Cutan Ocul Toxicol. 2012;31(2):148–50.
65. Templeton SF, Solomon AR, Swerlick RA. Intradermal bleomycin injections into normal human skin. A histopathologic and immunopathologic study. Arch Dermatol. 1994;130(5):577–83.
66. Shlapak D, Kerisit K, Lin C, Wang A, Stumpf B. Resident rounds. Part III: neutrophilic eccrine hidradenitis in the setting of acute myelogenous leukemia treated with cytarabine. J Drugs Dermatol. 2013;12(2):231–2.
67. Marini M, Wright D, Ropolo M, Abbruzzese M, Casas G. Neutrophilic eccrine hidradenitis secondary to topotecan. J Dermatol Treat. 2002;13(1):35–7.
68. Grahovac M, Maximiliane Ehmann L, Flaig M, Reibke R, Wollenberg A. Neutrophilic eccrine hidradenitis induced by cytarabine. Acta Dermatovenerol Croat. 2012;20(4):272–5.
69. Fitzpatrick JE, Bennion SD, Reed OM, Wilson T, Reddy VV, Golitz L. Neutrophilic eccrine hidradenitis associated with induction chemotherapy. J Cutan Pathol. 1987;14(5):272–8.
70. Burg G, Bieber T, Langecker P. [Localized neutrophilic eccrine hydradenitis in mitoxantrone therapy: a typical side-effect of cytostatic drugs]. Der Hautarzt; Zeitschrift fur Dermatologie, Venerologie, und verwandte Gebiete. 1988;39(4):233–6.
71. Herms F, Franck N, Kramkimel N, Fichel F, Delaval L, Laurent-Roussel S, et al. Neutrophilic eccrine hidradenitis in 2 patients treated with BRAF inhibitors: a new cutaneous adverse event. Br J Dermatol. 2016;176(6):1645–8.
72. Bhanu P, Santosh KV, Gondi S, Manjunath KG, Rajendaran SC, Raj N. Neutrophilic eccrine hidradenitis: a new culprit-carbamazepine. Indian J Pharmacol. 2013;45(1):91–2.

73. Brehler R, Reimann S, Bonsmann G, Metze D. Neutrophilic hidradenitis induced by chemotherapy involves eccrine and apocrine glands. Am J Dermatopathol. 1997;19(1):73–8.
74. Bachmeyer C, Chaibi P, Aractingi S. Neutrophilic eccrine hidradenitis induced by granulocyte colony-stimulating factor. Br J Dermatol. 1998;139(2):354–5.
75. EL Sayed F, Ammoury A, Chababi M, Dhaybi R, Bazex J. Neutrophilic eccrine hidradenitis to acetaminophen. J Eur Acad Dermatol Venereol. 2006;20(10):1338–40.
76. Smith KJ, Skelton HG III, James WD, Holland TT, Lupton GP, Angritt P. Neutrophilic eccrine hidradenitis in HIV-infected patients. Armed Forces Retrovirus Research Group. J Am Acad Dermatol. 1990;23(5 Pt 1):945–7.
77. Cohen PR. Neutrophilic dermatoses: a review of current treatment options. Am J Clin Dermatol. 2009;10(5):301–12.
78. Villarreal-Villarreal CD, Ocampo-Candiani J, Villarreal-Martinez A. Sweet syndrome: a review and update. Actas Dermosifiliogr. 2016;107(5):369–78.
79. Debol SM, Herron MJ, Nelson RD. Anti-inflammatory action of dapsone: inhibition of neutrophil adherence is associated with inhibition of chemoattractant-induced signal transduction. J Leukoc Biol. 1997;62(6):827–36.

The Neutrophil and Its Role in Skin Diseases

21

Antonio Costanzo and Alessandra Narcisi

Introduction

Neutrophils (or polymorphonuclear granulocytes [PMNs]) are the most abundant white blood cells in the human circulation. These cells have long been viewed as simple suicide killers, with a marginal role in immune response. This view has changed in the last 10 years, when accumulating evidences enlightened important and unexpected functions for these neglected cells. Their role as critical mediators of immune response and inflammation is now more and more clear. Indeed these cells participate in protection against both intracellular and extracellular pathogens, including viruses and mycobacteria and modulate the adaptive immune response by functional interaction with dendritic cells, B cells and T cells. In addition, neutrophils have been shown to activate an alternate pathway of systemic anaphylaxis and to mediate allergic skin reactions. Finally, neutrophils were found to be involved in several physiological and pathological processes beyond the immune system, such as diabetes, atherosclerosis, and thrombus formation. Many of these functions appear to be related to their unique ability to release neutrophil extracellular traps even in the absence of pathogens.

In this chapter we will explore neutrophil functions and how these functions are involved in the pathophysiology of skin diseases.

A. Costanzo (✉) • A. Narcisi
Department of Biomedical Sciences, Humanitas University and Skin Pathology Laboratory
Humanitas Research Hospital, Milan, Italy
e-mail: antonio.costanzo@hunimed.eu

D. Wallach et al. (eds.), *Neutrophilic Dermatoses*,
https://doi.org/10.1007/978-3-319-72649-6_21

Anti-bacterial Defense

Neutrophils play a pivotal role in antimicrobial host defense (primarily in innate immunity) by recognizing microorganisms through their various receptor systems and forming one of the first lines of defense against invading microbes. Neutrophils originate from the bone marrow where they develop from the common myeloid progenitor cells through the myeloblast–promyelocyte–myelocyte–metamyelocyte pathway [1]. After being released from the bone marrow, neutrophils circulate in vessels until being attracted to tissues by chemotactic signals (e.g., formyl peptides, lipid mediators and chemokines) (Fig. 21.1). When activated, these cells target their massive weaponry against the invading microbes. Neutrophils contain four different exocytic compartments (namely the primary/azurophilic, the secondary/specific and the tertiary/gelatinase granules, as well as the secretory vesicles) each of which contain antimicrobial enzymes and other proteins, as well as important membrane receptors (Fig. 21.1). Release of these compartments into extracellular space or phagosome through the process of degranulation results in the release of proteases that degrade the invading microbes, chelation of nutrients essential for microbial

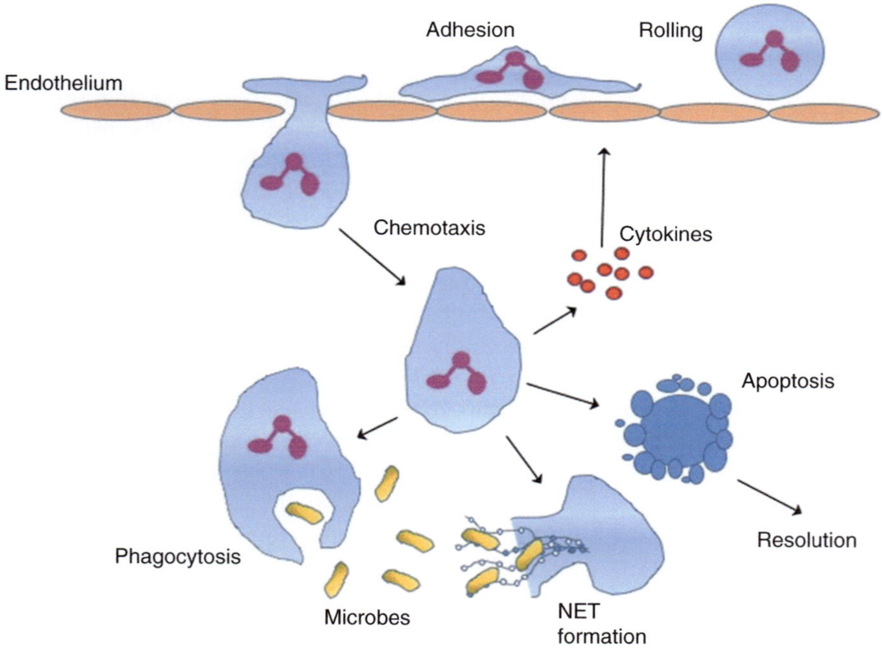

Fig. 21.1 Neutrophil functions: state of the art in the early 2000s. After migrating to the site of inflammation, neutrophils (PMN) phagocyte and digest the invading microbes; release NETs, which likely trap bacteria; and produce cytokines, which contribute to the inflammatory reaction. Once infection is cleared, neutrophils die by apoptosis and trigger an active program to resolve inflammation. Pathogen killing inside the phagosome occurs by ROS generated by the NADPH oxidase, as well as by granule enzymes released from intracellular granules

growth, modification of cytokines and endogenous enzyme inhibitors and increased sensitivity of the cells toward microbial and inflammatory signals. Neutrophils are also sources of toxic oxygen species that are produced as superoxide by the multi-unit NADPH oxidase and converted to more toxic materials by the enzyme myeloperoxidase [2].

Anti-viral Defense

Whereas neutrophils are critical for immunity against bacterial and fungi, their role in antiviral host defense is less appreciated. In a recent study, Saitoh et al. [3] proposed a role for Neutrophil extracellular traps (NETs) in the control of HIV-1 infection. HIV-1 triggered NET formation by human neutrophils and neutrophil-derived NETs were able to capture HIV-1 particles and reduce their efficiency to infect T cells. When neutrophils and T cells were co-cultured, neutrophils were able to reduce the infectivity of HIV-1. Pharmacological studies indicated that NET formation was dependent on Toll Like Receptor-7 (TLR-7) and TLR8 in endocytic compartments and that the effect of neutrophil-derived NETs on T cells could be inhibited by DNase treatment. In agreement with these findings, the neutrophil-mediated inhibition of HIV-1 infectivity on T cells required TLR7 and TLR8, and it was suspended by DNase treatment.

Another study provided evidence for the role of neutrophils and NETs in antiviral host defense [4]. Injection of viral TLR ligands or poxvirus infection led to dramatic accumulation of neutrophils in liver sinusoids that formed aggregates with platelets and released NETs inside the vessels. DNase treatment increased the percentage of liver cells infected with poxviruses, indicating that extracellular DNA exerts protective effects against viral infection [4].

Although these studies suggest a role for neutrophils and NETs in antiviral host defense, they also raise several questions. Studies on NET formation by neutrophils indicate critical roles for NADPH oxidase activity in this process [5] and it is difficult to imagine how viral particles would be able to trigger such a stimulation of neutrophils. However, because NET formation in the absence of NADPH oxidase activity has recently been shown to occur under more physiological conditions [6, 7], it may be possible that viral particles trigger NET formation. In addition, Jenne et al. [4] used systemic administration of LPS to induce protection from viral infection. Although additional studies in the field are warranted, these observations open up new light on the role of neutrophils in the host defense against viruses.

Cooperation with Adaptive Immune System

Neutrophils have until now been seen as effector cells that have little influence on the adaptive immune response. This view is being changed by several reports.

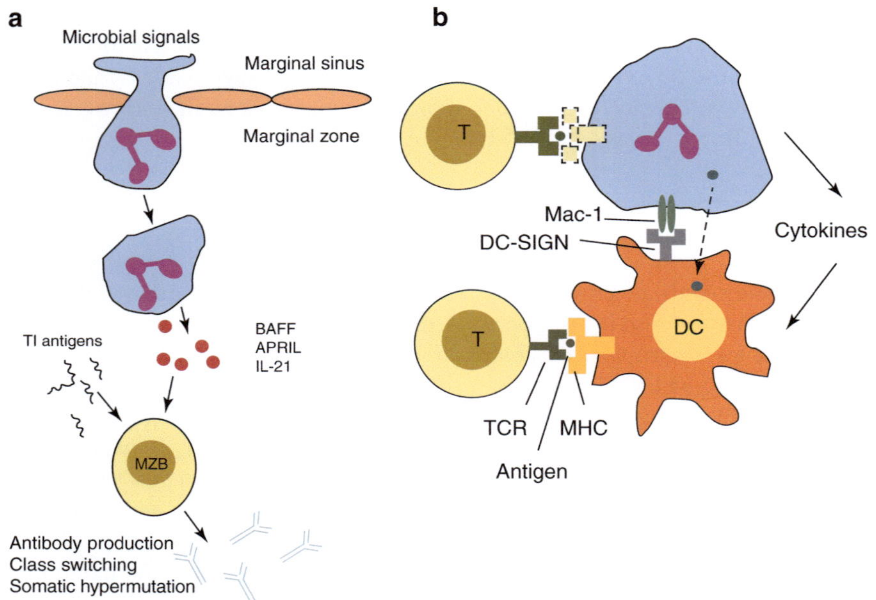

Fig. 21.2 Novel interactions of neutrophils with other immune cells. (**a**) Neutrophils (PMN) accumulate in the splenic marginal zone upon microbial challenge and facilitate the antibody production and maturation of marginal zone B cells (MZB) in response to T cell–independent (TI) antigens. (**b**) Neutrophils participate in a vicious cycle during autoimmune disease (e.g., SLE) pathogenesis by releasing NETs that trigger pDCs to release IFN-α, which then promotes antibody production by B cells (**b**)

Marginal zone B cells are B cells of the spleen located outside the germinal centers and close to marginal sinus, thus positioned closely to blood circulation. Their primary function is to trigger a rapid initiation of T cell–independent antibody responses to blood-borne microbes. Neutrophils are the major cell type responsible for capturing and transporting circulating bacteria to the splenic marginal zone [8]. In addition, human studies showed that activated neutrophils express B cell–activating factor (BAFF), the cytokine (also known as BLyS) and that neutrophils are a major source of A proliferation-inducing ligand (APRI)L, the BAFF-related, B cell–stimulating cytokine in B cell lymphomas [9] and mucosal plasma cell niches [10, 11]. In 2011, Puga et al. [12] revealed strict relationships between neutrophils and marginal zone B cells and hypothesized that this interaction can mediate T cell–independent antibody responses using BAFF and APRIL as mediators (Fig. 21.2a). They found a large number of neutrophils positioned around splenic marginal zone in humans, macaques, and mice. Splenic mice neutrophils activate marginal zone B cells, but they had limited stimulatory effect on follicular B cells. Splenic neutrophils could promote B cell survival, antibody production and class switching to IgG and IgA, qualifying to act as B helper cells. Splenic neutrophils express large amounts of marginal zone B cell stimulating cytokines such as APRIL, Interleukin-21 (IL-21) and BAFF. Circulating neutrophils can activate marginal zone B cells after exposure to splenic endothelial cells in the presence of microbial signals. Colonization of splenic marginal zones by neutrophils occurs soon after birth in humans, and marginal zone neutrophils were significantly less abundant in germ-free mice, indicating that microbial products, originating from the commensal flora, play an important role in the accumulation of splenic marginal zone neutrophils. Patients suffering from various defects of neutrophil development or function had normal circulating B cell numbers but strongly reduced marginal zone B cells circulating cells. The study of Puga et al. [12] revealed a potentially important immunological mechanism whereby splenic neutrophils may facilitate the antibody response of marginal zone B cells to T cell–independent microbial antigens.

The role of neutrophils in the regulation of T cell function is less well understood. Regulation of T cells by myeloid cells occurs via antigen presentation by DCs or macrophages, supported by the migration of antigen-carrying DCs to the lymph nodes. Neutrophils also appear to migrate in lymphatic vessels in a CC Chemokine Receptor-7 (CCR7)-dependent manner carrying antigens to the lymph nodes [13–15]. In a recent study Duffy et al. [16] showed that Vaccinia virus-specific CD8+ T cells appear in the bone marrow and identified neutrophils as the antigen transporting cells from the dermis to the bone marrow. Neutrophils express molecules required for antigen processing and presentation to T lymphocytes [17, 18]. Mouse neutrophils are able to present extracellular antigens on MHC class II molecules to CD8+ T cells [18], and also prime antigen-specific Th1 and Th17 cells [19]. The transport of antigens to the site of T cell priming and the direct priming/activation of antigen-specific T cells in an MHC-restricted manner raise the possibility that neutrophils may possibly even perform some level of classical antigen-presenting cell function (Fig. 21.2b).

These studies indicate that neutrophils positively regulate antigen-specific T cell responses. However, several works indicate a negative role for neutrophils in T cell function. Splenic neutrophils negatively regulate CD4+ T cell function [12]. A subset of human neutrophils also inhibits T cell responses during acute systemic inflammatory reactions such as bacterial sepsis [20].

Regulation of Dendritic Cells (DCs) by Neutrophils

Neutrophils act on adaptive immunity not only by directly acting on B and T cells, but also by modulating the function of DCs. Mouse neutrophils are capable of activating DCs during microbial infection [21, 22]. Neutrophils interaction with DCs leads to various responses including access to antigens captured by neutrophils, DC maturation and activation and consequently DC-mediated proliferation and TH1 polarization of T cells [23–25]. Dendritic Cell-Specific Intercellular adhesion molecule-3-Grabbing Non-integrin (DC-SIGN) and Mac-1, expressed on the surface of DCs and neutrophils, are the molecular mediators of neutrophils/DC interaction [24, 26–28] (Fig. 21.2b).

An additional role for neutrophils in DC activation was recently discovered in the pathogenesis of autoimmune diseases such as systemic lupus erythematosus (SLE).

Systemic lupus erythematosus (SLE) is an autoimmune disorder that affects approximatively 0.1% of the human population (mostly females) [29, 30]. SLE shows autoimmunity against nuclear antigens and can attack multiple organs, including the skin, the kidneys and the joints. One of the critical pathogenetic features of SLE is the presence of anti-DNA antibodies which form DNA-containing immune complexes and trigger interferon-α (IFNα) production from plasmacytoid dendritic cells (pDCs) [31]. It has been recently proposed that the source of extracellular DNA involved in pDC activation is the so-called neutrophil extracellular traps (NETs) [32, 33], complexes of cellular DNA with various antimicrobial peptides and other granule components released by neutrophils during a unique cell death pathway called NETosis [5]. The neutrophil antimicrobial peptide LL37 was found to be present in the circulating DNA-containing immune complexes of SLE patients and the molecule was shown to be essential in immune complex-mediated pDC activation leading to IFNα production [32]. DNA-containing immune complexes, on the other hand, trigger neutrophil activation and NET formation, leading to further pDC activation and IFNα production through a TLR9-dependent mechanism [32, 33] (Fig. 21.3).

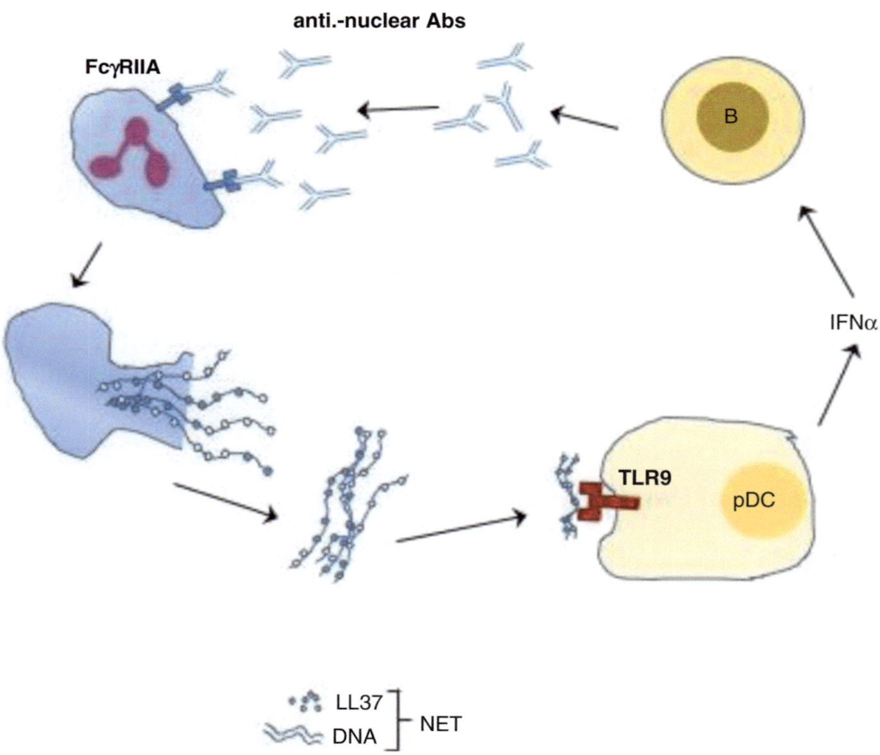

Fig. 21.3 Role of Neutrophils in SLE pathogenesis. Neutrophils may directly present antigens to T cells (T) and they also activate DCs and deliver antigens to them

In line with these findings, serum from SLE patients induces neutrophil aggregation [34]. These results indicate an important role for neutrophil activation and NET formation in the core of the pathogenesis of SLE in humans (Fig. 21.3).

This study suggests an unexpected role for neutrophils in early phases of autoimmune disease pathogenesis through triggering of type I interferon production by pDCs. There are, however, several open questions that need to be addressed. First, it is widely believed that NET formation requires NADPH oxidase [35]; therefore SLE pathogenesis would be expected to rely on the presence of this enzyme. However, deficiency of the NADPH oxidase component Nox2 exacerbated, rather than inhibited disease pathogenesis in lupus-prone mice [36], arguing against the role of NETs in SLE pathogenesis. This issue is further complicated by NADPH oxidase-independent NET formation proposed by other recent studies [6, 7].

Neutrophils in Autoimmune Skin Diseases

Given the expanding knowledge on neutrophils function in the regulation of immune diseases it is difficult to categorize skin diseases according to the role of neutrophils. Neutrophils are present in almost all inflammatory skin reactions and take part in many autoimmune disorders with skin involvement.

In this chapter, we will try to summarize the role of neutrophils in autoimmune and inflammatory skin diseases.

Up to now, the role of neutrophils in the neutrophilic dermatoses has not carefully been evaluated at a basic research level. However, the complex interplay between neutrophils, other immune system cells, cytokines and different effector molecules is discussed in the chapter on the pathophysiology of the neutrophilic dermatoses.

Bullous Pemphigoid and Epidermolysis Bullosa Acquisita

Both bullous pemphigoid (BP) and the rare epidermolysis bullosa acquisita (EBA) are subepidermal blistering skin diseases characterized (and likely caused) by autoimmunity to epidermal or dermal proteins. While the major autoantigens in BP are hemidesmosomal proteins such as BP180 or BP230, EBA is caused by autoimmunity against collagen VII (CVII), the major anchoring fibril in the skin.

Sera and purified IgG from human BP patients recruited neutrophils to the dermal–epidermal junction and induced ex vivo subepidermal separation in human skin cryosections [37]. This response was entirely dependent on the Fc portion of the autoantibodies [37], pointing to a likely pathogenetic role of Fc-receptor-mediated neutrophil activation by the autoantibodies present in BP patients.

An animal model resembling human BP can be triggered in neonatal BALB/c mice by the intradermal injection of rabbit polyclonal anti-BP180 antibodies [38]. Neutrophils were present in large quantities in the lesional skin sections of these animals and neutrophil depletion protected mice from disease development without affecting IgG and complement deposition at lesional sites [39, 40]. The recruitment of neutrophils to the inflamed skin was dependent on complement C5a fragment [39]. Gelatinase B (GB; also known as MMP9), an important granule protein of neutrophils, was shown to be present in the blister fluid of lesional skin and GB-deficient mice were resistant to disease development despite normal deposition of pathogenic IgG and mostly normal recruitment of neutrophils to the lesional skin [41]. Reconstitution of GB-deficient mice with intradermal injection of wild type neutrophils could restore the dermal–epidermal separation indicating an important role for neutrophil GB in the disease pathogenesis [42]. Neutrophil elastase (NE) could also be detected in the lesional skin in mouse models of bullous pemphigoid. NE-deficient mice were completely protected from experimental BP despite normal IgG and C3 deposition at the basal membrane zone [41] and NE inhibitors blocked disease development in the animals. Intradermal injection of wild type neutrophils into NE-deficient mice restored susceptibility to experimental bullous pemphigoid [41], again pointing to an important role for neutrophils in disease pathogenesis. In addition, GB was shown to activate neutrophil elastase by cleaving α1-proteinase inhibitor, the natural inhibitor of NE [43], providing a link between GB and NE in BP pathogenesis. NE was recently shown to directly cleave the BP180 autoantigen both in human and in mouse skin, generating peptides that were able to attract additional neutrophils [44]. Taken together, these results indicate a critical role for neutrophils in the effector phase of BP, whereby autoantibody deposition leads to Fc-receptor-mediated neutrophil activation triggering GB and NE release and activation, subsequent degradation of BP180, and as a result, tissue degradation and attraction of additional neutrophils.

In contrast to BP, the rare EBA is caused by autoantibodies against type VII collagen. The treatment of human skin cryosections with sera from EBA patients recruited neutrophils to the dermal–epidermal junction and triggered the separation of the two skin layers [45]. Animal models of EBA can be triggered by active immunization of mice with murine type VII collagen [46] or by injection (passive immunization) of mice with antibodies against mouse type VII collagen raised in rabbits [47]. Complement C5-deficient mice were totally resistant to the passive model of EBA [47], indicating a role for complement activation in the effector phase of the disease. Neutrophil depletion with anti-Gr1 antibodies also protected mice from disease induced by antibodies against type VII collagen despite normal deposition of the pathogenic antibodies at the dermal–epidermal junction [48]. One of the key enzymes in neutrophil effector functions is the NADPH oxidase, a multisubunit complex responsible for the generation of superoxide ($O_2^{\cdot -}$), the first component of reactive oxygen species cascades. Genetic deficiency of the p47phox (Ncf1) component of the NADPH oxidase protected mice from experimental EBA, while reconstitution of p47phox-deficient mice with wild type granulocytes restored skin inflammation [48]. In line with these findings, the pharmacological inhibition of the NADPH oxidase with diphenylene iodonium or the genetic deficiency of NADPH oxidase in neutrophils from CGD patients prevented the ex vivo separation of skin layers in human cryosections treated with sera from EBA patients in the presence of human neutrophils [48].

Psoriasis

Psoriasis is a chronic skin disease of supposedly autoimmune origin and a characteristic hyperplasia of epidermal keratinocytes. Neutrophils can be observed in the skin lesions of psoriatic patients and drug-induced agranulocytosis causes the disappearance of psoriasis vulgaris [49]. In line with this finding, generalized pustular psoriasis (which is one of the major complications of psoriasis), could be treated with granulocyte and monocyte adsorption apheresis [50]. Neutrophils appear early in new psoriasis lesions. Neutrophil function can be modulated by T lymphocytes and by monocytes. Neutrophils in turn can modulate the function of these cells. Many psoriasis associated pro-inflammatory molecules including angiopoetin- 1, cathelicidins, CCR6, CD15, CD40, CD40L, CD69, CXCL10, Fas ligand, folic acid pathways and associated molecules (homocysteine, NF-kappaB, VCAM-1 and VEGF), GM-CSF, IFN-gamma, interleukins 1beta, 4, 6, 8, 12, 15, 17, 20, 22 and 23, Leukotriene B4, S100A7-9 and S100A12, Sphingosine 1-Phosphate, TGF beta -1, and TNF-alpha all affect, are secreted by or are affected by neutrophils. Clinical triggers of psoriasis, drugs that induce psoriasis, drugs that flare psoriasis, psoriasis associated disorders, disorders treatable with therapies used to treat psoriasis, and side effects of many psoriasis therapies can be explained at least in part by the interplay between these disorders and drugs and neutrophils.

Neutrophils in Autoimmune Vasculitis

Anti-neutrophil cytoplasmic autoantibody (ANCA) associated vasculitis is a group of diseases characterized by systemic chronic inflammation of small blood vessels, with a frequency of one in 50,000 people [51]. The two main autoantigens are myeloperoxidase (MPO, its autoantibody is called perinuclear or p-ANCA) and proteinase 3 (PR3, its antibody is termed cytoplasmic or c-ANCA). Both of those autoantigens are components of the primary granules of neutrophils. Churg–Strauss syndrome, microscopic polyangiitis and crescentic glomerulonephritis are mainly characterized by p-ANCA, while 80% of patients with Wegener's granulomatosis have c-ANCA. ANCAs can induce human PMNs to produce superoxide, to release intracellular granules and to secrete proinflammatory cytokines in vitro [52]. It has been proposed that neutrophil extracellular traps (NETs) could also participate in vasculitis pathogenesis since ANCA-stimulated neutrophils could undergo NET formation and NETs containing chromatin fibers were shown to be present in the affected glomeruli of patients with small vessel vasculitis glomerulonephritis [53] .

Xiao and colleagues developed an experimental ANCA-model by sensitizing MPO-deficient mice with MPO and then transferring their splenocytes or purified IgG to healthy animals, thus provoking systemic vasculitis and necrotizing crescentic glomerulonephritis with a predominant neutrophil presence in lung lesions [54]. Neutrophil depletion resulted in a significant decrease of glomerulonephritis in α-MPO antibody-treated mice [55]. Acute lung injury, a fulminant form of Wegener's granulomatosis, could be provoked by the injection of TNFα-primed neutrophils into rats in the presence of monoclonal PR3 antibodies [56]. Lung abnormalities (like edema formation) were found to be dependent on the NADPH-oxidase and neutrophil elastase [56].

Neutrophils in Allergy and Anaphylaxis

Allergic and anaphylactic reactions are responses of the adaptive immune system triggered by repeated exposure to allergens, and are characterized by vascular reactions such as vasodilation and edema formation. Several recent studies suggest unexpected roles for neutrophils in these reactions.

The paradigm of anaphylaxis is that allergen-induced cross-linking of IgE molecules bound to Fcε-receptors on mast cells and basophils triggers histamine release and subsequent systemic vasodilation [57]. Although this mechanism is likely responsible for the majority of anaphylactic reactions, several observations indicate that alternative mechanisms, possibly mediated by IgG and cellular lineages other than mast cells and basophils, may also play a role [58–61]. Jönsson et al. [61] identified neutrophils as important players of active and IgG-induced passive systemic anaphylaxis in experimental mice (Fig. 21.4). Passive systemic anaphylaxis triggered by IgG antibodies was blocked by neutrophil depletion using the RB6-8C5

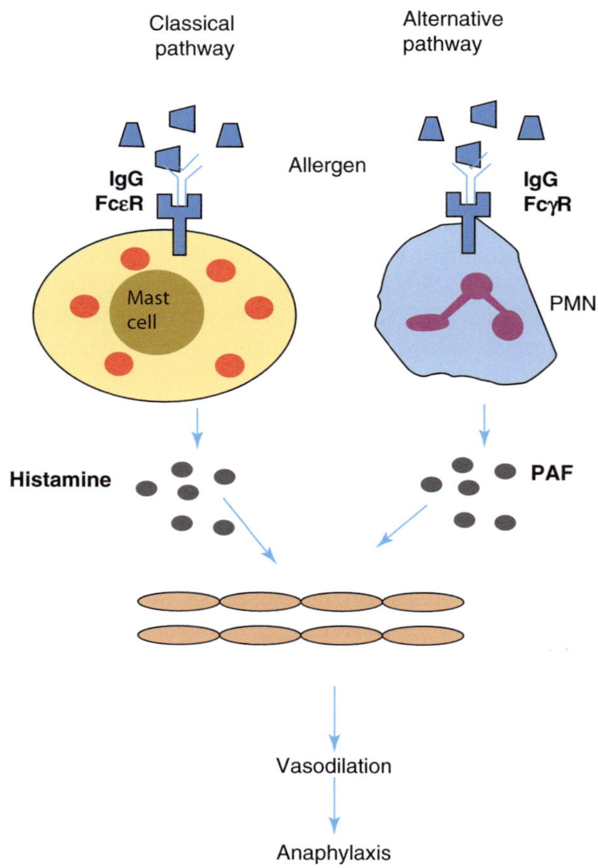

Fig. 21.4 Novel functions of neutrophils in vascular diseases. Neutrophils (PMN) mediate an alternative pathway of anaphylactic reaction which is distinct from the classical pathway mediated by mast cells or basophils

anti-Gr1 antibody. Active systemic anaphylaxis was partially reduced by anti-Gr1 antibodies alone, and it was nearly completely blocked by simultaneously depleting both neutrophils and basophils [61]. Interestingly, mice lacking all activating Fcγ- and Fcε-receptors except FcγRIV were able to mount normal active anaphylactic reactions which were, however, completely blocked by anti-Gr1 antibodies. Adoptive transfer of wild-type neutrophils rescued anaphylaxis development in FcR γ-chain-deficient animals (which lack all activating Fcγ- and Fcε-receptors including FcγRIV, and fail to mount active systemic anaphylaxis). Those results suggest that neutrophils are responsible for the FcγRIV-mediated component of active systemic anaphylaxis in mice and that this component is sufficient to trigger a full-blown anaphylaxis response. Additional experiments indicated that the neutrophil-dependent anaphylactic reaction was mediated primarily by PAF rather than histamine [61]. Importantly, active systemic anaphylaxis could be restored by adoptive transfer of human neutrophils to FcRγ−/− animals [61] or by transgenic expression of human FcγRIIA in FcRγ−/− mice [61], suggesting that human neutrophils may also be able to mediate systemic anaphylactic reactions.

The various forms of skin allergies comprise a major group of localized allergic diseases. As with other allergic diseases, their mechanism can also be divided into two conceptually different phases, the sensitization phase (leading to priming of the adaptive immune system) and the elicitation phase (causing local tissue damage through activation of the primed adaptive immune cells). They are also often complicated by additional inflammatory insults, such as chemically induced tissue damage in allergic contact dermatitis or mechanical damage caused by itching-induced scratching in atopic dermatitis. Several recent studies indicate an important role for neutrophils in skin allergies. Anti-Gr1 antibody treatment has been known to prevent ear swelling and T cell infiltration during contact hypersensitivity, a mouse model of allergic contact dermatitis [62]. In a recent study, neutrophils expressing the LTB4-receptor BLT1 were found to be required for inflammation and recruitment of allergen-primed T cells at the allergen challenge site in a novel mouse model of atopic dermatitis combining ovalbumin immunization and challenge with mechanical skin injury (reminiscent of itching-induced scratching; [63]).

Both of the aforementioned studies revealed important roles for neutrophils in the elicitation phase of allergic skin inflammation. However, although innate immune mechanisms likely also play important roles in DC activation and T cell priming during the earlier and conceptually different sensitization phase of allergic skin diseases [64], no studies on the role on neutrophils in that phase have been completed yet. Interestingly, our own recent studies (unpublished data; published in abstract form in Weber et al., [65] suggested an important role for neutrophils in the sensitization phase of contact hypersensitivity. In that study, we found that Ly6G antibody-mediated depletion of neutrophils, selectively during the sensitization phase, abrogated the contact hypersensitivity reaction, and diminished DC activation and priming of allergen-specific T cells. In addition, lymph node cells from allergen-sensitized mice that were previously treated with neutrophil-depleting anti-Ly6G antibodies or were genetically deficient of neutrophils because of a myeloid-specific deletion of the Mcl-1 protein [66] were unable to transfer sensitivity toward contact allergens to normal naive recipients [65]. Therefore, neutrophils appear to be critical players in both the sensitization and elicitation phases of allergic skin inflammatory reactions.

Conclusion

Besides being key players in innate immunity, increasing evidence indicates that neutrophils are also important in the molecular pathogenesis of various inflammatory and autoimmune skin diseases including SLE, blistering skin diseases, psoriasis or ANCA-mediated vasculitis. The emerging complexity of the function of these cells suggests that they are active participants, rather than just innocent bystanders in these diseases. Better understanding of neutrophil biology and of the contribution of neutrophils to in vivo autoimmune disease models (e.g., through further lineage-specific deletion studies) will provide additional information about the diseases where inhibition of neutrophil function may provide clinical benefit in human patients.

References

1. Eyles JL, Roberts AW, Metcalf D, Wicks IP. Granulocyte colony-stimulating factor and neutrophils—forgotten mediators of inflammatory disease. Nat Clin Pract Rheumatol. 2006;2:500–10.
2. Nathan C. Neutrophils and immunity: challenges and opportunities. Nat Rev Immunol. 2006;6:173–82.
3. Saitoh T, Komano J, Saitoh Y, et al. Neutrophil extracellular traps mediate a host defense response to human immunodeficiency virus-1. Cell Host Microbe. 2012;12:109–16.
4. Jenne CN, Wong CH, Zemp FJ, et al. Neutrophils recruited to sites of infection protect from virus challenge by releasing neutrophil extracellular traps. Cell Host Microbe. 2013;13:169–80.
5. Brinkmann V, Reichard U, Goosmann C, et al. Neutrophil extracellular traps kill bacteria. Science. 2004;303:1532–5.
6. Chen K, Nishi H, Travers R, et al. Endocytosis of soluble immune complexes leads to their clearance by FcγRIIIB but induces neutrophil extracellular traps via FcγRIIA in vivo. Blood. 2012;120:4421–31.
7. Parker H, Dragunow M, Hampton MB, Kettle AJ, Winterbourn CC. Requirements for NADPH oxidase and myeloperoxidase in neutrophil extracellular trap formation differ depending on the stimulus. J Leukoc Biol. 2012;92:841–9.
8. Balázs M, Martin F, Zhou T, Kearney J. Blood dendritic cells interact with splenic marginal zone B cells to initiate T-independent immune responses. Immunity. 2002;17:341–52.
9. Schwaller J, Schneider P, Mhawech-Fauceglia P, et al. Neutrophil-derived APRIL concentrated in tumor lesions by proteoglycans correlates with human B-cell lymphoma aggressiveness. Blood. 2007;109:331–8.
10. Scapini P, Bazzoni F, Cassatella MA. Regulation of B-cell-activating factor (BAFF)/B lymphocyte stimulator (BLyS) expression in human neutrophils. Immunol Lett. 2008;116:1–6.
11. Huard B, McKee T, Bosshard C, et al. APRIL secreted by neutrophils binds to heparan sulfate proteoglycans to create plasma cell niches in human mucosa. J Clin Invest. 2008;118:2887–95.
12. Puga I, Cols M, Barra CM, et al. B cell-helper neutrophils stimulate the diversification and production of immunoglobulin in the marginal zone of the spleen. Nat. Immunol. 2011;13: 170–80.

13. Abadie V, Badell E, Douillard P, et al. Neutrophils rapidly migrate via lymphatics after Mycobacterium bovis BCG intradermal vaccination and shuttle live bacilli to the draining lymph nodes. Blood. 2005;106:1843–50.
14. Maletto BA, Ropolo AS, Alignani DO, et al. Presence of neutrophil-bearing antigen in lymphoid organs of immune mice. Blood. 2006;108:3094–102.
15. Beauvillain C, Cunin P, Doni A, et al. CCR7 is involved in the migration of neutrophils to lymph nodes. Blood. 2011;117:1196–204.
16. Duffy D, Perrin H, Abadie V, et al. Neutrophils transport antigen from the dermis to the bone marrow, initiating a source of memory CD8+ T cells. Immunity. 2012;37:917–29.
17. Ashtekar AR, Saha B. Poly's plea: membership to the club of APCs. Trends Immunol. 2012;24:485–90.
18. Beauvillain C, Delneste Y, Scotet M, et al. Neutrophils efficiently cross-prime naive T cells in vivo. Blood. 2007;110:2965–73.
19. Abi Abdallah DS, Egan CE, Butcher BA, Denkers EY. Mouse neutrophils are professional antigen-presenting cells programmed to instruct Th1 and Th17 T-cell differentiation. Int Immunol. 2011;23:317–26.
20. Pillay J, Kamp VM, van Hoffen E, et al. A subset of neutrophils in human systemic inflammation inhibits T cell responses through Mac-1. J Clin Invest. 2012;122:327–36.
21. Bennouna S, Bliss SK, Curiel TJ, Denkers EY. Cross-talk in the innate immune system: neutrophils instruct recruitment and activation of dendritic cells during microbial infection. J Immunol. 2003;171:6052–8.
22. Charmoy M, Brunner-Agten S, Aebischer D, et al. Neutrophil-derived CCL3 is essential for the rapid recruitment of dendritic cells to the site of Leishmania major inoculation in resistant mice. PLoS Pathol. 2010;6(2):e1000755.
23. Bennouna S, Denkers EY. Microbial antigen triggers rapid mobilization of TNF-alpha to the surface of mouse neutrophils transforming them into inducers of high-level dendritic cell TNF-alpha production. J Immunol. 2005;174:4845–51.
24. van Gisbergen KP, Sanchez-Hernandez M, Geijtenbeek TB, van Kooyk Y. Neutrophils mediate immune modulation of dendritic cells through glycosylation-dependent interactions between Mac-1 and DC-SIGN. J Exp Med. 2005;201:1281–92.
25. Megiovanni AM, Sanchez F, Robledo-Sarmiento C, Morel C, Gluckman JC, Boudaly S. Polymorphonuclear neutrophils deliver activation signals and antigenic molecules to dendritic cells: a new link between leukocytes upstream of T lymphocytes. J Leukoc Biol. 2005;79:977–88.
26. van Gisbergen KP, Geijtenbeek TB, van Kooyk Y. Close encounters of neutrophils and DCs. Trends Immunol. 2005;26:626–31.
27. Boudaly S. Activation of dendritic cells by polymorphonuclear neutrophils. Front Biosci. 2005;14:1589–95.
28. Yang CT, Cambier CJ, Davis JM, Hall CJ, Crosier PS, Ramakrishnan L. Neutrophils exert protection in the early tuberculous granuloma by oxidative killing of mycobacteria phagocytosed from infected macrophages. Cell Host Microbe. 2012;12:301–12.
29. D'Cruz DP, Khamashta MA, Hughes GR. Systemic lupus erythematosus. Lancet. 2007;369:587–96.
30. Rahman A, Isenberg DA. Systemic lupus erythematosus. N Engl J Med. 2008;358:929–39.
31. Ronnblom L, Pascual V. The innate immune system in SLE: type I interferons and dendritic cells. Lupus. 2008;17:394–9.
32. Lande R, Ganguly D, Facchinetti V, et al. Neutrophils activate plasmacytoid dendritic cells by releasing self-DNA-peptide complexes in systemic lupus erythematosus. Sci Transl Med. 2012;3:73ra19.
33. Garcia-Romo GS, Caielli S, Vega B, Connolly J, Allantaz F, Xu Z, et al. Netting neutrophils are major inducers of type I IFN production in pediatric systemic lupus erythematosus. Sci Transl Med. 2011;3:73ra20.
34. Abramson SB, Given WP, Edelson HS, Weissmann G. Neutrophil aggregation induced by sera from patients with active systemic lupus erythematosus. Arthritis Rheum. 1983;26:630–6.

35. Fuchs TA, Abed U, Goosmann C, et al. Novel cell death program leads to neutrophil extracellular traps. J Cell Biol. 2007;176:231–41.
36. Campbell AM, Kashgarian M, Shlomchik MJ. NADPH oxidase inhibits the pathogenesis of systemic lupus erythematosus. Sci Transl Med. 2012;4:157ra141.
37. Sitaru C, Schmidt E, Petermann S, Munteanu LS, Bröcker EB, Zillikens D. Autoantibodies to bullous pemphigoid antigen 180 induce dermal–epidermal separation in cryosections of human skin. J Invest Dermatol. 2002;118:664–71.
38. Liu Z, Diaz LA, Troy JL, et al. A passive transfer model of the organ-specific autoimmune disease, bullous pemphigoid, using antibodies generated against the hemidesmosomal antigen, BP180. J Clin Invest. 1993;92:2480–8.
39. Liu Z, Giudice GJ, Zhou X, et al. A major role for neutrophils in experimental bullous pemphigoid. J Clin Invest. 1997;100:1256–63.
40. Chen R, Fairley JA, Zhao ML, et al. Macrophages, but not T and B lymphocytes, are critical for subepidermal blister formation in experimental bullous pemphigoid: macrophage-mediated neutrophil infiltration depends on mast cell activation. J Immunol. 2002;169:3987–92.
41. Liu Z, Shapiro SD, Zhou X, et al. A critical role for neutrophil elastase in experimental bullous pemphigoid. J Clin Invest. 2000;105:113–23.
42. Liu Z, Shipley JM, TH V, et al. Gelatinase B-deficient mice are resistant to experimental bullous pemphigoid. J Exp Med. 1998;188:475–82.
43. Liu Z, Zhou X, Shapiro SD, et al. The serpin α1-proteinase inhibitor is a critical substrate for gelatinase B/MMP-9 in vivo. Cell. 2000;102:647–55.
44. Lin L, Betsuyaku T, Heimbach L, et al. Neutrophil elastase cleaves the murine hemidesmosomal protein BP180/type XVII collagen and generates degradation products that modulate experimental bullous pemphigoid. Matrix Biol. 2012;31:38–44.
45. Sitaru C, Kromminga A, Hashimoto T, Brocker EB, Zillikens D. Autoantibodies to type VII collagen mediate Fcγ-dependent neutrophil activation and induce dermal–epidermal separation in cryosections of human skin. Am J Pathol. 2002;161:301–11.
46. Sitaru C, Chiriac MT, Mihai S, et al. Induction of complement-fixing autoantibodies against type VII collagen results in subepidermal blistering in mice. J Immunol. 2006;177:3461–8.
47. Sitaru C, Mihai S, Otto C, et al. Induction of dermal–epidermal separation in mice by passive transfer of antibodies specific to type VII collagen. J Clin Invest. 2005;115:870–8.
48. Chiriac MT, Roesler J, Sindrilaru A, Scharffetter-Kochanek K, Zillikens D, Sitaru C. NADPH oxidase is required for neutrophil-dependent autoantibody-induced tissue damage. J Pathol. 2007;212:56–65.
49. Toichi E, Tachibana T, Furukawa F. Rapid improvement of psoriasis vulgaris during drug-induced agranulocytosis. J Am Acad Dermatol. 2000;43:391–5.
50. Fujisawa T, Murase K, Okumura Y, et al. Generalized pustular psoriasis successfully treated with granulocyte and monocyte adsorption apheresis. Ther Apher Dial. 2011;15:374–8.
51. Rarok AA, Limburg PC, Kallenberg CG. Neutrophil-activating potential of antineutrophil cytoplasm autoantibodies. J Leukoc Biol. 2003;74:3–15.
52. Falk RJ, Terrell RS, Charles LA, Jennette JC. Anti-neutrophil cytoplasmic autoantibodies induce neutrophils to degranulate and produce oxygen radicals in vitro. Proc Natl Acad Sci U S A. 1990;87:4115–9.
53. Kessenbrock K, Krumbholz M, Schonermarck U, et al. Netting neutrophils in autoimmune small-vessel vasculitis. Nat Med. 2009;15:623–5.
54. Xiao H, Heeringa P, Hu P, et al. Antineutrophil cytoplasmic autoantibodies specific for myeloperoxidase cause glomerulonephritis and vasculitis in mice. J Clin Invest. 2002;110:955–63.
55. Xiao H, Heeringa P, Liu Z, et al. The role of neutrophils in the induction of glomerulonephritis by anti-myeloperoxidase antibodies. Am J Pathol. 2005;167:39–45.
56. Hattar K, Oppermann S, Ankele C, et al. c-ANCA-induced neutrophil-mediated lung injury: a model of acute Wegener's granulomatosis. Eur Respir J. 2010;36:187–95.
57. Khan BQ, Kemp SF. Pathophysiology of anaphylaxis. Curr Opin Allergy Clin Immunol. 2011;11:319–25.

58. Finkelman FD. Anaphylaxis: lessons from mouse models. J Allergy Clin Immunol. 2007;120:506–15.
59. Tsujimura Y, Obata K, Mukai K, et al. Basophils play a pivotal role in immunoglobulin-G-mediated but not immunoglobulin-E-mediated systemic anaphylaxis. Immunity. 2008;28:581–9.
60. Ohnmacht C, Schwartz C, Panzer M, Schiedewitz I, Naumann R, Voehringer D. Basophils orchestrate chronic allergic dermatitis and protective immunity against helminths. Immunity. 2010;33:364–74.
61. Jönsson F, Mancardi DA, Kita Y, et al. Mouse and human neutrophils induce anaphylaxis. J Clin Invest. 2011;121:1484–96.
62. Dilulio NA, Engeman T, Armstrong D, Tannenbaum C, Hamilton TA, Fairchild RL. Groalpha-mediated recruitment of neutrophils is required for elicitation of contact hypersensitivity. Eur J Immunol. 1999;29:3485–95.
63. Oyoshi MK, He R, Li Y, et al. Leukotriene B4-driven neutrophil recruitment to the skin is essential for allergic skin inflammation. Immunity. 2012;37:747–58.
64. Kaplan MJ. Neutrophils in the pathogenesis and manifestations of SLE. Nat Rev Rheumatol. 2011;7:691–9.
65. Weber FC, Nemeth T, Ozsvari B, et al. Neutrophils are crucial innate effector cells in contact hypersensitivity. Eur J Clin Invest. 2012;42(S1):17.
66. Dzhagalov I, St John A, He YW. The antiapoptotic protein Mcl-1 is essential for the survival of neutrophils but not macrophages. Blood. 2007;109:1620–6.

Genetics of the Neutrophilic Dermatoses 22

William W. Huang and Christine S. Ahn

Introduction

Neutrophilic dermatoses are a heterogeneous group of skin disorders linked together by overlapping histopathologic findings, pathophysiology, clinical features, and principles of management. Although many of the neutrophilic dermatoses are idiopathic, they can occur in association with systemic diseases and genetic factors. In-depth knowledge of the genetic basis of some of the neutrophilic dermatoses is important because it explains responsiveness to certain treatments and can help guide management. This chapter will discuss the neutrophilic dermatoses with known and emerging associated genetic alterations, which include Sweet syndrome, pyoderma gangrenosum, and pustular psoriasis, among others.

Sweet Syndrome

Sweet syndrome, also known as acute febrile neutrophilic dermatosis, is characterized by the presence of tender erythematous, often edematous, skin lesions, fever, and peripheral neutrophilia. It can be further characterized into three clinical subsets: idiopathic, drug-induced, and malignancy-induced Sweet syndrome, although it can also occur in association with infections, pregnancy, and autoimmune or inflammatory diseases [1, 2]. In the drug-induced form, Sweet syndrome has been most commonly associated with exposure to exogenous granulocyte colony-stimulating factor (G-CSF), likely related to the role that G-CSF plays in suppressing apoptosis and promoting survival of neutrophils [3]. Other drugs linked to Sweet syndrome include trimethoprim-sulfamethoxazole, minocycline, all-trans-retinoic

W. W. Huang (✉) • C. S. Ahn
Department of Dermatology, Wake Forest School of Medicine,
Winston-Salem, NC, USA
e-mail: whuang@wakehealth.edu; cahn@wakehealth.edu

D. Wallach et al. (eds.), *Neutrophilic Dermatoses*,
https://doi.org/10.1007/978-3-319-72649-6_22

acid, levonorgestrel/ethinyl estradiol, and bortezomib [2]. In malignancy-induced Sweet syndrome, the most commonly associated solid tumors and hematologic malignancies are genitourinary cancers and acute myeloid leukemia, respectively.

The pathogenesis of Sweet syndrome is not fully understood, although it is thought to be driven by T helper cells through the production of cytokines such as IL-1, IL-2, IFN-γ, and G-CSF [1]. In patients with acute myeloid leukemia, Sweet syndrome has been reported in up to 1% of patients, and gene mutations in FMS-related tyrosine kinase-3 (FLT3) was observed in 39% of patients in one study [4]. In patients with myelodysplastic syndrome, heterozygous mutations on alleles R202Q and G304R in the MEFV gene were described by Jo et al. MEFV, known to cause familial Mediterranean fever, is located on chromosome 16p and plays a role in the production of pyrin [5]. Defects in MEFV lead to a diminished ability of pyrin to control inflammation, leading to an inappropriate or uncontrolled inflammatory response [5].

Pyoderma Gangrenosum

Pyoderma gangrenosum (PG) is a painful, ulcerating inflammatory skin disease. There are several clinical variants but the classic lesion of PG is a rapidly progressive ulcer with a violaceous, undermined border. Histopathologically, a sterile dermal neutrophilic infiltrate, often with accompanying leukocytoclasia and necrosis, is observed. PG is a diagnosis of exclusion, as there are no laboratory tests or histopathologic features specific to this entity. In up to 70% of cases, PG is associated with a systemic disease, of which the most common are inflammatory bowel disease (IBD), autoimmune or autoinflammatory arthritis, and hematologic disorders such as monoclonal gammopathies, acute myelogenous leukemia, and myelodysplastic syndrome [6].

Although not fully understood, the pathogenesis of PG is thought to be multifactorial, with neutrophilic dysfunction, inflammatory mediators, and genetic predisposition each playing a role. Over the last several decades, several PG-associated genetic syndromes have been described. In one group of genetic syndromes, the constellation of findings result from mutations on chromosome 15q, which affect the proline-serine-threonine-phosphatase interactive protein (PSTPIP)-1 gene, also known as the CD2-binding protein (CD2BP)-1 (Table 22.1). PSTPIP1 is a

Table 22.1 Genetic syndromes with PSTPIP1-related mutations

Syndrome	Constellation of findings	Mutation
PAPA	Pyogenic arthritis, pyoderma gangrenosum, acne	A230T, E250Q, E250K, D266N
PASH	Pyoderma gangrenosum, acne, suppurative hidradenitis	CCTG microsatellite repeats NCSTN
PAPASH	Pyogenic sterile arthritis, pyoderma gangrenosum, acne, hidradenitis suppurativa	E277D
PAC	Pyoderma gangrenosum, acne, ulcerative colitis	G1207C

cytoskeleton-associated phosphatase protein that modulates T-cell activation, cytoskeletal organization, and production of IL-1β [6, 7]. The mutations lead to a hyperphosphorylated variant of PSTPIP1 that demonstrates a higher affinity to pyrin. Improper binding to pyrin is thought to cause increased assembly of the apoptosis/speck-like protein containing a caspase-recruitment domain (ASC) pyroptosome, which then recruits and activates procaspase-1, the precursor to caspase-1. Activation of caspase-1 leads to increased production of IL-1β and IL-18, leading to inflammation [8]. Due to the expression of pyrin on neutrophils and not lymphocytes, the downstream effects of PSTPIP1 binding to pyrin is a neutrophil-predominant inflammatory reaction [9] PAPA syndrome, characterized by the triad of pyogenic arthritis, pyoderma gangrenosum, and acne, was first described in 1975. Inherited in an autosomal dominant manner, PAPA syndrome results from mutations of A230T, E250Q, E250K, and D266N on chromosome 15q [8]. There are at least five families of PAPA syndrome reported in the literature, and penetrance can be as high as 100% based on available data [10]. PASH syndrome, which consists of PG, acne, and suppurative hidradenitis, results from an increased number of CCTG microsatellite repeats in the promoter region of PSTPIP1. More recently, Duchatelet et al. described a case of PASH syndrome with a nicastrin (NCSTN) mutation. Mutations in nicastrin, which is a γ-secretase gene, can lead to impaired Notch signaling and impact epidermal homeostasis. Loss-of-function mutations in nicastrin and other γ-secretase genes including presenilin enhancer gamma secretase subunit (PSENEN) and presenilin-1 (PSEN1) have been reported in a small number of hidradenitis suppurativa cases [11]. PAPASH syndrome, which consists of pyogenic sterile arthritis, PG, acne, and hidradenitis suppurativa, results from an E277D missense mutation on chromosome 15q [6]. In a recent report, a new mutation in PSTPIP1 (G > C transversion at cDNA position 1207) was identified in a patient with PG, acne, and ulcerative colitis, thus termed PAC syndrome [12]. Despite a growing understanding of PG in the setting of mutations in the PSTPIP1 gene, there are several reports of individuals with PAPA and other PG-related syndromes in the absence of any known mutations in the PSTPIP1 gene. This suggests that factors other than genetic mutations play a role in creating a pro-inflammatory state that predisposes individuals to developing the constellation of findings in these syndromes [9].

In patients with inflammatory bowel disease, several genetic loci have been linked to susceptibility to PG. In a genome-wide association study, three single nucleotide polymorphisms (SNPs) of the gene TRAF3IP2 were found to confer a higher risk to develop cutaneous manifestations in IBD, including pyoderma gangrenosum [13]. In a large case control study, Weizman et al. identified several known IBD susceptibility loci which also demonstrated a significant association with PG including IL8RA, MUC17, MMP24, WNK2, DOCK9, PRDM1, and NDIFIP1 [14].

Pyoderma gangrenosum has also been described in the presence of a Janus kinase (JAK) 2 mutation. In two reports, JAK2V617F mutations were identified in association with PG [15]. The JAK-STAT (signal transducer and activator of transcription) pathway is essential for cell proliferation, differentiation, and apoptosis during hematopoiesis and defects can lead to inflammatory and myeloproliferative disorders. The pathway can be activated by a number of cytokines, including granulocyte colony-stimulating factor (G-CSF), tumor necrosis factor-α, as well as interleukins and interferons. Although the relationship between JAK and causation of PG is not fully understood, G-CSF plays a known role in neutrophilic dermatoses and in PG in particular, as it mediates adhesion and proliferation of neutrophils at sites of inflammation and tissue injury [15].

Lastly, there are reports of PG in the context of disorders of immunodeficiency including common variable immunodeficiency (CVID), severe combined immunodeficiency (SCID) with a mutation in RAG1, and leukocyte adhesion deficiency (LAD)-1 with mutations in ITGB2 [16–19].

Pustular Psoriasis

Generalized pustular psoriasis is a potentially life-threatening, uncommon variant of psoriasis. There are four different clinical variants of generalized pustular psoriasis, which include the von Zumbusch, annular, exanthematic, and localized patterns. On histology, the presence of neutrophilic infiltrates is the predominant feature of this subtype of psoriasis. Neutrophils can be seen in large accumulations in the stratum corneum with surrounding parakeratosis.

Various mutations on the IL36RN gene have been identified as causally associated with generalized pustular psoriasis and other pustular skin disorders such as palmoplantar psoriasis, acute generalized exanthematous pustular eruption, and acrodermatitis continua of Hallopeau. IL36RN, which encodes IL-36 receptor antagonist, is a protein that plays a key role in activating intracellular NF-kB and the mitogen-activated protein kinase pathway. The loss of function mutations in IL36RN are thought to be a critical component to the pathogenesis of psoriasis or psoriatic lesions in both mice and humans [20].

Other Neutrophilic Dermatoses

Neutrophilic urticarial dermatosis (NUD) occurs as an urticarial eruption in cryopyrin-associated periodic syndromes (CAPS) and Still's disease. It is a relatively recently described condition that is characterized histologically by the presence of intact neutrophils, with eosinophils and nuclear dust lacking [21]. In one report of a patient with NUD, genetic testing revealed a mutation in the NLRP3 gene, indicative of concomitant CAPS. In this case, the patient's father, paternal aunt, and brother all carried the same mutation. The gain-of-function mutation of NLRP3 in patients with CAPS leads to overproduction of IL-1β, which explains responsiveness to anti-IL-1 agents such as anakinra [21].

Conclusions

There is continued emphasis on elucidating the pathogenic mechanisms behind neutrophilic dermatoses as many of these diseases are undoubtedly connected. Understanding the pathogenesis of the neutrophilic dermatoses as well as the underlying genetic factors can help clinicians determine which medications may be most efficacious and also shed light on further directions in management.

References

1. Rochet NM, Chavan RN, Cappel MA, Wada DA, Gibson LE. Sweet syndrome: clinical presentation, associations, and response to treatment in 77 patients. J Am Acad Dermatol. 2013;69(4):557–64.
2. Casarin Costa JR, Virgens AR, Mestre LO, et al. Sweet syndrome. J Cutan Med Surg. 2017;21(3):211–6. https://doi.org/10.1177/1203475417690719.
3. Marzano AV, Ishak RS, Saibeni S, et al. Autoinflammatory skin disorders in inflammatory bowel diseases, pyoderma gangrenosum and Sweet's syndrome: a comprehensive review and disease classification criteria. Clin Rev Allergy Immunol. 2013;45(2):202–10.
4. Kazmi SM, Pemmaraju N, Patel KP, et al. Characteristics of Sweet syndrome in patients with acute myeloid leukemia. Clin Lymphoma Myeloma Leuk. 2015;15(6):358–63.
5. Jo T, Horio K, Migita K. Sweet's syndrome in patients with MDS and MEFV mutations. N Engl J Med. 2015;372(7):686–8.
6. Braswell SF, Kostopoulos TC, Ortega-Loayza AG. Pathophysiology of pyoderma gangrenosum (PG): an updated review. J Am Acad Dermatol. 2015;73(4):691–8.
7. Campbell L, Raheem I, Malemud CJ, Askari AD. The relationship between NALP3 and autoinflammatory syndromes. Int J Mol Sci. 2016;17(5):E725.
8. Lindwall E, Singla S, Davis WE, Quinet RJ. Novel PSTPIP1 gene mutation in a patient with pyogenic arthritis, pyoderma gangrenosum and acne (PAPA) syndrome. Semin Arthritis Rheum. 2015;45(1):91–3.
9. Park BM, Yun SJ, Lee SC, Lee JB. A sporadic case of pyogenic arthritis, pyoderma gangrenosum and acne syndrome without an identifiable mutation. Clin Exp Dermatol. 2014;39(1):73–5.
10. Hong JB, Su YN, Chiu HC. Pyogenic arthritis, pyoderma gangrenosum, and acne syndrome (PAPA syndrome): report of a sporadic case without an identifiable mutation in the CD2BP1 gene. J Am Acad Dermatol. 2009;61(3):533–5.
11. Duchatelet S, Miskinyte S, Join-Lambert O, et al. First nicastrin mutation in PASH (pyoderma gangrenosum, acne and suppurative hidradenitis) syndrome. Br J Dermatol. 2015;173(2):610–2.
12. Zeeli T, Padalon-Brauch G, Ellenbogen E, et al. Pyoderma gangrenosum, acne and ulcerative colitis in a patient with a novel mutation in the PSTPIP1 gene. Clin Exp Dermatol. 2015;40(4):367–72.
13. Ciccacci C, Biancone L, Di Fusco D, et al. TRAF3IP2 gene is associated with cutaneous extraintestinal manifestations in inflammatory bowel disease. J Crohns Colitis. 2013;7(1):44–52.
14. Weizman A, Huang B, Berel D, et al. Clinical, serologic, and genetic factors associated with pyoderma gangrenosum and erythema nodosum in inflammatory bowel disease patients. Inflamm Bowel Dis. 2014;20(3):525–33.
15. Palanivel JA, Macbeth AE, Levell NJ. Pyoderma gangrenosum in association with Janus kinase 2 (JAK2V617F) mutation. Clin Exp Dermatol. 2013;38(1):44–6.
16. Boussofara L, Gammoudi R, Ghariani N, et al. Familial pyoderma gangrenosum in association with common variable immunodeficiency. Br J Dermatol. 2013;169(4):944–6.

17. Vahlquist A, Håkansson LD, Rönnblom L, et al. Recurrent pyoderma gangrenosum and cystic acne associated with leucocyte adhesion deficiency due to novel mutations in ITGB2: successful treatment with infliximab and adalimumab. Acta Derm Venereol. 2015;95(3):349–51.
18. Patiroglu T, Akar HH, Gilmour K, et al. Atypical severe combined immunodeficiency caused by a novel homozygous mutation in Rag1 gene in a girl who presented with pyoderma gangrenosum: a case report and literature review. J Clin Immunol. 2014;34(7):792–5.
19. Madkaikar M, Italia K, Gupta M, et al. Leukocyte adhesion deficiency-I with a novel intronic mutation presenting with pyoderma gangrenosum-like lesions. J Clin Immunol. 2015;35(4):431–4.
20. Tauber M, Bal E, Pei XY, et al. IL36RN mutations affect protein expression and function: a basis for genotype-phenotype correlation in pustular diseases. J Invest Dermatol. 2016;136(9):1811–9.
21. Herbert VG, Ahmadi-Simab K, Reich K, Böer-Auer A. Neutrophilic urticarial dermatosis (NUD) indicating Cryopyrin-associated periodic syndrome associated with a novel mutation of the NLRP3 gene. J Eur Acad Dermatol Venereol. 2016;30(5):852–3.

Mechanisms of Inflammation in the Neutrophilic Dermatoses

23

Angelo Valerio Marzano and Massimo Cugno

Introduction

Neutrophilic dermatoses are a heterogenous group of conditions characterized by accumulation of neutrophils in the skin and, rarely, the internal organs [1, 2]. The cutaneous manifestations of neutrophilic dermatoses are polymorphic, including pustules, bullae, abscesses, papules, nodules, plaques and ulcers, and almost any organ system can be involved, giving rise to the term 'neutrophilic disease' [2]. The definition of neutrophilic dermatoses is similar to that of autoinflammatory diseases, which encompass a wide spectrum of conditions that are hallmarked by recurrent episodes of inflammation in the affected organs, in the absence of infection, allergy and high titer of circulating autoantibodies or autoreactive T cells [3]. The prototype of neutrophilic dermatoses is pyoderma gangrenosum, which typically manifests as a skin ulcer with undermined erythematous-violaceous borders, but it may also present with pustular, bullous and vegetating plaque-type lesions [1, 4]. Pyoderma gangrenosum may be isolated or associated with systemic conditions (i.e. inflammatory bowel diseases, rheumatological disorders and lymphoproliferation as well as other blood disorders), or occur in the context of autoinflammatory syndromes such as PAPA (pyogenic arthritis, PG and acne) [5], PASH (PG, acne and suppurative hidradenitis [also known as hidradenitis suppurativa; HS] [4, 6, 7] or other more recently described syndromes such as

A. V. Marzano (✉)
Dipartimento di Fisiopatologia Medico-Chirurgica e dei Trapianti, Università degli Studi di Milano, Unità Operativa di Dermatologia, IRCCS Fondazione Ca' Granda, Ospedale Maggiore Policlinico, Milano, Italy
e-mail: angelo.marzano@unimi.it

M. Cugno
Dipartimento di Fisiopatologia Medico-Chirurgica e dei Trapianti, Università degli Studi di Milano, Medicina Interna, IRCCS Fondazione Ca' Granda, Ospedale Maggiore Policlinico, Milano, Italy
e-mail: massimo.cugno@unimi.it

D. Wallach et al. (eds.), *Neutrophilic Dermatoses*,
https://doi.org/10.1007/978-3-319-72649-6_23

PAPASH (pyogenic arthritis, acne, PG and suppurative hidradenitis) [8]. The classic monogenic autoinflammatory syndromes such as PAPA are due to mutations of single genes regulating the innate immunity [5, 9]; however, there is increasing evidence that mutations in different genes involved in autoinflammation are associated with other neutrophilic dermatoses [7, 8, 10]. Here we review the pathophysiology of neutrophilic dermatoses focusing on the expression of cytokines and other effector molecules involved in autoinflammation as well as on their genetic profile, in order to support the inclusion of pyoderma gangrenosum and the other neutrophilic dermatoses in the spectrum of autoinflammatory diseases. This inclusion may provide the rationale for treatment aimed at blocking the cytokines crucially involved in autoinflammation.

Cytokines and Effector Molecules in Neutrophilic Dermatoses

An increasing body of evidence supports the role of pro-inflammatory cytokines in the pathophysiology of neutrophilic dermatoses. Recent studies have defined the cytokine expression pattern in lesional skin of different neutrophilic dermatoses [11–15]. In particular, a comprehensive immunological investigation on 13 patients with PG and 7 patients with the recently described PG-associated syndrome PASH showed in lesional skin of both PG and PASH a constant inflammatory profile with overexpression of interleukin (IL)-1-beta, IL17, tumor necrosis factor (TNF)-alpha, IL8 and the other chemokines C-X-C motif ligand (CXCL)1,2,3 and CXCL16 [10]. The overexpression of IL-1-beta and its receptor suggests the role of autoinflammation through the activation of inflammasome in PG similarly to the PG-associated syndromes, like the classic monogenic autoinflammatory syndrome PAPA [16]. The inflammasome is a molecular platform activated by infection or stress, which promotes the release of a number of proinflammatory cytokines. Dysfunction or activation of the inflammasome in the absence of infection depends on genetic changes, usually gene mutations as occurring in the syndromes, and can trigger the autoinflammatory cascade, leading to the onset of PG [17].

IL-17 is a pivotal cytokine in regulating the innate immune response, but it is also crucial in autoinflammation recruiting neutrophils, activating them and stimulating their production of IL-8 [17]. IL-8 is the main chemoattractor of neutrophils and acts synergically with TNFα in maintaining the pro-inflammmtory profile. In line with these findings, our group has previously described an imbalance of T- regulatory cells and T helper 17 effector cells in patients with PG, proposing the use of an IL-17 antagonist as a possible treatment in refractory cases of the disease [18].

IL-1 β, IL-17 and TNFα are also elevated in the lesional skin of other neutrophilic dermatoses such as Sweet's syndrome (an acute febrile neutrophilic dermatosis presenting with tender erythematous papules or plaques usually on the upper limbs, face and neck) [13], HS (a rare chronic disease of the follicular unit in areas bearing apocrine sweat glands, such as the axillary, inguinal and anogenital regions manifesting as nodules, abscesses and fistulas) [15, 19, 20] and amicrobial pustulosis of the folds (a rare entity characterized by relapsing pustular lesions mainly in the cutaneous folds including the axillary and inguinal folds as well the anogenital area) [14, 21, 22]. IL-1 β, IL-17 and TNFα increase both production and activation of matrix metalloproteinases, like MMP-2 and MMP-9, responsible for tissue damage. MMP9 is overexpressed in inflammatory infiltrate of PG, whilst MMP-2 is commonly involved in several neutrophilic dermatoses. The overproduction of MMPs is partially balanced by the overproduction of tissue inhibitor metalloproteinases, either way the final result is equally a great inflammatory insult and the consequent destruction of the targeted tissue [12, 13].

Genetics of Neutrophilic Dermatoses

Recently, various mutations have been described in genes encoding signalling molecules, including germline-encoded pattern recognition receptors, which are involved in triggering innate immune responses [23]. In particular, gain-of-function mutations in the nucleotide-binding domain, leucine-rich repeat-containing receptor protein 3 gene (NLRP3) have been recognized as an aetiological factor of cryopyrin-associated periodic syndromes (CAPS), which are characterized by neutrophil-rich urticarial skin lesions. These NLRP3 mutations result in overproduction of the proinflammatory cytokine interleukin (IL)-1beta due to the activation of a cytoplasmic innate immune protein complex called inflammasome [24]. Inflammasomes are cytoplasmic molecular platforms that regulate the processing and activation of the proinflammatory cytokines IL-1-beta and IL-18 [25]. Two signals are needed for the secretion of bioactive IL-1-beta: the first one occurs upon stimulation of Toll-like receptors inducing the expression of IL-1-alpha and IL-1-beta as pro-proteins (pro-IL-1-alpha and pro-IL-1-beta), the second one occurs upon sensing of pathogen-associated molecular patterns and/or damage-associated molecular patterns by receptors such as NLRP3, leading to the subsequent assembly and activation of the inflammasome composed of NLRP3, ASC [apoptosis-associated speck-like protein containing a caspase recruitment domain (CARD)] and caspase-1. As a consequence, activated caspase-1 can cleave pro-IL-1-beta and the proinflammatory cytokine pro-IL-18 to their active forms. IL-1-beta binds to IL-1R1 and IL-1R accessory protein (IL-1RAcP), and IL-18 binds to IL-18R-alpha and IL-18R-beta to initiate effector functions on target cells [25].

In neutrophilic dermatoses, such as PG, Sweet's syndrome and amicrobial pustulosis of the folds, there is increasing evidence on the cytokine expression profile confirming the important autoinflammatory component in their pathogenesis [12–14]. This theory is enriched by the genetic findings on the main genes of classic autoinflammatory monogenic diseases in syndromic PG like PASH [7]. Based on this fact, our group evaluated, not only in PASH but also in isolated PG, ten genes most commonly defective in classic autoinflammatory diseases [10]. The paradigmatic autoinflammatory syndrome presenting with PG, PAPA syndrome, is inherited in an autosomal dominant fashion as result of two main mutations, A230T and E250Q, involving the proline-serine-threonine-phosphatase interactive protein (PSTPIP)-1 gene [5, 26–30]. Mutated PSTPIP-1 leads to decreased inhibition of the inflammasome and consequent activation of caspase-1; this enzyme proteolytically cleaves pro-IL-1-beta into its active isoform, IL-1-beta, with increased production of this cytokine that drives the autoinflammation associated with the PAPA triad [26]. In non syndromic PG, mutations in Janus kinase 2 (JAK2) gene [30, 31] as well as in methylene tetrahydrofolate reductase (MTHFR) [32] have been found, which are associated with hematological disorders. Nesterovitch et al. [33], studying 14 PG patients, found the G258A mutation involving the PSTPIP1 gene in a patient with a history of mild arthralgia and acne, thus suggesting a mild form of PAPA syndrome. Moreover, PG has been described in familial cases in different settings [34–38]. In the recent study of our group, a comprehensive analysis of the main genes involved in autoinflammation has been made, demonstrating that both PG and PASH are associated with mutations in classic autoinflammatory genes [10]. Based on these findings, it is possible to hypothesize that PG and PASH are different phenotypes of a spectrum of autoinflammatory polygenic conditions. In particular, we found a number of mutations in Mediterranean Fever (MEFV), NLRP3, NLRP12, nucleotide-binding oligomerization domain-containing protein 2 (NOD2) and Lipin 2 (LPIN2) in PG and its syndromic form. Mutations of MEFV gene are associated with familial mediterranean fever that can be considered a prototypic example of monogenic autoinflammatory disease with neutrophil dysfunction [39]. Mutations in the NLRP3 and rarely NLRP12 genes are characteristic of the cryopyrin-associated periodic syndrome (CAPS), which is a spectrum of conditions presenting with recurrent episodes of systemic inflammation due to an uncontrolled activation of the innate immunity. The skin involvement in CAPS usually consists of urticaria-like lesions, histologically characterized by neutrophil-rich inflammatory infiltrates [40, 41]. Concerning NOD2 and LPIN2, loss-of-function mutations involving NOD2 gene are regarded as genetic risk factors for Crohn's disease [42, 43], while mutations of both genes, NOD2 and LPIN2, have been described in SAPHO (synovitis, acne, pustulosis, hyperostosis, and osteitis) syndrome, a rare autoinflammatory disorder that mainly affects bone and skin. [44]. Finally, a single mutation of the PSTPIP1 gene was observed in one patient with PASH syndrome [10].

Model of Autoinflammation in Neutrophilic Dermatoses

The term 'autoinflammatory syndrome' was initially introduced after the identification of the genetic causes of the most prevalent monogenic autoinflammatory disease worldwide—the autosomal recessive disease familial Mediterranean fever—and the discovery of TNF receptor mutations in the autosomal dominant disorder, TNF receptor-associated periodic syndrome, in 1999 [45]. Since then, the number of identified autoinflammatory diseases has increased substantially. Several of the mutations associated with autoinflammatory disorders occur in the IL-1-beta pathway [46]. Inflammasomes are involved in the activation of caspase 1, a protease that cleaves the functionally inactive pro-IL-1-beta to its active isoform IL-1-beta

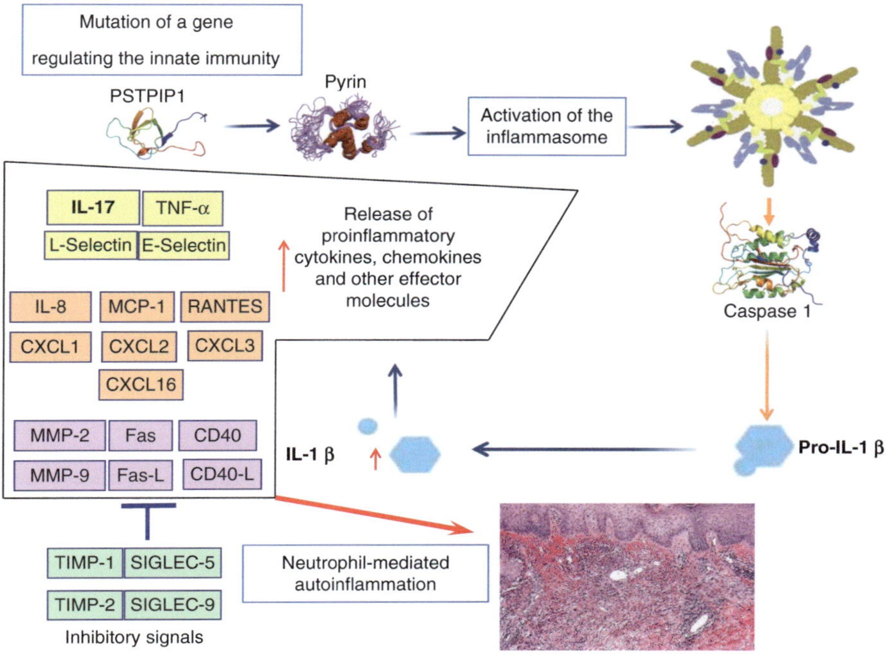

Fig. 23.1 Pathophysiological model of autoinflammation. Mutations of a gene regulating innate immunity such as *PSTPIP1* (proline–serine–threonine phosphatase-interacting protein (1) induce activation of the inflammasome via increased binding affinity to pyrin. This molecular platform is responsible for the activation of caspase-1, an enzyme that proteolytically cleaves pro-IL (prointerleukin)-1-beta to its active isoform IL-1-beta. This pivotal cytokine is thus overproduced, leading to an uncontrolled release of a number of proinflammatory cytokines (particularly IL-17), chemokines and other effector molecules responsible for neutrophil-mediated autoinflammation. Inhibitory signals carried by molecules such as TIMP-1 (tissue inhibitor of metalloproteinase-1), TIMP-2, Siglec-5 (sialic acid-binding immunoglobulin-type lectin-5) and Siglec-9 represent an attempt to dampen inflammation. *CXCL* chemokine (CXC motif) ligand; *E-selectin* endothelial selectin; *L-selectin* leucocyte selectin; *MCP* monocyte chemotactic protein; *MMP* matrix metalloproteinase; *RANTES* regulated on activation, normal T cell expressed and secreted; *TNF* tumour necrosis factor

[47]. The inflammasome activation is triggered by molecules associated with cell damage or pathogen infections, recognized by specific receptors [48]. The overproduction of IL-1-beta triggers the release of a number of proinflammatory cytokines, particularly TNF-alpha, and chemokines such as IL-8, CXCL1,2,3 and CXCL16, which are responsible for the recruitment and activation of neutrophils, leading to a neutrophil-mediated inflammation (Fig. 23.1) [12, 49, 50].

An important contributing role in autoinflammation is played by IL-17, which is also a leading actor in neutrophil recruitment and activation [15].

The pathophysiological model of autoinflammation in neutrophilic dermatoses is summarized in Fig. 23.1 [51].

Conclusions

Neutrophils are essential players in inflammatory responses and are the first line of defense against harmful stimuli. However, dysregulation of neutrophil homeostasis can result in excessive inflammation and subsequent tissue damage. Neutrophilic dermatoses are a spectrum of inflammatory disorders characterized by polymorphic cutaneous lesions resulting from a neutrophil-rich inflammatory infiltrate in the absence of infection. Skin lesions in autoinflammatory diseases also involve neutrophil infiltrates and clinically mimic clinical features of neutrophilic dermatoses. Molecular mechanisms causing autoinflammatory monogenic diseases are also potentially relevant in neutrophilic dermatoses, which may be regarded as a spectrum of polygenic autoinflammatory conditions. Indeed, mutations of PSTPIP1, the gene of PAPA, as well as of a number of other genes involved in classic autoinflammatory diseases are likely to play a role in the pathogenesis of both isolated PG and its syndromic, non-monogenic form PASH. Both inherited autoinflammatory syndromes and neutrophilic dermatoses share the overactivation of the innate immune system leading to increased production of IL-1 family members and sterile neutrophil-rich inflammation groups, giving rise to consider them as "innate immune disorders".

References

1. Ahronowitz I, Harp J, Shinkai K. Etiology and management of pyoderma gangrenosum: a comprehensive review. Am J Clin Dermatol. 2012;13:191–211.
2. Wallach D, Vignon-Pennamen MD. From acute febrile neutrophilic dermatosis to neutrophilic disease: forty years of clinical research. J Am Acad Dermatol. 2006;55:1066–71.
3. Kastner DL, Aksentijevich I, Goldbach-Mansky R. Autoinflammatory disease reloaded: a clinical perspective. Cell. 2010;140:784–90.
4. Marzano AV, Ishak RS, Saibeni S, et al. Autoinflammatory skin disorders in inflammatory bowel diseases, pyoderma gangrenosum and Sweet's syndrome: a comprehensive review and disease classification criteria. Clin Rev Allergy Immunol. 2013;45:202–10.
5. Wise CA, Gillum JD, Seidman CE, Lindor NM, Veile R, Bashiardes S, Lovett M. Mutations in CD2BP1 disrupt binding to PTP PEST and are responsible for PAPA syndrome, an autoinflammatory disorder. Hum Mol Genet. 2002;11(8):961–9.
6. Braun-Falco M, Kovnerystyy O, Lohse P, Ruzicka T. Pyoderma gangrenosum, acne, and suppurative hidradenitis (PASH)—a new autoinflammatory syndrome distinct from PAPA syndrome. J Am Acad Dermatol. 2012;66(3):409–15.
7. Marzano AV, Ceccherini I, Gattorno M, Fanoni D, Caroli F, Rusmini M, Grossi A, De Simone C, Borghi OM, Meroni PL, Crosti C, Cugno M. Association of pyoderma gangrenosum, acne, and suppurative hidradenitis (PASH) shares genetic and cytokine profiles with other autoinflammatory diseases. Medicine. 2014;93(27):e187.
8. Marzano AV, Trevisan V, Gattorno M, Ceccherini I, De Simone C, Crosti C. Pyogenic arthritis, pyoderma gangrenosum, acne, and hidradenitis suppurativa (PAPASH): a new autoinflammatory syndrome associated with a novel mutation of the PSTPIP1 gene. JAMA Dermatol. 2013;149(6):762–4.
9. Smith EJ, Allantaz F, Bennett L, et al. Clinical, molecular, and genetic characteristics of PAPA syndrome: a review. Curr Genomics. 2010;11:519–27.

10. Marzano A, Damiani G, Ceccherini I, Berti E, Gattorno M, Cugno M. Autoinflammation in pyoderma gangrenosum and its syndromic form PASH. Br J Dermatol. 2017;176(6):1588–98. https://doi.org/10.1111/bjd.15226.
11. DeFilippis EM, Feldman SR, Huang WW. The genetics of pyoderma gangrenosum and implications for treatment: a systematic review. Br J Dermatol. 2015;172:1487–97.
12. Marzano AV, Cugno M, Trevisan V, et al. Role of inflammatory cells, cytokines and matrix metalloproteinases in neutrophil-mediated skin diseases. Clin Exp Immunol. 2010;162:100–7.
13. Marzano AV, Fanoni D, Antiga E, et al. Expression of cytokines, chemokines and other effector molecules in two prototypic autoinflammatory skin diseases, pyoderma gangrenosum and Sweet's syndrome. Clin Exp Immunol. 2014;178:48–56.
14. Marzano AV, Tavecchio S, Berti E, Gelmetti C, Cugno M. Cytokine and chemokine profile in amicrobial pustulosis of the folds: evidence for autoinflammation. Medicine. 2015;94:e2301.
15. Lima AL, Karl I, Giner T, et al. Keratinocytes and neutrophils are important sources of proinflammatory molecules in hidradenitis suppurativa. Br J Dermatol. 2016;174:514–21.
16. Shoham NG, Centola M, Mansfield E, Hull KM, Wood G, Wise CA, Kastner DL. Pyrin binds the PSTPIP1/CD2BP1 protein, defining familial Mediterranean fever and PAPA syndrome as disorders in the same pathway. Proc Natl Acad Sci U S A. 2003;100(23):13501–6.
17. Braswell SF, Kostopoulos TC, Ortega-Loayza AG. Pathophysiology of pyoderma gangrenosum (PG): an updated review. J Am Acad Dermatol. 2015;73:691–8.
18. Caproni M, Antiga E, Volpi W, et al. The Treg/Th17 cell ratio is reduced in the skin lesions of patients with pyoderma gangrenosum. Br J Dermatol. 2015;173:275–8.
19. van der Zee HH, de Ruiter L, van den Broecke DG, Dik WA, Laman JD, Prens EP. Elevated levels of tumour necrosis factor (TNF)-α, interleukin (IL)-1β and IL-10 in hidradenitis suppurativa skin: a rationale for targeting TNF-α and IL-1β. Br J Dermatol. 2011;164:1292–8.
20. Mozeika E, Pilmane M, Nürnberg BM, Jemec GB. Tumour necrosis factor-alpha and matrix metalloproteinase-2 are expressed strongly in hidradenitis suppurativa. Acta Derm Venereol. 2013;93:301–4.
21. Amazan E, Ezzedine K, Mossalayi MD, Taieb A, Boniface K, Seneschal J. Expression of interleukin-1 alpha in amicrobial pustulosis of the skin folds with complete response to anakinra. J Am Acad Dermatol. 2014;71:e53–6.
22. Marzano AV, Cugno M, Trevisan V, Lazzari R, Fanoni D, Berti E, Crosti C. Inflammatory cells, cytokines and matrix metalloproteinases in amicrobialpustulosis of the folds and other neutrophilic dermatoses. Int J Immunopathol Pharmacol. 2011;24:451–60.
23. Broderick L, De Nardo D, Franklin BS, et al. The inflammasomes and autoinflammatory syndromes. Annu Rev Pathol. 2015;10:395–424.
24. Hoffman HM, Mueller JL, Broide DH, et al. Mutation of a new gene encoding a putative pyrin-like protein causes familial cold autoinflammatory syndrome and Muckle-Wells syndrome. Nat Genet. 2001;29:301–5.
25. Martinon F, Burns K, Tschopp J. The inflammasome: a molecular platform triggering activation of inflammatory caspases and processing of proIL-b. Mol Cell. 2002;10:417–26.
26. Yeon HB, Lindor NM, Seidman JG, et al. Pyogenic arthritis, pyoderma gangrenosum, and acne syndrome maps to chromosome 15q. Am J Hum Genet. 2000;66:1443–8.
27. Heymann MC, Rosen-Wolff A. Contribution of the inflammasomes to autoinflammatory diseases and recent mouse models as research tools. Clin Immunol. 2013;147:175–84.
28. Wollina U, Tchernev G. Pyoderma gangrenosum: pathogenetic oriented treatment approaches. Wien Med Wochenschr. 2014;164:263–73.
29. Wollina U, Haroske G. Pyoderma gangraenosum. Curr Opin Rheumatol. 2011;23:50–6.
30. Palanivel JA, Macbeth AE, Levell NJ. Pyoderma gangrenosum in association with Janus kinase 2 (JAK2V617F) mutation. Clin Exp Dermatol. 2013;38:44–6.
31. Hideki M, Tetsurou T, Sakae F, et al. Idiopathic myelofibrosis and pyoderma gangrenosum involving a mutation of Janus kinase 2 (JAK2V617F), showing poor prognosis. Eur J Dermatol. 2013;23:256–7.

32. Crittenden SC, Gilbert JE, Callen JP. Hydroxyurea-induced leg ulceration in a patient with a omozygous MTHFR polymorphism misdiagnosed as pyoderma gangrenosum. JAMA Dermatol. 2014;150:780–1.
33. Nesterovitch AB, Hoffman MD, Simon M, et al. Mutations in the PSTPIP1 gene and aberrant splicing variants in patients with pyoderma gangrenosum. Clin Exp Dermatol. 2011;36:889–95.
34. al-Rimawi HS, Abuekteish FM, Daoud AS, Oboosi MM. Familial pyoderma gangrenosum presenting in infancy. Eur J Pediatr. 1996;155:759–62.
35. Alberts JH, Sams HH, Miller JL, King LE Jr. Familial ulcerative pyoderma gangrenosum: a report of 2 kindred. Cutis. 2002;69:427–30.
36. Boussofara L, Gammoudi R, Ghariani N, et al. Familial pyoderma gangrenosum in association with common variable immunodeficiency. Br J Dermatol. 2013;169:944–6.
37. Khandpur S, Mehta S, Reddy BS. Pyoderma gangrenosum in two siblings: a familial predisposition. Pediatr Dermatol. 2001;18:308–12.
38. Shands JW Jr, Flowers FP, Hill HM, Smith JO. Pyoderma gangrenosum in a kindred. Precipitation by surgery or mild physical trauma. J Am Acad Dermatol. 1987;16:931–4.
39. Ozen S, Demirkaya E, Amaryan G, et al. Results from a multicentre international registry of familial Mediterranean fever: impact of environment on the expression of a monogenic disease in children. Ann Rheum Dis. 2014;73:662–7.
40. Borghini S, Tassi S, Chiesa S, et al. Clinical presentation and pathogenesis of cold-induced autoinflammatory disease in a family with recurrence of an NLRP12 mutation. Arthritis Rheum. 2011;63:830–9.
41. Levy R, Gérard L, Kuemmerle-Deschner J, Lachmann HJ. Phenotypic and genotypic characteristics of cryopyrin-associated periodic syndrome: a series of 136 patients from the Eurofever Registry. Ann Rheum Dis. 2015;74:2043–9.
42. Hugot JP, Chamaillard M, Zouali H, et al. Association of NOD2 leucine-rich repeat variants with susceptibility to Crohn's disease. Nature. 2001;411:599–603.
43. Ogura Y, Bonen DK, Inohara N, et al. A frameshift mutation in NOD2 associated with susceptibility to Crohn's disease. Nature. 2001;411:603–6.
44. Hurtado-Nedelec M, Chollet-Martin S, Chapeton D, et al. Genetic susceptibility factors in a cohort of 38 patients with SAPHO syndrome: a study of PSTPIP2, NOD2, and LPIN2 genes. J Rheumatol. 2010;37:401–9.
45. McDermott MF, Aksentijevich I, Galon J, et al. Germline mutations in the extracellular domains of the 55 kDa TNF receptor, TNFR1, define a family of dominantly inherited autoinflammatory syndromes. Cell. 1999;97:133–44.
46. Dinarello CA. Interleukin-1 in the pathogenesis and treatment of inflammatory diseases. Blood. 2011;117:3720–32.
47. Ozkurede VU, Franchi L. Immunology in clinic review series; focus on autoinflammatory diseases: role of inflammasomes in autoinflammatory syndromes. Clin Exp Immunol. 2012;167:382–90.
48. Saïd-Sadier N, Ojcius DM. Alarmins, inflammasomes and immunity. Biomed J. 2012;35:437–49.
49. Dinarello CA. A clinical perspective of IL-1β as the gatekeeper of inflammation. Eur J Immunol. 2011;41:1203–17.
50. Dinarello CA, van der Meer JW. Treating inflammation by blocking interleukin-1 in humans. Semin Immunol. 2013;25:469–84.
51. Marzano AV, Borghi A, Meroni PL, Cugno M. Pyoderma gangrenosum and its syndromic forms: evidence for a link with autoinflammation. Br J Dermatol. 2016;175:882–91.

24 Auto-inflammation and the Skin

Ramtin Lichtenberger, Emmanuel Contassot, Lars E. French, and Alexander A. Navarini

Introduction

Inflammation is a complex response of tissues to harmful influences. These can be trauma, pathogens or irritants [1]. This mechanism is in principle beneficial and aims to remove problematic stimuli from the body, with the goal of restoring tissue homeostasis.

The type of the full inflammatory response, as well as the intensity, are very much dependent on the initial stimulus. The very first steps however are invariably the same, we know them as the innate immune response. Since the classical ages, inflammation was characterized *by rubor, dolor, calor, tumor* and *functio laesa*, translated as the cardinal signs redness, pain, heat, swelling and loss of function of the inflamed tissue [2]. However, inflammation can also become chronic and destructive thus contributing to the pathogenesis of chronic inflammatory diseases [3–5]. Several diseases that we did not expect to be immune mediated were discovered to be dependent on smoldering inflammation, namely type 2 diabetes, Alzheimer's disease, atherosclerosis, and cancer [1, 6].

The skin is our largest organ that covers, together with the hair follicles, at least 100 m^2 [7]. It is our largest surface where we encounter myriads of microbes, pathogens, irritants, toxins and physical great influences. Most of these situations are answered by raising an inflammatory response, which is clearly meant to be a protective local response, even if that goal is not always achieved [8]. In fact, the skin can also be a site of excessive immune responses and immunopathology. This can entail subsequent chronic inflammation, autoimmunity or autoinflammation [9]. During the last 15 years progress was made in understanding the molecular and cellular mechanisms underlying the initiation of an inflammatory response as part of the innate immune response, be it beneficial or undesirable. Among cytokines that

R. Lichtenberger • E. Contassot • L. E. French • A. A. Navarini (✉)
Department of Dermatology, University Hospital Zurich, Zurich, Switzerland
e-mail: Alexander.Navarini@usz.ch

D. Wallach et al. (eds.), *Neutrophilic Dermatoses*,
https://doi.org/10.1007/978-3-319-72649-6_24

have proven essential at the onset of inflammation and during an innate immune response is the proinflammatory cytokine interleukin-1 (IL-1). This cytokine plays a fundamental role in regulating systemic but also certain cutaneous inflammatory responses, and recently acquired knowledge regarding the processing and activation of IL-1 beta (IL-1β) has taught us that it is implicated in the pathogenesis of an emerging family of autoinflammatory diseases and fever syndromes [8, 10].

We describe the key advances in the understanding of biology and pathophysiological role of IL-1 with special focus on its contribution to autoinflammation [3–5] and its function in the skin.

Interleukin-1 (IL-1)

IL-1 is an essential proinflammatory cytokine, which possesses multiple properties and affects almost all cell types [10, 11]. IL-1 mediates the acute phase of inflammation perhaps like no other cytokine, resulting in both local and systemic responses. For example, IL-1 can induce the expression of adhesion molecules on endothelial cells. Once upregulated, the tissue expressing IL-1 is quickly infiltrated by inflammatory and immunocompetent cells [10]. It also induces pain sensitivity, fever, vasodilation and hypotension. The expression of IL-1 and related cytokines can be found on keratinocytes, epithelial cells, monocytes, macrophages, dendritic cells and endothelial cells [8, 10] (Fig. 24.1). IL-1α and IL1β-activities are regulated by the ubiquitous expressed IL-1 receptor type I (IL-1RI). As Dinarello et al. presented, IL-1RI and Toll-like receptors share both the Toll/interleukin-1 receptor domain (TIR) demonstrating a significant role of IL-1 regarding to inflammation and the innate immunity. IL1-F6, a cytokine of the IL-1 family, forms a heterodimer by recruiting the IL-1R accessory protein (IL-1RAcP) and binding to the IL-1R related protein (IL-1Rrp2). The heterodimer activates finally the nuclear factor κB (NF-κB), the C-Jun-N.terminal kinase (JNK) and the p38 mitogen-activated protein kinase (MAPK) pathway [12]. IL-1R type II (IL-1RII) is a decoy receptor, which lacks the TIR domain and cannot signal. This receptor is also released from cells and can thus block the activity of IL-1 also for neighboring cells.

Agonists of IL-1RI are IL-1α and IL-1β, which are transcribed from separate genes. In contrast, binding of IL-1R antagonist (IL-1Ra) to IL-1RI, which prevents binding of IL-1α and IL-1β, does not result in recruitment of IL-1RAcP and consequently leads to blockade of IL-1RI signaling [13]. Recombinant IL-1Ra (anakinra) is used as a therapeutic in humans and has been approved for the treatment of rheumatoid arthritis [14]. During the last years it turned out that anakinra shows clinical efficacy in the treatment of a relatively broad spectrum of inflammatory diseases without causing significant side effects demonstrating the central role IL-1 plays in these conditions [11]. A disadvantage of anakinra is however its short half-life in vivo, which requires daily injection of the drug. This has been overcome by additional inhibitors of IL-1 signaling including a soluble receptor for IL-1 (rilonacept), and a monoclonal antibody to IL-1α (canakinumab).

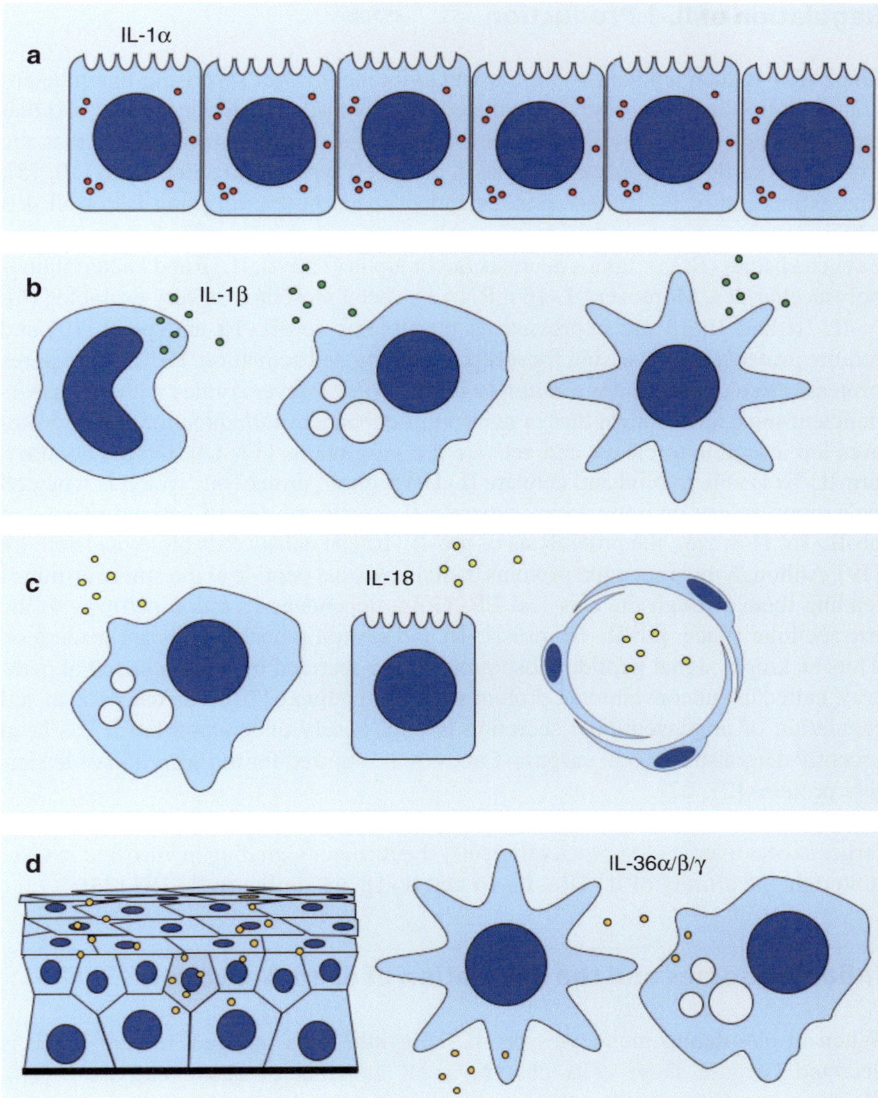

Fig. 24.1 (**a**) IL-1-alpha precursor in all epithelial cells including epidermis and stratum corneum, as well as in the gastrointestinal, lung, liver, kidney, endothelium. It is released upon tissue damage. (**b**) IL-1-beta is actively produced by blood monocytes, tissue macrophages, skin dendritic cells and brain microglia. Triggers are inflammatory factors such as pattern recognition receptor signalling or other cytokines. (**c**) IL-18 is released from macrophages, epithelial cells and endothelial cells. It can be constitutively or inducibly expressed. It is pro-inflammatory, is also known as IFN-y inducing factor and therefore a Th1 inductor. (**d**) IL-36-alpha/beta/gamma is expressed in epithelial cells, dendritic cells, macrophages; triggered by inflammatory stimuli. IL-36 mirrors IL-1. It is pro-inflammatory and induces neutrophils, Th17 and Th1

Regulation of IL-1 Production

Since IL-1 is such a potent and important cytokine it is not surprising that the generation of IL-1 activity is tightly regulated at different levels. Evidence suggests that the expression of IL-1α exists to some extent at a constitutive level, whereas the expression of IL-1β is only detectable in most cell types upon stimulation [10, 15]. The expression of IL-1α and -β is dependent from the transcription factor NF-κB which acts in regulating the immune responses and can be activated by reactive oxygen species (ROS), tumor necrosis factor alpha (TNFα), IL1β and bacterial lipopolysaccharides. Moreover, IL-1β mRNA has been presented as very unstable [16].

IL-1α and IL-1β are expressed as proproteins (proIL-1α and proIL-1β) and require proteolytic processing for receptor binding and activation. ProIL-1β requires proteases like caspase-1 for binding to IL1-RI [6], however studies with caspase-1-deficient mice have shown that in neutrophil-dependent inflammation, other proteases are also able to cleave and activate the proproteins [17, 18]. On the contrary, pro-IL-1α is able to bind and activate IL-1RI without proteolysis which is why cell lysis upon injury or trauma can generate IL-1 activity due to passive release of proIL-1α. However, the proteolysis of pro-IL-1α can enhance its biological activity [19]. Although most secreted proteins contain a signal peptide at the amino terminus leading them through the classical ER-/Golgi-dependent secretion pathway to the extracellular space, pro-IL-1α, pro-IL-1β and several other proteins are leaderless. Thus lacking a signal peptide those proteins are secreted by a non-canonical pathway, called the unconventional protein secretion pathway [20]. The mechanism and regulation of unconventional secretion is only poorly understood but it has been recently demonstrated that caspase-1 activity is required for the secretion of leaderless proteins [21, 22].

As mentioned above IL-1Ra blocks IL-1 activity. However, IL-1Ra needs a much larger excess over IL-1 to block efficiently the receptor signaling in vitro and in vivo, although, the affinity of IL-1Ra, IL-1α and IL-1β are similar to IL-1RI [23].

Inflammasomes and the Regulation of IL-1α Activation

When in circulating monocytes pro-IL-1β synthesis is induced, mature IL-1β is secreted because these cells contain small amounts of active caspase-1 [18]. However, in all other cell types caspase-1 is inactive in the absence of activation signals since this protease is synthesized as an inactive proenzyme. Activation of the protease takes place in recently identified innate immune complexes called inflammasomes [6]. The NLRP1 (nucleotide-binding domain, leucine-rich repeat-containing receptor protein, also called NALP1) inflammasome was identified in 2002 in a cell-free system of the myeloid cell line THP1 [24]. NLRP1 is the large backbone protein of the complex, which binds upon assembly of the inflammasome complex to caspase-5 and to ASC (apoptosis-associated speck-like protein containing a caspase recruitment domain (CARD)). The latter interacts with caspase-1, which brings both proteases into close proximity resulting in their activation [24].

NLRP3, NLRP6 and AIM2 (absent in melanoma 2) can also bind caspase-1 via binding to the adaptor protein ASC, whereas NLRC4 (Nod-like receptor family CARD domain-containing proteins) interacts directly with caspase-1 [25]. Assembly of these complexes results in oligomerization and subsequent activation of caspase-1. As a consequence, active caspase-1 cleaves and activates proIL-1β, but also the proinflammatory cytokine proIL-18 (Fig. 24.1).

The assembly and activation of caspase-1 is regulated by inflammasomes in response to selected proinflammatory stimuli. This includes pathogen-associated molecular patterns (PAMPs) like LPS and endogenous damage-associated molecular patterns (DAMPs) like ATP. Four types of inflammasome complexes have been identified to be activated through interaction with distinct types of DAMPs and/or PAMPs. These are the Aim2, NLRP1, NLRP3 and NLRC4 inflammasomes. The Aim2 inflammasome is activated by binding to viral and bacterial double-stranded DNA resulting from intracellular pathogens, the NLRP1 inflammasome by muramyl dipeptide, and the NLRC4 inflammasome by flagellin [25]. NLRP3, as one of the most important inflammasomes, assembles in response to a large variety of PAMPs and DAMPs, and its deficiency is identified to be associated with immunological dysfunction in mice and disease states in men. Since a direct interaction of any of these activators with NLRP3 could not be shown, indirect activation mechanisms have been suggested. Particulates such as asbestos or crystals such as gout-causing monosodium urate (MSU) or cholesterol are phagocytosed by macrophages [26, 27]. However, their clearance is not efficient and this results in lysosomal rupture, which, in turn, activates the NLRP3 inflammasome by an unknown mechanism perhaps involving cathepsins [27, 28]. As all NLRP3 activators induce the generation of reactive oxygen species (ROS), it has been reported that this ROS production triggers NLRP inflammasome activation [28]. In exchange, ROS induces the dissociation of thioredoxin from thioredoxin-interacting protein which is then able to bind NLRP3 inducing the inflammasome activation [29]. Mitochondria represent the main source of ROS generated by dangers signals and also regulates the inflammasome activation through the release of mitochondrial DNA [30, 31].

Next to IL-1β and of IL-18-secretion, Inflammasome-dependent activation of caspase-1 also triggers a lytic form of cell death called pyroptosis [32–34]. In pyroptotic cells caspase-1-dependent DNA fragmentation occurs, however, this does not require classical apoptotic caspases. Pyroptosis is characterized by osmotic swelling of the cell, which results in rupture of the plasma membrane. Due to the rupture, proinflammatory cytokines induce a strong inflammatory reaction by release of proIL-1α, other proinflammatory molecules and through spreading of ATP [35]. In contrast, apoptosis is immunologically silent.

The Skin

At the body's surface the skin prevents the loss of essential body fluids and invasion of microbes and irritants. Its outer layer is the epidermis, which consists mainly of keratinocytes and contains few Langerhans cells, a specialized form of DCs (dendritic cells), and some pigment-producing melanocytes [8, 9]. Keratinocytes express several types of keratins. These proteins which are expressed only in epithelia, form intermediate filaments through assembly into bundles and generate the toughness of the epidermis [36]. The underlying dermis contains several types of immune cells like macrophages, T cells and mast cells. They are embedded in connective tissue, which is made up by a mixture of extracellular matrix proteins produced by fibroblasts. The supply of nutrients of the whole skin is guaranteed by blood vessels in the dermis, the latter also containing lymphatic vessels and nerve endings. In contrast to the dermis, the epidermis is a constantly renewing tissue. Proliferation of keratinocytes is restricted to the basal cell layer, where stem cells and transit amplifying cells are located. During an apoptosis-like process of terminal differentiation, keratinocytes change their expression profile and properties and migrate to the outer surface of the epidermis. This generates several densely-packed layers of keratinocytes with dead, flat and keratin-filled corneocytes at the surface, which form a protective envelope.

Under homeostatic conditions, the skin is colonized by a certain number and diversity of microorganisms on its surface. The dynamic equilibrium between the epidermis and microorganisms is regulated amongst others by sebocytes, which are located in sebaceous glands within the dermis and produce anti-microbial lipids, as well as by the microbes themselves, which produce antibiotic and antifungal substances as well as bacteriolytic enzymes. Moreover, in case of injury or infection, keratinocytes can trigger TLRs through PAMPs and DAMPs leading to the release of antimicrobial substances [37]. Certain keratinocyte-derived antimicrobial peptides as well as cytokines can influence the immunological properties of dendritic cells and T cells, which are also influenced by the stimulation of their own TLRs and can activate adaptive immunity [8, 9]. Hereby, the skin must ensure an efficient defense against pathogens and immunosurveillance, but also minimize an excessive immune response leading otherwise to disease states such as allergy, chronic inflammation and autoimmunity.

IL-1 and Inflammasomes in Keratinocytes

Human primary keratinocytes constitutively express inflammasome proteins as proIL-1α, proIL-1β, and IL-1Ra, contrary to macrophages and DCs [38, 39]. The amount of secreted proIL-1α as well as mature and active IL-1β has been shown by irradiation with a physiological dose of UVB similar to the activated macrophages [38]. This secretion requires expression of NLRP1, NLRP3, ASC, caspase-4 and caspase-1 as well as caspase-1 and -4 activity [40]. The assembly of the inflammasome is dependent on an increase of the concentration of cytoplasmic Ca^{2+}. Most importantly, caspase-1 expression is also required in vivo in mice for the induction of an inflammatory response upon UVB irradiation [38]. This highlights the dependency of keratinocytes to inflammasome and IL-1 for the induction of sunburn and the innate immune responses.

Contact hypersensitivity (CH) is a frequent inflammatory skin disease also called eczema which can be studied in established mouse models of allergic contact dermatitis, and is based on an adaptive immune response to haptens [39]. In the first phase, application of haptens to the skin primes T cells. A second hapten stimulus induces a local inflammatory response. This inflammation is most likely dependent on the migration of Langerhans cells to lymph nodes, subsequent antigen presentation and recruitment of expanded T cells to the site of hapten application [9, 41]. Recent evidence provided by our group and others has now shown that the earliest phase of sensitization in CH critically depends on IL-1, ASC and NLRP3 expression and can be inhibited by administration of IL-1Ra [39, 42–44]. IL-1 and the inflammasome are involved in sensing contact sensitizers in the skin and triggering an innate immune response to these, which subsequently also very likely plays a role in helping trigger the adaptive immune response to contact sensitizers in the skin.

Keratinocytes express the inflammasome component Aim2 in vitro and in vivo, a molecule which is important for sensing intracellular double stranded DNA. Accordingly, transfection of keratinocytes with double-stranded DNA in vitro induces secretion of mature IL-1β in an Aim2- and caspase-1-dependent manner [45, 46]. Whether Aim2 expression is increased in skin biopsies of patients suffering from psoriasis, a chronic inflammatory skin disease is controversially discussed. Interestingly, cytosolic DNA was detected in keratinocytes of psoriatic lesions in contrast to healthy skin suggesting that cytosolic DNA may act as a DAMP in psoriasis via activation of the Aim2 inflammasome [45]. The antimicrobial peptide LL-37, which can interact with DNA and induce interferon alpha production by plasmacytoid dendritic cells in psoriatic skin, can also block activation of the Aim2 inflammasome by binding to and neutralizing cytosolic DNA. These data suggest that the generation of IL-1 activity by the Aim2 inflammasome in keratinocytes may contribute to the pathogenesis of psoriasis.

Recent studies with NLRP3 gene mutated mice causing CAPS (cryopyrin-associated periodic syndromes) indicates the consequences of dysregulated control of inflammasome activation for the skin and inflammatory disease. These mice that have a hyperactive inflammasome spontaneously develop a neutrophil rich inflammation of the skin with a Th_{17} dominant immune response [47]. Interestingly, a redundant feature of inflammasome activation and IL-1α release in tissues thus appears to be the neutrophilic nature of the inflammatory infiltrates at sites of tissue inflammation. This feature is also observed in several human autoinflammatory diseases.

Autoinflammatory Diseases with Skin Involvement

Autoinflammatory diseases differ from allergic and autoimmune diseases by seemingly unprovoked recurrent inflammation in the absence of evidence for circulated auto-antibodies or antigen-specific T cell response [48]. Recently it has been shown that several mutations in proteins of the inflammasome complex or proteins that regulate the function of the inflammasome are associated with autoinflammatory disease, including the cryopyrin-associated periodic syndromes such as Muckle-Wells syndrome, but also other diseases such as Schnitzler's syndrome and Behçet's disease in which IL-1 also appears to play a critical role.

Cryopyrin-Associated Periodic Syndromes

Cryopyrin-Associated Periodic Syndromes (CAPS, OMIM/606416) belong to a group of rare inherited inflammatory disorders. These syndromes appear by different autosomal dominant mutations in the cryopyrin-coding gene NLRP3 (nucleotide-binding domain, leucine-rich repeat containing gene family, pyrin domain containing protein 3) on chromosome 1q44 which is also known as CIAS1, PYPAF1 or NALP3. Currently, more than 90 mutations associated with CAPS have been reported. CAPS activates caspase-1 and leads to subsequent abnormal IL-1α secretion. CAPS contains a spectrum of hereditary periodic fever syndromes including familial cold autoinflammatory syndrome (FCAS; OMIM/120100), Muckle-Wells Syndrome (MWS; OMIM/191900), and chronic infantile neurological cutaneous and articular syndrome (CINCA; OMIM/607115). The latter is also known as neonatal-onset multisystem inflammatory disease (NOMID). Characteristic symptoms are described as clinically periodic fever and urticaria-like skin lesions are the characteristic symptoms. Dependent to severity, they can be associated with one or several following symptoms: arthritis, conjunctivitis, amyloidosis, sensorineural hearing loss, aseptic meningitis and/or cerebral atrophy.

A very good therapeutic efficacy has been shown with Interleukin-1 blockade leading to rapid resolution of clinical symptoms and complete remission of inflammatory markers like CRP. The recombinant IL-1 receptor antagonist anakinra is the current medication for CAPS, although canakinumab and rilonacept can be also considered as effective alternative IL-1 inhibitors. Canakinumab is a recombinant, fully human, monoclonal, anti-IL-1β antibody whereas rilonacept obtains, as a dimeric fusion protein, the extracellular domains of IL-1R1 and IL-1RAP with a combined Fc domain of human IgG1 [49, 50].

Familial Cold Autoinflammatory Syndrome

FCAS is the mildest form of CAPS and typically starts in the first year of life. FCAS presents with recurrent attacks of a maculopapular, painful, non-pruritic urticarial exanthema accompanied by fever, chills, joint stiffness, conjunctivitis, and headache after exposure to cold [51]. The urticarial rash begins 1–3 h after cold stimulus, peaks at 2–6 h and is accompanied by sweating. The intensity of the urticarial exanthema in FCAS is comparable to common urticaria. Furthermore, the seemingly unprovoked sterile inflammation can also result in neurosensory deafness, intellectual impairment and meningitis [52]. An amyloidosis can be found in fewer than 5% of the cases.

However, unlike in common urticaria, anti-IL-1 therapy—rather than antihistamines—results in a complete remission of symptoms in patients suffering from FCAS as long as the treatment is given.

Muckle-Wells Syndrome

Muckle-Wells syndrome (MWS), also known as urticaria-deafness-amyloidosis syndrome, has an intermediate severity among CAPS and was first reported in 1962. MWS is a hereditary disease related to FCAS with recurrent episodes of urticaria-like skin lesions appearing without cold exposure [53]. MWS is also associated with late-onset neurosensory deafness and renal amyloidosis occurring in 25% of patients.

Chronic Infantile Neurological Cutaneous and Articular Syndrome

CINCA was first described in 1981 and is the most severe form of CAPS. It occurs sporadically without a family history and typically starts during the neonatal period. Symptoms of CINCA include high fever, maculopapular or urticaria-like, non-pruritic migratory exanthemas, arthropathy, lymphadenopathy, hepatosplenomegaly and chronic meningitis. CINCA is also associated to a progressive loss of vision and neurosensory deafness, mental and growth retardation. The mortality of CINCA patients is reported by 20% within the first two decades.

About 50–60% of examined patients harbor de novo mutations in NLRP3 [54, 55]. Long-term efficacy of anakinra treatment of patients suffering from CINCA has been reported [56].

Other Autoinflammatory Diseases and the Overlap with Neutrophilic Diseases

Deficiency of Interleukin-1 Receptor Antagonist

The recently reported deficiency of interleukin-1 receptor antagonist (DIRA; OMIM/147679) is an autosomal recessive mutation in IL1RN on chromosome 2 leading to the absence of IL-1RA and subsequent to an IL-1 overactivity [57, 58]. DIRA manifests itself clinically with perinatal-onset pustular dermatitis, joint swelling, painful osteolytic lesions, and periosteitis. Contrary to CINCA, fever is rare and neurologic inflammation is absent.

Treatment with anakinra—substituting the missing protein in patients with its recombinant form—leads to a rapid clinical improvement [59].

Pyogenic Arthritis-Pyoderma Gangrenosum-Acne Syndrome

Pyogenic arthritis-pyoderma gangrenosum-acne syndrome (OMIM/604416), known as PAPA syndrome is a rare, inherited disorder. The responsible gene mutation has been identified on chromosome 15q24-q25.1. It affects the proline-serine-threonine phosphatase-interactive protein 1 (PSTPIP1) gene, also referred as CD2-binding protein 1 (CD2BP1) [60]. Despite the divergent clinical symptoms, the pathophysiology of PAPA and FMF is related.

Sterile erosive arthritis especially of the knees, elbows and ankles, usually starts in early childhood. During adulthood, severe cystic acne can persist whereas the arthritic symptoms tend to regress compared to the puberty. Pyoderma gangrenosum shows a clinical heterogenous expression and presents itself as a poorly healing ulcer. The ulcers are typically located on the distal limbs, but pyoderma gangrenosum can present as a multifocal fashion on the entire skin. In PAPA syndrome patients, the regulation of caspase-1 activation is lacking and increased production of IL-1α as well as tumor necrosis factor (TNF) in peripheral blood mononuclear cells has been reported [61, 62].

The treatment of PAPA syndrome is dependent from clinical severity. Anakinra has been shown to be effective in the control of inflammatory lesions in PAPA syndrome patients [63, 64]. Infliximab (anti-TNF antibody) has been reported to be successful [65]. Although, arthritis episodes can be successfully treated with corticosteroids, pyoderma gangrenosum often responds poorly. Therefore, treatment with immunosuppressants is usually indicated.

Schnitzler Syndrome

This condition arises invariably in combination with an IgM gammopathy. Adults are affected, and these patients suffer from non-pruritic urticaria-like exanthemas that can also arise together with fever, lymphadenopathy, arthritis or simply joint pain, bone pain, and hepato- and/or splenomegaly [66]. Both the exact etiology and pathogenesis of Schnitzler syndrome remain to be clarified.

Therapies using antihistamines, non-steroidal anti-inflammatory drugs, corticosteroids, immunosuppressive drugs, colchicine, dapsone or thalidomide have shown very limited effects. TNF blockers have been shown to be ineffective. A mutation in NLRP3 has been reported in a single case suggesting a possible implication of the inflammasome in the pathogenesis [67]. Peripheral mononuclear cells produce high amounts of IL-1 in Schnitzler's syndrome. As the efficacy of IL-1 blockade has been proven in this condition, it is highly likely that IL-1α plays a crucial role in this disease [68].

Sweet's Syndrome

Sweet's syndrome was first reported in 1964 as an acute febrile neutrophilic dermatosis [69]. Sweet's syndrome (OMIM/608068) is a neutrophilic skin disease characterized by fever, an elevated neutrophil count, and painful erythematous cutaneous nodules or plaques constituted histologically by a diffuse dense infiltrate of mature neutrophils in the upper dermis. Sweet's syndrome is frequently associated with hematological malignancies or chronic inflammatory disorders such as rheumatoid arthritis and inflammatory bowel disease, but may also occur in the absence of coexisting disease and is to date considered as a hypersensitivity reaction. A possible link with HLA-Bw54 is suspected in patients with Sweet's syndrome, and high levels of the cytokine G-CSF (granulocyte-colony stimulating factor) have been demonstrated in the serum of patients. Furthermore, the report of cases where exogenous G-CSF has triggered the disease, suggests that this cytokine which promotes the production and survival of neutrophils plays a role in the pathogenesis of Sweet's syndrome. Sweet's syndrome does fulfil the current criteria for being classified as an autoinflammatory disease, notably the seemingly unprovoked inflammation in the absence of detectable autoantibodies and evidence of an antigen specific T-cell response.

So far, perhaps because the response is quick and reliable, systemic corticosteroids remain the mainstay for treatment of Sweet's syndrome. Another strategy that may make more sense from the pathogenesis' perspective would be blocking of IL-1.

Behçet's Disease

This condition (BD, OMIM/109650) is defined by bipolar aphthous ulcers (recurrent oral and genital ulcers) as well as uveitis [70]. BD is quite frequent in the Middle East, but considered a rare condition in Western countries. This chronic inflammatory disease can touch many organ systems. Besides the mucocutaneous tissues (oral and genital ulceration, pseudofolliculitis, acne- and erythema nodosum-like skin lesions), it can affect the eyes, the blood vessels, the digestive and/or nervous system. The pathogenesis of BD, which is incompletely understood, is suggested to be of autoimmune etiology, although strong evidence for a causative autoantigen and respective autoantibodies is lacking to date. Triggering of such an immune reaction by certain infectious agents that may inhabit the oral cavity (Streptococcus and Staphylococcus species, herpes simplex virus (HSV) and/or Escherichia coli) has been suggested to play a role in BD [71, 72]. The systemic involvement of multiple organs, which can be observed in BD, is based histopathologically on the development of vasculitic lesions due to tissue infiltration with both T cells and neutrophils. The presence of neutrophils and the fact that BD is characterized by recurrent episodes of inflammation without apparent cause open the possibility that BD may be an autoinflammatory disease. Perhaps not surprisingly, IL-1α gene variants are found in BD cohorts and are thought to increase the risk of BD in the Turkish population [73, 74]. In addition, IL-1 blocking with anakinra has been found to be of excellent utility in several BD patients, which underlines the probably role of IL-1 in this disease [75, 76].

Generalized Pustular Psoriasis, Also Known as Deficiency of IL-36 Receptor Antagonist (DITRA)

Homozygous or compound heterozygous damaging mutations in IL36RN [77, 78] cause this syndrome of generalized pustular rashes and systemic inflammation. IL36RN encodes IL-36Ra, which inhibits binding of IL-36α, -β, and -γ by occupying the IL-36 receptor. This leads to blocking of NF-κB activation further downstream. IL36Ra is highly expressed in keratinocytes that also show enhanced IL36R signaling when a damaging mutation is present. It is presumed that the enhanced signaling directly or indirectly attracts immune cells, especially neutrophils, that give rise to the pustular rashes. Although IL-36 and IL-1 are closely related, antagonism of IL-1 does not seem to be a very effective therapeutic strategy. Recently, autosomal dominant AP1S3 mutations [79] were described with a closely-related phenotype. The pathogenesis remains to be functionally investigated.

Merging Pathways of Auto-inflammation and Neutrophilic Disease

In most auto-inflammatory conditions, the IL-1 pathway is overactivated and can be inhibited for efficient therapy (Table 24.1). Interestingly enough, the cytokine expression pattern in skin biopsies of pyoderma gangrenosum and Sweet's syndrome also show IL-1 overexpression, together with the IL-1 receptor, IL-17 and TNF-α [80, 81]. In the serum of Sweet's syndrome patients, another study has shown that Th1 cytokines including IL-2 and IL-1 β are elevated [82]. Even in amicrobial intertriginous pustulosis, IL-1α was overexpressed and IL-1 receptor antagonists resulted in rapid control of this condition [83]. In a recent case of Sweet's syndrome triggered by azathioprine, we also found IL-1β greatly overexpressed [84]. Further, in an ongoing study on pyoderma gangrenosum, IL-1β was also upregulated both in biopsies as well as in serum [85]. Both Sweet's syndrome and pyoderma gangrenosum can respond quickly to steroids, which may also derive from a direct involvement of the IL-1 pathway. Corticosteroids reduce the production of IL-1α and 1β partially by lowering greatly the stability of their mRNA [86, 87]. Sweet's syndrome has been successfully treated with anakinra, as has pyoderma gangrenosum [88]. The classical disease groups probably contain defined subsets with a more uniform pathogenesis. In 20 children with suspected Sweet syndrome, a subset of three patients were found to suffer of a novel neutrophilic disease with lipodystrophy and elevated temperature which is now recognized as the CANDLE syndrome, an official auto-inflammatory condition. It includes lipodystrophy, periorbital erythema, finger- or toe-swelling, hepatomegaly, fever, failure to thrive and recurrent reddish cutaneous plaques. These patients have a *PSMB8*-mutation that causes a clinical phenotype by mutilating the immunoproteasome [89, 90].

Table 24.1 Autoinflammatory disorders with skin involvement

Disease	Affected tissues	Deficient molecule	IL-1-targeting treatment	Target molecule
CAPS				
FCAS	Skin, joints, eyes	NLRP3	Anakinra Rilonacept Canakinumab	IL-1R1 IL-1 IL-1α
MWS	Skin, joints, eyes, ears, meninges	NLRP3	Anakinra Rilonacept Canakinumab	IL-1R1 IL-1α IL-1α
CINCA	Skin, joints, eyes, ears, meninges and bones	NLRP3	Anakinra Canakinumab	IL-1R1 IL-1α
Other inflammatory disorders				
DIRA	Skin, bones, lungs, blood vessels	IL-1RA	Anakinra	IL-1R1
PAPA syndrome	Skin, joints	PSTPIP1	Anakinra	IL-1R1
Schnitzler syndrome	Skin, joints, bones	?	Anakinra	IL-1R1
Sweet's syndrome	Skin	?	Anakinra	IL-1R1
Behçet's disease	Skin, eyes, mucosa, gastro-intestinal tract, nervous system, blood vessels	IL-1α	Anakinra	IL-1R1
Generalized pustular psoriasis	Skin, mucosa	IL-36α/β/γ	Anakinra	IL1-R1 (not always successful)

Further Considerations on the Neutrophilic Auto-inflammatory Spectrum

Many aspects of diseases within the two groups of ND and AD seem quite compatible when seen as parts of a spectrum (Fig. 24.2). For instance, the focal intensity of granulocyte infiltration varies among ND and AD. Pyoderma gangrenosum is a highly focused, local infiltration of neutrophil granulocytes. Sweet's syndrome or erythema elevatum diutinum are normally multifocal but still consist of well demarcated regions with neutrophil infiltration adjacent to skin which remains uninvolved. Generalized pustular psoriasis, AGEP and subcorneal pustulosis Sneddon-Wilkinson are disseminated but still show microfocal accumulations of neutrophil granulocytes. Lastly, the wheals and fleeting infiltrations of neutrophils that are found in the urticarial rash of CAPS and other auto-inflammatory conditions could be interpreted as diffuse, unfocused neutrophil infiltration.

From a temporal perspective, pyoderma gangrenosum has a very slow dynamic with lesions that persist for a long period of time, whilst already Sweet's syndrome and even more so pustular eruptions are much more dynamic and can occur and regress over a period of days. The most temporally unstable skin lesions however

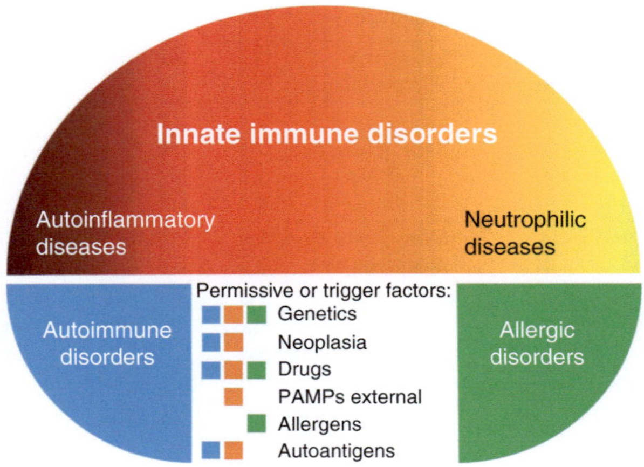

Fig. 24.2 Autoinflammatory disorders are very close to the neutrophilic diseases and could be summed up as innate immune disorders

are clearly CAPS and other auto-inflammatory conditions that can appear and wane within a few hours.

Conclusion

Both auto-inflammatory conditions as well as neutrophilic diseases include long lists of various conditions that partially show overlapping clinical features. Set against auto-immune conditions, both AD and ND find themselves on the same side. We believe that in many ways, neutrophilic and auto-inflammatory diseases are part of a spectrum with often overlapping pathogenesis that could be grouped as *innate immune disorders*. In many instances, auto-inflammation might also represent a predisposing state that allows to then develop additional neutrophilic diseases. However, these pathogenetic connections are difficult to investigate. As studies investigating rare and damaging genetic variants in both groups of conditions continue to yield more answers and information of relevance to pathogenesis, we expect that many of these connections will become clear in the future. As the field is evolving, we believe it may be more rigorous to refer to an open group of *innate immune disorders* as the counterpart of autoimmune disorders, rather than to create small subclassifications that rapidly reach their limits.

References

1. Medzhitov R. Origin and physiological roles of inflammation. Nature. 2008;454:428–35.
2. May S, Lees P, Higgins A, Sedgwick A. Inflammation: a clinical perspective. The Ciba-Geigy Prize for Research in Animal Health. Vet Rec. 1987;120:514–7.
3. Fenini G, Contassot E, French LE. Potential of IL-1, IL-18 and inflammasome inhibition for the treatment of inflammatory skin diseases. Front Pharmacol. 2017;8:278.
4. Beer HD, Contassot E, French LE. The inflammasomes in autoinflammatory diseases with skin involvement. J Invest Dermatol. 2014;134:1805–10.
5. Contassot E, Beer HD, French LE. Interleukin-1, inflammasomes, autoinflammation and the skin. Swiss Med Wkly. 2012;142:w13590.

6. Martinon F, Mayor A, Tschopp J. The inflammasomes: guardians of the body. Annu Rev Immunol. 2009;27:229–65.
7. Gallo RL. Human skin is the largest epithelial surface for interaction with microbes. J Invest Dermatol. 2017;137:1213–4.
8. Feldmeyer L, Werner S, French LE, Beer H-D. Interleukin-1, inflammasomes and the skin. Eur J Cell Biol. 2010;89:638–44.
9. Nestle FO, Di Meglio P, Qin JZ, Nickoloff BJ. Skin immune sentinels in health and disease. Nat Rev Immunol. 2009;9:679–91.
10. Dinarello CA. Immunological and inflammatory functions of the interleukin-1 family. Annu Rev Immunol. 2009;27:519–50.
11. Dinarello CA. Interleukin-1 in the pathogenesis and treatment of inflammatory diseases. Blood. 2011;117:3720–32.
12. Weber A, Wasiliew P, Kracht M. Interleukin-1 (IL-1) pathway. Sci Signal. 2010;3:cm1.
13. Dinarello CA. Interleukin-1, interleukin-1 receptors and interleukin-1 receptor antagonist. Int Rev Immunol. 1998;16:457–99.
14. Dinarello C. Therapeutic strategies to reduce IL-1 activity in treating local and systemic inflammation. Curr Opin Pharmacol. 2004;4:378–85.
15. Hacham M, Argov S, White RM, Segal S, Apte RN. Distinct patterns of IL-1α; and IL-1β; organ distribution—a possible basis for organ mechanisms of innate immunity. In: Keisari Y, Ofek I, editors. The biology and pathology of innate immunity mechanisms. Advances in experimental medicine and biology. Boston: Springer; 2002. p. 185–202.
16. Schindler R, Lonnemann G, Shaldon S, Koch K-M, Dinarello CA. Transcription, not synthesis, of interleukin-1 and tumor necrosis factor by complement. Kidney Int. 1990;37:85–93.
17. Guma M, Ronacher L, Liu-Bryan R, Takai S, Karin M, Corr M. Caspase 1-independent activation of interleukin-1beta in neutrophil-predominant inflammation. Arthritis Rheum. 2009;60:3642–50.
18. Joosten LAB, Netea MG, Fantuzzi G, et al. Inflammatory arthritis in caspase-1 gene-deficient mice: contribution of proteinase 3 to caspase 1-independent production of bioactive interleukin-1beta. Arthritis Rheum. 2009;60:3651–62.
19. Afonina Inna S, Tynan Graham A, Logue Susan E, et al. Granzyme B-dependent proteolysis acts as a switch to enhance the proinflammatory activity of IL-1α. Mol Cell. 2011;44:265–78.
20. Nickel W. The mystery of nonclassical protein secretion. Eur J Biochem. 2003;270:2109–19.
21. Keller M, Rüegg A, Werner S, Beer H-D. Active caspase-1 is a regulator of unconventional protein secretion. Cell. 2008;132:818–31.
22. Nickel W, Rabouille C. Mechanisms of regulated unconventional protein secretion. Nat Rev Mol Cell Biol. 2008;10:148–55.
23. Gabay C, Lamacchia C, Palmer G. IL-1 pathways in inflammation and human diseases. Nat Rev Rheumatol. 2010;6:232–41.
24. Martinon F, Burns K, Tschopp J. The inflammasome. Mol Cell. 2002;10:417–26.
25. Strowig T, Henao-Mejia J, Elinav E, Flavell R. Inflammasomes in health and disease. Nature. 2012;481:278–86.
26. Duewell P, Kono H, Rayner KJ, et al. NLRP3 inflammasomes are required for atherogenesis and activated by cholesterol crystals. Nature. 2010;464:1357–61.
27. Hornung V, Latz E. Critical functions of priming and lysosomal damage for NLRP3 activation. Eur J Immunol. 2010;40:620–3.
28. Tschopp J, Schroder K. NLRP3 inflammasome activation: the convergence of multiple signalling pathways on ROS production? Nat Rev Immunol. 2010;10:210–5.
29. Zhou Q, Lee G-S, Brady J, et al. A hypermorphic missense mutation in PLCG2, encoding phospholipase Cγ2, causes a dominantly inherited autoinflammatory sisease with immunodeficiency. Am J Hum Genet. 2012;91:713–20.
30. Nakahira K, Haspel JA, Rathinam VA, et al. Autophagy proteins regulate innate immune responses by inhibiting the release of mitochondrial DNA mediated by the NALP3 inflammasome. Nat Immunol. 2011;12:222–30.

31. Shimada K, Crother TR, Karlin J, et al. Oxidized mitochondrial DNA activates the NLRP3 inflammasome during apoptosis. Immunity. 2012;36(3):401–14.
32. Bergsbaken T, Fink SL, Cookson BT. Pyroptosis: host cell death and inflammation. Nat Rev Microbiol. 2009;7:99–109.
33. Ting JP, Willingham SB, Bergstralh DT. NLRs at the intersection of cell death and immunity. Nat Rev Immunol. 2008;8:372–9.
34. Yeretssian G, Labbe K, Saleh M. Molecular regulation of inflammation and cell death. Cytokine. 2008;43:380–90.
35. Miao EA, Leaf IA, Treuting PM, et al. Caspase-1-induced pyroptosis is an innate immune effector mechanism against intracellular bacteria. Nat Immunol. 2010;11:1136–42.
36. Fuchs E, Raghavan S. Getting under the skin of epidermal morphogenesis. Nat Rev Genet. 2002;3:199–209.
37. Glaser R, Harder J, Lange H, Bartels J, Christophers E, Schroder JM. Antimicrobial psoriasin (S100A7) protects human skin from Escherichia coli infection. Nat Immunol. 2005;6:57–64.
38. Feldmeyer L, Keller M, Niklaus G, Hohl D, Werner S, Beer H-D. The inflammasome mediates UVB-induced activation and secretion of interleukin-1β by keratinocytes. Curr Biol. 2007;17:1140–5.
39. Watanabe H, Gaide O, Petrilli V, et al. Activation of the IL-1beta-processing inflammasome is involved in contact hypersensitivity. J Invest Dermatol. 2007;127:1956–63.
40. Sollberger G, Strittmatter GE, Kistowska M, French LE, Beer HD. Caspase-4 is required for activation of inflammasomes. J Immunol. 2012;188:1992–2000.
41. O'Leary JG, Goodarzi M, Drayton DL, von Andrian UH. T cell– and B cell–independent adaptive immunity mediated by natural killer cells. Nat Immunol. 2006;7:507–16.
42. Kondo S, Pastore S, Fujisawa H, et al. Interleukin-1 receptor antagonist suppresses contact hypersensitivity. J Invest Dermatol. 1995;105:334–8.
43. Shornick LP. Mice deficient in IL-1beta manifest impaired contact hypersensitivity to trinitrochlorobenzone. J Exp Med. 1996;183:1427–36.
44. Sutterwala FS, Ogura Y, Szczepanik M, et al. Critical role for NALP3/CIAS1/cryopyrin in innate and adaptive immunity through its regulation of caspase-1. Immunity. 2006;24:317–27.
45. Dombrowski Y, Peric M, Koglin S, et al. Cytosolic DNA triggers inflammasome activation in keratinocytes in psoriatic lesions. Sci Transl Med. 2011;3:82ra38.
46. Kopfnagel V, Wittmann M, Werfel T. Human keratinocytes express AIM2 and respond to dsDNA with IL-1β secretion. Exp Dermatol. 2011;20:1027–9.
47. Meng G, Zhang F, Fuss I, Kitani A, Strober WA. Mutation in the Nlrp3 gene causing inflammasome hyperactivation potentiates Th17 cell-dominant immune responses. Immunity. 2009;30:860–74.
48. Masters SL, Simon A, Aksentijevich I, Kastner DL. Horror autoinflammaticus: the molecular pathophysiology of autoinflammatory disease (*). Annu Rev Immunol. 2009;27:621–68.
49. Hoffman HM, Throne ML, Amar NJ, et al. Efficacy and safety of rilonacept (interleukin-1 trap) in patients with cryopyrin-associated periodic syndromes: Results from two sequential placebo-controlled studies. Arthritis Rheum. 2008;58:2443–52.
50. Kuemmerle-Deschner JB, Hachulla E, Cartwright R, et al. Two-year results from an open-label, multicentre, phase III study evaluating the safety and efficacy of canakinumab in patients with cryopyrin-associated periodic syndrome across different severity phenotypes. Ann Rheum Dis. 2011;70:2095–102.
51. Glaser RL, Goldbach-Mansky R. The spectrum of monogenic autoinflammatory syndromes: understanding disease mechanisms and use of targeted therapies. Curr Allergy Asthma Rep. 2008;8:288–98.
52. Goldbach-Mansky R, Dailey NJ, Canna SW, et al. Neonatal-onset multisystem inflammatory disease responsive to interleukin-1β inhibition. N Engl J Med. 2006;355:581–92.
53. Hawkins PN, Lachmann HJ, Aganna E, McDermott MF. Spectrum of clinical features in Muckle-Wells syndrome and response to anakinra. Arthritis Rheum. 2004;50:607–12.

54. Agostini L, Martinon F, Burns K, McDermott MF, Hawkins PN, Tschopp J. NALP3 forms an IL-1β-processing inflammasome with increased activity in Muckle-Wells autoinflammatory disorder. Immunity. 2004;20:319–25.
55. Aksentijevich I, Nowak M, Mallah M, et al. De novo CIAS1 mutations, cytokine activation, and evidence for genetic heterogeneity in patients with neonatal-onset multisystem inflammatory disease (NOMID): a new member of the expanding family of pyrin-associated autoinflammatory diseases. Arthritis Rheum. 2002;46:3340–8.
56. Neven B, Marvillet I, Terrada C, et al. Long-term efficacy of the interleukin-1 receptor antagonist anakinra in ten patients with neonatal-onset multisystem inflammatory disease/chronic infantile neurologic, cutaneous, articular syndrome. Arthritis Rheum. 2010;62:258–67.
57. Aksentijevich I, Masters SL, Ferguson PJ, et al. An autoinflammatory disease with deficiency of the interleukin-1-receptor antagonist. N Engl J Med. 2009;360:2426–37.
58. Reddy S, Jia S, Geoffrey R, et al. An autoinflammatory disease due to homozygous deletion of the IL1RN locus. N Engl J Med. 2009;360:2438–44.
59. Schnellbacher C, Ciocca G, Menendez R, et al. Deficiency of interleukin-1 receptor antagonist responsive to anakinra. Pediatr Dermatol. 2012;30:758–60.
60. Nesterovitch AB, Gyorfy Z, Hoffman MD, et al. Alteration in the gene encoding protein tyrosine phosphatase nonreceptor type 6 (PTPN6/SHP1) may contribute to neutrophilic dermatoses. Am J Pathol. 2011;178:1434–41.
61. Cortis E, De Benedetti F, Insalaco A, et al. Abnormal production of the tumor necrosis factor inhibitor etanercept and clinical efficacy of tumor in a patient with PAPA syndrome. J Pediatr. 2004;145:851–5.
62. Shoham NG, Centola M, Mansfield E, et al. Pyrin binds the PSTPIP1/CD2BP1 protein, defining familial Mediterranean fever and PAPA syndrome as disorders in the same pathway. Proc Natl Acad Sci U S A. 2003;100:13501–6.
63. Brenner M, Molin S, Ruebsam K, Weisenseel P, Ruzicka T, Prinz JC. Generalized pustular psoriasis induced by systemic glucocorticosteroids: four cases and recommendations for treatment. Br J Dermatol. 2009;161:964–6.
64. Dierselhuis MP. Anakinra for flares of pyogenic arthritis in PAPA syndrome. Rheumatology. 2005;44:406–8.
65. Stichweh DS, Punaro M, Pascual V. Dramatic improvement of pyoderma gangrenosum with infliximab in a patient with PAPA syndrome. Pediatr Dermatol. 2005;22:262–5.
66. Asahina A, Sakurai N, Suzuki Y, Narushima K. Schnitzler's syndrome with prominent neutrophil infiltration misdiagnosed as Sweet's syndrome: a typical example of urticarial neutrophilic dermatosis. Clin Exp Dermatol. 2010;35:e123–e6.
67. Loock J, Lamprecht P, Timmann C, Mrowietz U, Csernok E, Gross WL. Genetic predisposition (NLRP3 V198M mutation) for IL-1–mediated inflammation in a patient with Schnitzler syndrome. J Allergy Clin Immunol. 2010;125:500–2.
68. de Koning HD, Schalkwijk J, van der Meer JW, Simon A. Successful canakinumab treatment identifies IL-1beta as a pivotal mediator in Schnitzler syndrome. J Allergy Clin Immunol. 2011;128:1352–4.
69. Sweet RD. An acute febrile neutrophilic dermatosis. Br J Dermatol. 1964;76:349–56.
70. Mendes D, Correia M, Barbedo M, et al. Behcet's disease—a contemporary review. J Autoimmun. 2009;32:178–88.
71. Direskeneli H. Behcet's disease: infectious aetiology, new autoantigens, and HLA-B51. Ann Rheum Dis. 2001;60:996–1002.
72. Lehner T. The role of heat shock protein, microbial and autoimmune agents in the aetiology of Behget's disease. Int Rev Immunol. 1997;14:21–32.
73. Coskun M, Bacanli A, Sallakci N, Alpsoy E, Yavuzer U, Yegin O. Specific interleukin-1 gene polymorphisms in Turkish patients with Behcet's disease. Exp Dermatol. 2005;14:124–9.
74. Ozcimen AA, Dilek K, Bingol U, et al. IL-1 cluster gene polymorphisms in Turkish patients with Behcet's disease. Int J Immunogenet. 2011;38:295–301.
75. Bilginer Y, Ayaz NA, Ozen S. Anti-IL-1 treatment for secondary amyloidosis in an adolescent with FMF and Behcet's disease. Clin Rheumatol. 2010;29:209–10.

76. Botsios C, Sfriso P, Furlan A, Punzi L, Dinarello CA. Resistant Behçet disease responsive to anakinra. Ann Intern Med. 2008;149:284.
77. Onoufriadis A, Simpson MA, Pink AE, et al. Mutations in IL36RN/IL1F5 are associated with the severe episodic inflammatory skin disease known as generalized pustular psoriasis. Am J Hum Genet. 2011;89:432–7.
78. Marrakchi S, Guigue P, Renshaw BR, et al. Interleukin-36–receptor antagonist deficiency and generalized pustular psoriasis. N Engl J Med. 2011;365:620–8.
79. Setta-Kaffetzi N, Simpson Michael A, Navarini Alexander A, et al. AP1S3 mutations are associated with pustular psoriasis and impaired toll-like receptor 3 trafficking. Am J Hum Genet. 2014;94:790–7.
80. Marzano AV, Cugno M, Trevisan V, et al. Role of inflammatory cells, cytokines and matrix metalloproteinases in neutrophil-mediated skin diseases. Clin Exp Immunol. 2010;162:100–7.
81. Marzano AV, Fanoni D, Antiga E, et al. Expression of cytokines, chemokines and other effector molecules in two prototypic autoinflammatory skin diseases, pyoderma gangrenosum and Sweet's syndrome. Clin Exp Immunol. 2014;178:48–56.
82. Giasuddin AS, El-Orfi AH, Ziu MM, El-Barnawi NY. Sweet's syndrome: is the pathogenesis mediated by helper T cell type 1 cytokines? J Am Acad Dermatol. 1998;39:940–3.
83. Amazan E, Ezzedine K, Mossalayi MD, Taieb A, Boniface K, Seneschal J. Expression of interleukin-1 alpha in amicrobial pustulosis of the skin folds with complete response to anakinra. J Am Acad Dermatol. 2014;71:e53–6.
84. Imhof L, Meier B, Frei P, et al. Severe Sweet's syndrome with elevated cutaneous interleukin-1beta after azathioprine exposure: case report and review of the literature. Dermatology. 2015;230:293–8.
85. Kolios AG, Maul JT, Meier B, et al. Canakinumab in adults with steroid-refractory pyoderma gangrenosum. Br J Dermatol. 2015;173:1216–23.
86. Amano Y, Lee SW, Allison AC. Inhibition by glucocorticoids of the formation of interleukin-1 alpha, interleukin-1 beta, and interleukin-6: mediation by decreased mRNA stability. Mol Pharmacol. 1993;43:176–82.
87. Lundberg I, Kratz AK, Alexanderson H, Patarroyo M. Decreased expression of interleukin-1alpha, interleukin-1beta, and cell adhesion molecules in muscle tissue following corticosteroid treatment in patients with polymyositis and dermatomyositis. Arthritis Rheum. 2000;43:336–48.
88. Acquitter M, Plantin P, Kupfer I, Auvinet H, Marhadour T. Anakinra improves pyoderma gangrenosum in psoriatic arthritis: a case report. Ann Intern Med. 2015;163:70–1.
89. Torrelo A, Patel S, Colmenero I, et al. Chronic atypical neutrophilic dermatosis with lipodystrophy and elevated temperature (CANDLE) syndrome. J Am Acad Dermatol. 2010;62:489–95.
90. Liu Y, Ramot Y, Torrelo A, et al. Mutations in proteasome subunit beta type 8 cause chronic atypical neutrophilic dermatosis with lipodystrophy and elevated temperature with evidence of genetic and phenotypic heterogeneity. Arthritis Rheum. 2012;64:895–907.

Therapeutic Strategies

25

Courtney R. Schadt and Jeffrey P. Callen

There is significant overlap among the therapeutic strategies of neutrophilic dermatoses given the targeting of neutrophils. In addition, there is a paucity of quality, randomized controlled trials. Most treatments have been reported through case series and reports. Systemic corticosteroids are effective for most neutrophilic conditions. However, side effects limit long-term use.

Sweet Syndrome, Pyoderma Gangrenosum

This group of conditions can be associated with underlying malignancy, particularly leukemia or preleukemic states or inflammatory/autoimmune conditions, including inflammatory bowel disease or inflammatory arthritis. Any underlying conditions need to be treated.

Limited Disease

Wound care in pyoderma gangrenosum (PG) includes bland occlusive dressings, such as Vaseline. Debridement should be avoided because of pathergy except in rare circumstances where necrotic tissue could increase infection risk. There are reports of successful graft and flap placement in exceptional cases of pyoderma gangrenosum, but maximal medical therapy is necessary to prevent recurrence or pathergy [1]. Use of vacuum assisted closure with split-thickness skin graft of refractory PG has also been reported [2].

C. R. Schadt, M.D. (✉) • J. P. Callen, M.D.
Division of Dermatology, University of Louisville School of Medicine,
Louisville, KY, USA

D. Wallach et al. (eds.), *Neutrophilic Dermatoses*,
https://doi.org/10.1007/978-3-319-72649-6_25

Application of topical high potency steroids (such as clobetasol ointment) once or twice daily can be effective for limited involvement of any of these conditions. This have been reported to be efficacious in Sweet syndrome [3], PG [4], and aseptic pustulosis of the folds in combination with other therapies [5] (although high potency topical steroids should be used for a very limited duration in the folds). While intralesional corticosteroids have been reported to be effective in some patients with Sweet Syndrome [3] and PG [4], pathergy is a concern, and these treatments should be used with extreme caution. Atrophy and dyspigmentation are potential side effects of topical steroids, so should be used with caution in the folds and facial skin.

Topical calcineurin inhibitors are an additional option for limited skin disease involvement. They are generally well tolerated with minimal burning at the site of application, and offer the advantage of no atrophy or dyspigmentation. One small open study suggests that tacrolimus 0.3% in a carmellose sodium base is more effective than clobetasol 0.05% for peristomal PG [6].

Widespread/Refractory Local Disease

First Line Treatment

Systemic corticosteroids are first line therapy in Sweet's syndrome and PG. These conditions have a rapid response to systemic corticosteroids, and this feature is also included amongst their diagnostic criteria [7, 8]. Dosing prednisone at 0.5–1 mg/kg/day or a maximum of 60 mg a day with a taper over weeks is recommended. In PG, pain may improve quickly, and tapering should be initiated with initial healing of the ulcer and pain reduction. Ulcers may require months of therapy to fully heal, so a steroid-sparing agent should be utilized given the side effects of long-term systemic corticosteroids. In patients with very severe, painful disease, intravenous pulse corticosteroids can be administered (1 g/day methylprednisolone for 1–5 days) [9].

Cyclosporine

Cyclosporine is also a first line agent in PG. A randomized controlled, observer blind trial comparing oral prednisolone 0.75 mg/kg/day to cyclosporine 4 mg/kg/day showed similar efficacy (47% healed in both groups at 6 months) [10]. However, the prednisolone group suffered more serious adverse reactions, including infections. Cyclosporine should be dosed at 4–5 mg/kg/day, and tapered as improvement of the ulcer occurs. Long-term treatment may be complicated by hypertension and renal toxicity, so therapy should be limited to less than a year if possible with close monitoring of blood pressure and renal function.

Other First Line Therapies: Sweet Syndrome

Antibiotics: Dapsone/Minocycline

In patients with less severe PG and Sweet syndrome, dapsone may offer benefit as monotherapy or as a steroid sparing agent prior to use of immunosuppressive agents. Dapsone has been shown to be effective in numerous case series and reports for both conditions, in doses typically ranging from 50 to 200 mg/day [11–14]. After confirming normal G6PD levels, dapsone can be started at 50 mg/day and titrated as needed up to 200 mg/day with close monitoring for anemia, symptomatic methemoglobinemia, liver toxicity, and peripheral motor neuropathy. There are also numerous case reports of efficacy with minocycline in PG, both as a mono and adjunctive therapy [11, 15, 16]. It is dosed at 100 mg twice daily, should be avoided in children under 9 years of age secondary to tooth discoloration, and other side effects include skin discoloration, vertigo, and rare allergic reactions. Minocycline, however, has been reported to induce Sweet syndrome, and should be used with caution in this condition [17, 18].

Colchicine

Numerous case reports and a small retrospective study have demonstrated efficacy of colchicine in Sweet Syndrome [19, 20]. It can have rapid onset with minimal side effects, most notably gastrointestinal distress. It can be dosed at 0.6 mg once to twice a day. It has only anecdotally been reported to be effective in PG [21], so would not be a first or second line therapy for this condition.

Potassium Iodide

Potassium iodide can effectively treat Sweet Syndrome, as reported in many case series [22–24]. Rapid response can be seen, with resolution of systemic and cutaneous symptoms and skin lesions within days. It is available as a 300 mg tablet or supersaturated 1000 mg/mL solution. The capsule should not be crushed or opened and should be taken with plenty of fluid to avoid intestinal ulceration. Typical dosing is a 300 mg capsule three times a day. The liquid solution should be initiated at 3 drops (150 mg) three times a day and increased by 1 drop per day as needed to a maximum dose of 7–10 drops a day [13]. Potential side effects include nausea, vomiting, lacrimal duct swelling, hypothyroidism, metallic taste, and a hypersensitivity reaction [25]. It can be taken with juice to improve the taste.

Refractory Disease: Sweet Syndrome

Several other therapies may be effective in refractory Sweet Syndrome. In one open label study of 18 patients, 17 had a rapid and lasting response to indomethacin (150 mg/day for 1 week, then 100 mg/day for 2 weeks) [26]. Other case reports have demonstrated efficacy with cyclosporine [27, 28], methotrexate [29], anakinra [30], cyclosphosphamide [29], thalidomide [31], chlorambucil [32], rixuximab [33], infliximab [34], etanercept [35], and azacitidine (although has also been reported to induce Sweet syndrome) [36, 37]. There are numerous case reports of azathioprine-induced Sweet Syndrome, so this medication should potentially be avoided in this condition [38]. It is possible that these patients may have a variant of azathioprine-hypersensitivity reaction that resembles Sweet syndrome clinically, but in most cases is not classic histologically for Sweet syndrome [39]. Sweet syndrome has also been reported with adalimumab [40].

Second Line Therapies: Pyoderma gangrenosum

Biologics

Infliximab is an effective treatment for PG, as demonstrated in a placebo-controlled randomized trial [41]. In this study, 69% of the thirty patients had a clinical response after 2 doses (at week 0 and 2) of 5 mg/kg of infliximab, and the remission rate at week 6 was 21%. Infliximab (5 mg/kg) should be administered intravenously at week 0, week 2, week 6, and every 6–8 weeks [42]. Cost can be a limiting factor, and adverse events include infusion reactions, infections, and rare hypersensitivity reactions. Many other case series and reports have shown benefit with infliximab for PG, most in patients with underlying inflammatory bowel disease and rheumatoid arthritis, but there are also some reports in idiopathic PG [41, 43, 44].

Other biologic agents, including adalimumab (40 mg weekly, twice a month) and etanercept (25 and 50 mg weekly), can be effective in PG, and most frequently in patients with underlying inflammatory bowel disease and rheumatoid arthritis [45–50]. In our personal experience, adalimumab is more efficacious than etanercept.

Other Immunosuppressants

More conventional immunosuppressants, including mycophenolate mofetil (MMF), methotrexate, and azathioprine can be effective in PG. However, onset of action is slower than prednisone or cyclosporine. These are typically used as steroid sparing and adjunctive therapies.

MMF has the most evidence to support efficacy of this group of medications. In one retrospective chart review of 26 patients with PG, 22 patients achieved clinical improvement on mycophenolate mofetil (average treatment duration of 12.1 months), and 13 patients achieved complete ulcer healing [51]. MMF dosing in PG is 1–1.5 g twice daily. It has a slow onset of action, and side effects include cytopenias, nausea/vomiting, and infections.

Methotrexate and azathioprine have been reported efficacious in individual patients [12, 52, 53], in addition to intravenous immune globulin [11, 54, 55]. Anecdotal therapies include certolizumab [56], ustekinumb [57], chlorambucil [58], cyclophosphamide [59], melphalan [60], thalidomide [11], and canakinumab [61].

Aseptic abscesses can be treated in a similar fashion to Sweet syndrome and PG. In the largest series of 30 patients with aseptic abscesses, all were treated with systemic corticosteroids, and 13 required additional immunosuppressant therapy, including cyclophosphamide, azathioprine, anti-TNF agents, and methotrexate [62]. While aseptic abscesses may rapidly respond to glucocorticoids [63, 64], relapse occurred in 60% of patients in the large series [62], so a steroid sparing agent needs to be started early.

Treatment of neutrophil panniciulitis is in the same spectrum as Sweet Syndrome and PG and demonstrates rapid responsiveness to systemic corticosteroids [65, 66].

Erythema Elevatum Diutinum (EED)

EED, like many other neutrophilic dermatoses, can be associated with underlying systemic conditions that need to be treated. The most effective therapy for EED is dapsone based on numerous case reports and small series [67–70]. In a review of 66 cases in the literature, dapsone monotherapy was effective in 80% of patients [70]. Efficacy was seen as an adjunctive treatment (systemic glucocorticoids, colchicine, excision, anti-retroviral, gluten free diet) in 11%. Dapsone may be less effective in nodular lesions because of extensive fibrosis, so early initiation and/or concomitant therapy may be needed [70]. Dapsone may also reduce some of the extracutaneous symptoms of EED, including arthralgias and ocular symptoms [70, 71]. Recurrence is very common after cessation of dapsone therapy [72, 73].

Other therapies for EED reported in individual patients include colchicine [74, 75], topical dapsone 5% gel [76], excision in combination with dapsone [77], excision alone [78], methotrexate [70], cyclosporine [69], cyclophosphamide [70], thalidomide and plasma exchange [79], and chloroquine [72]. Prompt recurrence with excision alone has been reported and should be avoided as a monotherapy [80].

Subcorneal Pustular Dermatosis (SPD)

Dapsone, at doses of 50–200 mg a day, is first line treatment for SPD, and response is typically seen within weeks. Numerous case reports have shown efficacy both in adult [81, 82] and pediatric patients [83, 84].

Other treatment options that have been reported in individual cases include acitretin [85, 86], etanercept [87], adalimumab [88], infliximab [89]; colchicine [90], narrow band UVB phototherapy [91], PUVA [92], cyclosporine and prednisolone [93, 94], and the topical vitamin D derivatives maxicalcitol [95] and tacalcitol [96].

IgA Pemphigus

IgA pemphigus is a chronic disease requiring use of a steroid-sparing agent. Dapsone is considered first line therapy for IgA pemphigus, and has been described in case reports and series [28, 97, 98]. In one study of 25 patients, it was effective in 16; etretinate was effective in four patients [99]. In a review of 49 cases, dapsone was first line therapy for both the subcorneal pustular dermatosis and intraepidermal neutrophilic subtypes [100]. Some patients may not respond to dapsone, and alternatives include acitretin, which has been reported in individual cases, in addition to its precursor, etretinate, which is no longer available in the United States [97, 100–103]. Isotretinoin has also been reported as effective, supporting the use of this class of medications in this condition [104].

Additional therapeutic options include colchicine [100, 105] and adalimumab as monotherapy [97], and in one case, in combination with mycophenolate mofetil [106]. Anecdotal reports include sulfapyridine [100], cyclophosphamide [100, 107], plasmapheresis [100, 107], IVIG [108], sulfamethoxazole [100], PUVA [100], and azithromycin [109].

Pustular Psoriasis

In pustular psoriasis, patients need to be assessed for hemodynamic instability and may require hospitalization. Patients should be categorized as severe acute disease vs. stable disease.

Stable Disease

The retinoid acitretin is an excellent choice in this disease if patients are not of childbearing age, although controlled trials are lacking. A large questionnaire based study of 385 patients in Japan with pustular psoriasis determined that 84.1% of patients responded to etretinate 1 mg/kg/day and tapered as tolerated [110]. In another review of 63 patients, 6 patients with acute disease responded to etretinate. Given lack of availability of etretinate, less clinical use of isotretinoin for this condition, acitretin is the preferred agent [111] at a dose of 25–50 mg/day. In a recent series of juvenile patients with pustular psoriasis, acitretin was effective in all 16 patients treated [112]. Methotrexate is another therapeutic option [111, 113] with a typical dose ranging from 15 to 25 mg once a week. Topical steroids can be used as adjunctive therapy, although application to a large body surface area is less feasible.

Biologics

Tumor necrosis factor antagonists, such as adalimumab and etanercept are therapeutic options in pustular psoriasis [114, 115]. Their onset of action is slower than infliximab, so these agents should be used for maintenance or less acute disease. These agents can also induce pustular psoriasis [116].

There are some small open label studies suggesting efficacy with agents targeting the Th17 pathway, including secukinumab [117] and ixekizumab [118], both anti-IL17A monoclonal antibodies, and brodalumab [119], an anti-IL17A receptor monoclonal antibody.

Psoralen Plus Ultraviolet A (PUVA)

PUVA phototherapy has shown efficacy in numerous case reports and an uncontrolled prospective study [120, 121]. Frequent office visits may be a limiting factor for some patients. Acute side effects include nausea and skin discomfort, and long term adverse reactions include photoaging, skin cancer, and cataracts.

Severe Acute Disease

Cyclosporine has a known rapid effect on severe pustular psoriasis with improvement within days [110, 112, 122]. Cyclosporine for severe disease should be dosed at 4–5 mg/kg/day with tapering over 2–3 months. Side effects include hypertension, hepatic and nephrotoxicity, and cytopenias, and use over year should be avoided.

Infliximab is also efficacious in severe acute pustular psoriasis. In a large post-marketing surveillance of patients with pustular psoriasis treated with infliximab, 19.4% had clearance and 68.4% had improvement of their disease [123]. Its use is supported in numerous cases series and reports, including pediatric patients [113, 114]. Dosing is intravenous 5 mg/kg on week 0, 2, 6, and 8 weeks thereafter. In addition, infliximab has been reported to induce pustular psoriasis [116].

PAPA (Pyogenic Sterile Arthritis, Pyoderma Gangrenosum, and Acne) and Related Syndromes

The known mutation in PAPA syndrome of the PSTPIP1 gene leads to increased binding of the PSTPIP1 protein to pyrin, thus interfering with pyrin's inhibitory effect on interleukin-1 (IL-1) secretion [124]. This has allowed for targeted therapy with the recombinant IL-1 antagonist, anakinra, demonstrating efficacy in several case reports [125–127]. Other reported treatments include systemic corticosteroids [126, 128], adalimumab [126, 127, 129], etanercept [130], infliximab [127], and isotretinoin [126]. Canakinumab, a human anti-interleukin-1B monoclonal antibody was efficacious in one patient with a PAPA-like syndrome [131]. PASH (pyoderma gangrenosum, acne, and suppurative hidradenitis) has been recently described with individual patients reported responding to adalimumab [132], glucocorticoids [133, 134], and infliximab [134], and combination of infliximab, cyclosporine, and dapsone [135].

References

1. Rozen SM, Nahabedian MY, Manson PN. Management strategies for pyoderma gangrenosum: case studies and review of literature. Ann Plast Surg. 2001;47:310–5.
2. Aydin S, Aydin CA, Ugurlucan FG, Yasa C, Dural O. Recurrent pyoderma gangrenosum after cesarean delivery successfully treated with vacuum-assisted closure and split thickness skin graft: a case report. J Obstet Gynaecol Res. 2015;41:635–9.
3. Cohen PR, Kurzrock R. Sweet's syndrome and cancer. Clin Dermatol. 1993;11:149–57.
4. Reichrath J, Bens G, Bonowitz A, Tilgen W. Treatment recommendations for pyoderma gangrenosum: an evidence-based review of the literature based on more than 350 patients. J Am Acad Dermatol. 2005;53:273–83.
5. Wang MZ, Camilleri MJ, Guo R, Wieland CN. Amicrobial pustulosis of the folds: report of 4 cases. J Cutan Pathol. 2016;44(4):367–72.
6. Lyon CC, Stapleton M, Smith AJ, Mendelsohn S, Beck MH, Griffiths CE. Topical tacrolimus in the management of peristomal pyoderma gangrenosum. J Dermatol Treat. 2001;12:13–7.
7. Walker DC, Cohen PR. Trimethoprim-sulfamethoxazole-associated acute febrile neutrophilic dermatosis: case report and review of drug-induced Sweet's syndrome. J Am Acad Dermatol. 1996;34:918–23.
8. Su WP, Davis MD, Weenig RH, Powell FC, Perry HO. Pyoderma gangrenosum: clinicopathologic correlation and proposed diagnostic criteria. Int J Dermatol. 2004;43:790–800.
9. Aseni P, Di Sandro S, Mihaylov P, Lamperti L, De Carlis LG. Atypical presentation of pioderma gangrenosum complicating ulcerative colitis: rapid disappearance with methylprednisolone. World J Gastroenterol. 2008;14:5471–3.
10. Ormerod AD, Thomas KS, Craig FE, et al. Comparison of the two most commonly used treatments for pyoderma gangrenosum: results of the STOP GAP randomised controlled trial. BMJ. 2015;350:h2958.
11. Binus AM, Qureshi AA, Li VW, Winterfield LS. Pyoderma gangrenosum: a retrospective review of patient characteristics, comorbidities and therapy in 103 patients. Br J Dermatol. 2011;165:1244–50.
12. von den Driesch P. Pyoderma gangrenosum: a report of 44 cases with follow-up. Br J Dermatol. 1997;137:1000–5.
13. Cohen PR, Kurzrock R. Sweet's syndrome: a review of current treatment options. Am J Clin Dermatol. 2002;3:117–31.

14. el Sherif AI, Bharija SC, Belhaj MS, Singh G. Dapsone in Sweet syndrome. Int J Dermatol. 1990;29:737.
15. Yamanaka K, Murota H, Goto H, et al. Pyoderma gangrenosum and annular erythema associated with Sjogren's syndrome controlled with minocycline. J Dermatol. 2015;42:834–6.
16. Sau M, Hill NC. Pyoderma gangrenosum of the vulva. BJOG. 2001;108:1197–8.
17. Thibault MJ, Billick RC, Srolovitz H. Minocycline-induced Sweet's syndrome. J Am Acad Dermatol. 1992;27:801–4.
18. Khan Durani B, Jappe U. Drug-induced Sweet's syndrome in acne caused by different tetracyclines: case report and review of the literature. Br J Dermatol. 2002;147:558–62.
19. Ritter S, George R, Serwatka LM, Elston DM. Long-term suppression of chronic Sweet's syndrome with colchicine. J Am Acad Dermatol. 2002;47:323–4.
20. Maillard H, Leclech C, Peria P, Avenel-Audran M, Verret JL. Colchicine for Sweet's syndrome. A study of 20 cases. Br J Dermatol. 1999;140:565–6.
21. Paolini O, Hebuterne X, Flory P, Charles F, Rampal P. Treatment of pyoderma gangrenosum with colchicine. Lancet. 1995;345:1057–8.
22. von den Driesch P. Sweet's syndrome (acute febrile neutrophilic dermatosis). J Am Acad Dermatol. 1994;31:535–56; quiz 57–60.
23. Cohen PR, Holder WR, Tucker SB, Kono S, Kurzrock R. Sweet syndrome in patients with solid tumors. Cancer. 1993;72:2723–31.
24. Horio T, Danno K, Okamoto H, Miyachi Y, Imamura S. Potassium iodide in erythema nodosum and other erythematous dermatoses. J Am Acad Dermatol. 1983;9:77–81.
25. Sanchez MR. Miscellaneous treatments: thalidomide, potassium iodide, levamisole, clofazimine, colchicine, and D-penicillamine. Clin Dermatol. 2000;18:131–45.
26. Jeanfils S, Joly P, Young P, Le Corvaisier-Pieto C, Thomine E, Lauret P. Indomethacin treatment of eighteen patients with Sweet's syndrome. J Am Acad Dermatol. 1997;36:436–9.
27. von den Driesch P, Steffan C, Zobe A, Hornstein OP. Sweet's syndrome—therapy with cyclosporin. Clin Exp Dermatol. 1994;19:274–7.
28. Yasuda F, Fujio Y, Kakuta R, Funakoshi T, Amagai M, Ohyama M. Use of cyclosporin A for successful management of steroid-resistant Sweet's syndrome patient with possible myelodysplastic syndrome. J Dermatol. 2014;41:465–6.
29. Ma EH, Akikusa JD, MacGregor D, Ng J, Su JC. Sweet's syndrome with postinflammatory elastolysis and Takayasu arteritis in a child: a case report and literature review. Pediatr Dermatol. 2012;29:645–50.
30. Kluger N, Gil-Bistes D, Guillot B, Bessis D. Efficacy of anti-interleukin-1 receptor antagonist anakinra (Kineret(R)) in a case of refractory Sweet's syndrome. Dermatology. 2011;222:123–7.
31. Browning CE, Dixon JE, Malone JC, Callen JP. Thalidomide in the treatment of recalcitrant Sweet's syndrome associated with myelodysplasia. J Am Acad Dermatol. 2005;53:S135–8.
32. Case JD, Smith SZ, Callen JP. The use of pulse methylprednisolone and chlorambucil in the treatment of Sweet's syndrome. Cutis. 1989;44:125–9.
33. Seminario-Vidal L, Guerrero C, Sami N. Refractory Sweet's syndrome successfully treated with rituximab. JAAD Case Rep. 2015;1:123–5.
34. Karamlou K, Gorn AH. Refractory sweet syndrome with autoimmune organizing pneumonia treated with monoclonal antibodies to tumor necrosis factor. J Clin Rheumatol. 2004;10:331–5.
35. Ambrose NL, Tobin AM, Howard D. Etanercept treatment in Sweet's syndrome with inflammatory arthritis. J Rheumatol. 2009;36:1348–9.
36. Yaghmour G, Wiedower E, Yaghmour B, Nunnery S, Duncavage E, Martin MG. Sweet's syndrome associated with clonal hematopoiesis of indeterminate potential responsive to 5-azacitidine. Ther Adv Hematol. 2017;8:91–5.
37. Trickett HB, Cumpston A, Craig M. Azacitidine-associated Sweet's syndrome. Am J Health Syst Pharm. 2012;69:869–71.

38. Biswas SN, Chakraborty PP, Gantait K, Bar C. Azathioprine-induced bullous Sweet's syndrome: a rare association. BMJ Case Rep. 2016;2016:10.1136/bcr-2016-215192. https://doi.org/10.1136/bcr-2016-215192.
39. Cyrus N, Stavert R, Mason AR, Ko CJ, Choi JN. Neutrophilic dermatosis after azathioprine exposure. JAMA Dermatol. 2013;149:592–7.
40. Banse C, Sobocinski V, Savoye G, Avenel G, Vittecoq O. Occurrence of Sweet syndrome under anti-TNF. Clin Rheumatol. 2015;34:1993–4.
41. Brooklyn TN, Dunnill MG, Shetty A, et al. Infliximab for the treatment of pyoderma gangrenosum: a randomised, double blind, placebo controlled trial. Gut. 2006;55:505–9.
42. Callen JP, Jackson JM. Pyoderma gangrenosum: an update. Rheum Dis Clin North Am. 2007;33:787–802, vi.
43. Del Giacco SR, Firinu D, Lorrai MM, et al. Idiopathic pyoderma gangrenosum: successful resolution with infliximab therapy and pro-inflammatory cytokines assessment. Acta Derm Venereol. 2012;92:439–40.
44. Kaur MR, Lewis HM. Severe recalcitrant pyoderma gangrenosum treated with infliximab. Br J Dermatol. 2005;153:689–91.
45. Alkhouri N, Hupertz V, Mahajan L. Adalimumab treatment for peristomal pyoderma gangrenosum associated with Crohn's disease. Inflamm Bowel Dis. 2009;15:803–6.
46. Hubbard VG, Friedmann AC, Goldsmith P. Systemic pyoderma gangrenosum responding to infliximab and adalimumab. Br J Dermatol. 2005;152:1059–61.
47. Sagami S, Ueno Y, Tanaka S, Nagai K, Hayashi R, Chayama K. Successful use of adalimumab for treating pyoderma gangrenosum with ulcerative colitis under corticosteroid-tapering conditions. Intern Med. 2015;54:2167–72.
48. Campanati A, Brisigotti V, Ganzetti G, et al. Finally, recurrent pyoderma gangrenosum treated with Adalimumab: case report and review of the literature. J Eur Acad Dermatol Venereol. 2015;29:1245–7.
49. Kim FS, Pandya AG. The use of etanercept in the treatment of peristomal pyoderma gangrenosum. Clin Exp Dermatol. 2012;37:442–3.
50. Rogge FJ, Pacifico M, Kang N. Treatment of pyoderma gangrenosum with the anti-TNFalpha drug—etanercept. J Plast Reconstr Aesthet Surg. 2008;61:431–3.
51. Li J, Kelly R. Treatment of pyoderma gangrenosum with mycophenolate mofetil as a steroid-sparing agent. J Am Acad Dermatol. 2013;69:565–9.
52. Teitel AD. Treatment of pyoderma gangrenosum with methotrexate. Cutis. 1996;57:326–8.
53. Duffill MB. Cyclosporine, azathioprine and local therapy for pyoderma gangrenosum. Australas J Dermatol. 1994;35:15–8.
54. Behm K, Larson DW, Colibaseanu D. Intravenous immunoglobulin use in managing severe, perioperative peristomal pyoderma gangrenosum following subtotal colectomy with end ileostomy for medically refractory chronic ulcerative colitis. J Surg Case Rep. 2015;2015(3). pii: rjv019.
55. Gupta AK, Shear NH, Sauder DN. Efficacy of human intravenous immune globulin in pyoderma gangrenosum. J Am Acad Dermatol. 1995;32:140–2.
56. Hurabielle C, Schneider P, Baudry C, Bagot M, Allez M, Viguier M. Certolizumab pegol—a new therapeutic option for refractory disseminated pyoderma gangrenosum associated with Crohn's disease. J Dermatolog Treat. 2016;27:67–9.
57. Goldminz AM, Botto NC, Gottlieb AB. Severely recalcitrant pyoderma gangrenosum successfully treated with ustekinumab. J Am Acad Dermatol. 2012;67:e237–8.
58. Burruss JB, Farmer ER, Callen JP. Chlorambucil is an effective corticosteroid-sparing agent for recalcitrant pyoderma gangrenosum. J Am Acad Dermatol. 1996;35:720–4.
59. Kaminska R, Ikaheimo R, Hollmen A. Plasmapheresis and cyclophosphamide as successful treatments for pyoderma gangrenosum. Clin Exp Dermatol. 1999;24:81–5.
60. Jones RR, Kobza Black A, Donaghy M, Moshtael O, Pinching AJ. Defective monocyte function in pyoderma gangrenosum with IgG kappa paraproteinaemia. Clin Exp Immunol. 1983;52:685–92.

61. Kolios AG, Maul JT, Meier B, et al. Canakinumab in adults with steroid-refractory pyoderma gangrenosum. Br J Dermatol. 2015;173:1216–23.
62. Andre MF, Piette JC, Kemeny JL, et al. Aseptic abscesses: a study of 30 patients with or without inflammatory bowel disease and review of the literature. Medicine. 2007;86:145–61.
63. Yildiz H, Munting A, Komuta M, Danse E, Lefebvre C. Aseptic lung and liver abscesses: a diagnostic challenge. Acta Clin Belg. 2016;72(4):1–5.
64. Fukuda S, Nanki T, Morio T, Hasegawa H, Koike R, Miyasaka N. Recurrent mitral valve regurgitation with neutrophil infiltration in a patient with multiple aseptic abscesses. Mod Rheumatol. 2014;24:537–9.
65. Nakanishi K, Kinjo M. Mimicker of necrotising fasciitis with systemic inflammatory response syndrome: recurrent necrotising Sweet's syndrome associated with chronic myelogenous leukaemia. BMJ Case Rep. 2016;2016. pii: bcr2016214461. https://doi.org/10.1136/bcr-2016-214461.
66. Qian L, Shen J, Cen J, Yin W, Ma Y. Myelodysplastic syndrome with neutrophilic panniculitis: a report of two cases and a literature review. Oncol Lett. 2015;9:1954–6.
67. Katz SI, Gallin JI, Hertz KC, Fauci AS, Lawley TJ. Erythema elevatum diutinum: skin and systemic manifestations, immunologic studies, and successful treatment with dapsone. Medicine. 1977;56:443–55.
68. Chan Y, Mok CC, Tang WY. Erythema elevatum diutinum in systemic lupus erythematosus. Rheumatol Int. 2011;31:259–62.
69. Takahashi H, Fukami Y, Honma M, Ishida-Yamamoto A, Iizuka H. Successful combination therapy with dapsone and cyclosporine for erythema elevatum diutinum with unusual appearance. J Dermatol. 2012;39:486–7.
70. Momen SE, Jorizzo J, Al-Niaimi F. Erythema elevatum diutinum: a review of presentation and treatment. J Eur Acad Dermatol Venereol. 2014;28:1594–602.
71. Jiao T, Wang M, Zhu X. A case of erythema elevatum diutinum associated with peripheral ulcerative keratitis. Australas J Dermatol. 2012;53:78–80.
72. Wilkinson SM, English JS, Smith NP, Wilson-Jones E, Winkelmann RK. Erythema elevatum diutinum: a clinicopathological study. Clin Exp Dermatol. 1992;17:87–93.
73. Gibson LE, el-Azhary RA. Erythema elevatum diutinum. Clin Dermatol. 2000;18:295–9.
74. Kocaturk E, Memet B, Topal IO, Yuksel T, Ulkumen PK, Kiziltac U. A case of erythema elevatum diutinum with pancytopenia: focus on dapsone-induced hematologic side effects and colchicine as a safe treatment option. J Drugs Dermatol. 2015;14:1090–2.
75. Henriksson R, Hofer PA, Hornqvist R. Erythema elevatum diutinum—a case successfully treated with colchicine. Clin Exp Dermatol. 1989;14:451–3.
76. Frieling GW, Williams NL, Lim SJ, Rosenthal SI. Novel use of topical dapsone 5% gel for erythema elevatum diutinum: safer and effective. J Drugs Dermatol. 2013;12:481–4.
77. Zacaron LH, Goncalves JC, Curty VM, D'Acri AM, Lima RB, Martins CJ. Clinical and surgical therapeutic approach in erithema elevatum diutinum—case report. An Bras Dermatol. 2013;88:15–8.
78. Thomas CL, Ffolkes L, Akhras V. A case of mistaken identity: unilateral erythema elevatum diutinum associated with IgA paraproteinaemia. Clin Exp Dermatol. 2015;40:761–4.
79. Manni E, Cervadoro E, Papineschi F. Case of erythema elevatum diutinum associated with IgA paraproteinemia successfully controlled with thalidomide and plasma exchange. Ther Apher Dial. 2015;19:195–6.
80. Atallah J, Garces JC, Loayza E, Carlson JA. Chronic localized fibrosing leukocytoclastic vasculitis associated with lymphedema, intralymphatic and intravascular lymphocytosis, and chronic myelogenous leukemia: a case report of unilateral erythema elevatum diutinum. Am J Dermatopathol. 2016;39(6):479–84.
81. Sandhu K, Saraswat A, Gupta S. Inverse subcorneal pustular dermatosis. J Eur Acad Dermatol Venereol. 2003;17:348–9.
82. Roger H, Thevenet JP, Souteyrand P, Sauvezie B. Subcorneal pustular dermatosis associated with rheumatoid arthritis and raised IgA: simultaneous remission of skin and joint involvements with dapsone treatment. Ann Rheum Dis. 1990;49:190–1.

83. Scalvenzi M, Palmisano F, Annunziata MC, Mezza E, Cozzolino I, Costa C. Subcorneal pustular dermatosis in childhood: a case report and review of the literature. Case Rep Dermatol Med. 2013;2013:424797.
84. Kocak M, Birol A, Erkek E, Bozdogan O, Atasoy P. Juvenile subcorneal pustular dermatosis: a case report. Pediatr Dermatol. 2003;20:57–9.
85. Marliere V, Beylot-Barry M, Beylot C, Doutre M. Successful treatment of subcorneal pustular dermatosis (Sneddon-wilkinson disease) by acitretin: report of a case. Dermatology. 1999;199:153–5.
86. Canpolat F, Akpinar H, Cemil BC, Eskioglu F, Ozturk E. A case of subcorneal pustular dermatosis in association with monoclonal IgA gammopathy successfully treated with acitretin. J Dermatol Treat. 2010;21:114–6.
87. Berk DR, Hurt MA, Mann C, Sheinbein D. Sneddon-Wilkinson disease treated with etanercept: report of two cases. Clin Exp Dermatol. 2009;34:347–51.
88. de Encarnacao Roque Diamantino F, Dias Coelho JM, Macedo Ferreira AM, Fidalgo AI. Subcorneal pustular dermatosis treated successfully with adalimumab. Eur J Dermatol. 2010;20:512–4.
89. Voigtlander C, Luftl M, Schuler G, Hertl M. Infliximab (anti-tumor necrosis factor alpha antibody): a novel, highly effective treatment of recalcitrant subcorneal pustular dermatosis (Sneddon-Wilkinson disease). Arch Dermatol. 2001;137:1571–4.
90. Pavithran K. Colchicine in the treatment of subcorneal pustular dermatosis. Indian J Dermatol Venereol Leprol. 1995;61:56–7.
91. Cameron H, Dawe RS. Subcorneal pustular dermatosis (Sneddon-Wilkinson disease) treated with narrowband (TL-01) UVB phototherapy. Br J Dermatol. 1997;137:150–1.
92. Bauwens M, De Coninck A, Roseeuw D. Subcorneal pustular dermatosis treated with PUVA therapy. A case report and review of the literature. Dermatology. 1999;198:203–5.
93. Karadogan SK, Aydogan K, Baskan EB, Tunali S. A case of subcorneal pustular dermatosis treated successfully with a combination of cyclosporin and prednisolone. J Eur Acad Dermatol Venereol. 2007;21:536–7.
94. Zachariae CO, Rossen K, Weismann K. An unusual severe case of subcorneal pustular dermatosis treated with cyclosporine and prednisolone. Acta Derm Venereol. 2000;80:386–7.
95. Hoshina D, Tsujiwaki M, Furuya K. Successful treatment of subcorneal pustular dermatosis with maxacalcitol. Clin Exp Dermatol. 2016;41:102–3.
96. Kawaguchi M, Mitsuhashi Y, Kondo S. A case of subcorneal pustular dermatosis treated with tacalcitol (1alpha,24-dihydroxyvitamin D3). J Dermatol. 2000;27:669–72.
97. Moreno AC, Santi CG, Gabbi TV, Aoki V, Hashimoto T, Maruta CW. IgA pemphigus: case series with emphasis on therapeutic response. J Am Acad Dermatol. 2014;70:200–1.
98. Niimi Y, Kawana S, Kusunoki T. IgA pemphigus: a case report and its characteristic clinical features compared with subcorneal pustular dermatosis. J Am Acad Dermatol. 2000;43:546–9.
99. Wallach D. Intraepidermal IgA pustulosis. J Am Acad Dermatol. 1992;27:993–1000.
100. Yasuda H, Kobayashi H, Hashimoto T, Itoh K, Yamane M, Nakamura J. Subcorneal pustular dermatosis type of IgA pemphigus: demonstration of autoantibodies to desmocollin-1 and clinical review. Br J Dermatol. 2000;143:144–8.
101. Ruiz-Genao DP, Hernandez-Nunez A, Hashimoto T, Amagai M, Fernandez-Herrera J, Garcia-Diez A. A case of IgA pemphigus successfully treated with acitretin. Br J Dermatol. 2002;147:1040–2.
102. Tagami H, Iwatsuki K, Iwase Y, Yamada M. Subcorneal pustular dermatosis with vesiculo-bullous eruption. Demonstration of subcorneal IgA deposits and a leukocyte chemotactic factor. Br J Dermatol. 1983;109:581–7.
103. Zillikens D, Miller K, Hartmann AA, Burg G. IgA pemphigus foliaceus: a case report. Dermatologica. 1990;181:304–7.
104. Gruss C, Zillikens D, Hashimoto T, et al. Rapid response of IgA pemphigus of subcorneal pustular dermatosis type to treatment with isotretinoin. J Am Acad Dermatol. 2000;43:923–6.
105. Hodak E, Lapidoth M, David M. Effect of colchicine in the subcorneal pustular dermatosis type of IgA pemphigus. J Am Acad Dermatol. 1999;40:91–4.

106. Howell SM, Bessinger GT, Altman CE, Belnap CM. Rapid response of IgA pemphigus of the subcorneal pustular dermatosis subtype to treatment with adalimumab and mycophenolate mofetil. J Am Acad Dermatol. 2005;53:541–3.
107. Sibley Hash K, Rencic A, Hernandez MI, Hashimoto T, Nousari HC. Aggressive immunosuppressive therapy for a refractory case of IgA pemphigus. Arch Dermatol. 2002;138:744–6.
108. Iskandarli M, Gerceker Turk B, Ertam I, Yaman B, Ozturk G. Successful treatment of Wilson disease-associated IgA pemphigus with IVIG. J Eur Acad Dermatol Venereol. 2016;30:1055–6.
109. Bliziotis I, Rafailidis P, Vergidis P, Falagas ME. Regression of subcorneal pustular dermatosis type of IgA pemphigus lesions with azithromycin. J Infect. 2005;51:E31–4.
110. Ozawa A, Ohkido M, Haruki Y, et al. Treatments of generalized pustular psoriasis: a multicenter study in Japan. J Dermatol. 1999;26:141–9.
111. Zelickson BD, Muller SA. Generalized pustular psoriasis. A review of 63 cases. Arch Dermatol. 1991;127:1339–45.
112. Lau BW, Lim DZ, Capon F, Barker JN, Choon SE. Juvenile generalized pustular psoriasis is a chronic recalcitrant disease: an analysis of 27 patients seen in a tertiary hospital in Johor, Malaysia. Int J Dermatol. 2017;56(4):392–9.
113. Tsang V, Dvorakova V, Enright F, Murphy M, Gleeson C. Successful use of infliximab as first line treatment for severe childhood generalized pustular psoriasis. J Eur Acad Dermatol Venereol. 2016;30:e117–e9.
114. Viguier M, Aubin F, Delaporte E, et al. Efficacy and safety of tumor necrosis factor inhibitors in acute generalized pustular psoriasis. Arch Dermatol. 2012;148:1423–5.
115. Matsumoto A, Komine M, Karakawa M, Kishimoto M, Ohtsuki M. Adalimumab administration after infliximab therapy is a successful treatment strategy for generalized pustular psoriasis. J Dermatol. 2016;44(2):202–4.
116. Collamer AN, Battafarano DF. Psoriatic skin lesions induced by tumor necrosis factor antagonist therapy: clinical features and possible immunopathogenesis. Semin Arthritis Rheum. 2010;40:233–40.
117. Imafuku S, Honma M, Okubo Y, et al. Efficacy and safety of secukinumab in patients with generalized pustular psoriasis: a 52-week analysis from phase III open-label multicenter Japanese study. J Dermatol. 2016;43:1011–7.
118. Saeki H, Nakagawa H, Ishii T, et al. Efficacy and safety of open-label ixekizumab treatment in Japanese patients with moderate-to-severe plaque psoriasis, erythrodermic psoriasis and generalized pustular psoriasis. J Eur Acad Dermatol Venereol. 2015;29:1148–55.
119. Yamasaki K, Nakagawa H, Kubo Y, Ootaki K, Japanese Brodalumab Study Group. Efficacy and safety of brodalumab in patients with generalized pustular psoriasis and psoriatic erythroderma: results from a 52-week, open-label study. Br J Dermatol. 2016;176(3):741–51.
120. Honigsmann H, Gschnait F, Konrad K, Wolff K. Photochemotherapy for pustular psoriasis (von Zumbusch). Br J Dermatol. 1977;97:119–26.
121. Hunt MJ, Lee SH, Salisbury EL, Wills EJ, Armati R. Generalized pustular psoriasis responsive to PUVA and oral cyclosporin therapy. Australas J Dermatol. 1997;38:199–201.
122. Varman KM, Namias N, Schulman CI, Pizano LR. Acute generalized pustular psoriasis, von Zumbusch type, treated in the burn unit. A review of clinical features and new therapeutics. Burns. 2014;40:e35–9.
123. Torii H, Terui T, Matsukawa M, et al. Safety profiles and efficacy of infliximab therapy in Japanese patients with plaque psoriasis with or without psoriatic arthritis, pustular psoriasis or psoriatic erythroderma: results from the prospective post-marketing surveillance. J Dermatol. 2016;43:767–78.
124. Shoham NG, Centola M, Mansfield E, et al. Pyrin binds the PSTPIP1/CD2BP1 protein, defining familial Mediterranean fever and PAPA syndrome as disorders in the same pathway. Proc Natl Acad Sci U S A. 2003;100:13501–6.
125. Caorsi R, Picco P, Buoncompagni A, Martini A, Gattorno M. Osteolytic lesion in PAPA syndrome responding to anti-interleukin 1 treatment. J Rheumatol. 2014;41:2333–4.

126. Ter Haar N, Lachmann H, Ozen S, et al. Treatment of autoinflammatory diseases: results from the Eurofever Registry and a literature review. Ann Rheum Dis. 2013;72:678–85.
127. Demidowich AP, Freeman AF, Kuhns DB, et al. Brief report: genotype, phenotype, and clinical course in five patients with PAPA syndrome (pyogenic sterile arthritis, pyoderma gangrenosum, and acne). Arthritis Rheum. 2012;64:2022–7.
128. Fathalla BM, Al-Wahadneh AM, Al-Mutawa M, Kambouris M, El-Shanti H. A novel de novo PSTPIP1 mutation in a boy with pyogenic arthritis, pyoderma gangrenosum, acne (PAPA) syndrome. Clin Exp Rheumatol. 2014;32:956–8.
129. Lee H, Park SH, Kim SK, Choe JY, Park JS. Pyogenic arthritis, pyoderma gangrenosum, and acne syndrome (PAPA syndrome) with E250K mutation in CD2BP1 gene treated with the tumor necrosis factor inhibitor adalimumab. Clin Exp Rheumatol. 2012;30:452.
130. Tofteland ND, Shaver TS. Clinical efficacy of etanercept for treatment of PAPA syndrome. J Clin Rheumatol. 2010;16:244–5.
131. Geusau A, Mothes-Luksch N, Nahavandi H, et al. Identification of a homozygous PSTPIP1 mutation in a patient with a PAPA-like syndrome responding to canakinumab treatment. JAMA Dermatol. 2013;149:209–15.
132. Murphy B, Morrison G, Podmore P. Successful use of adalimumab to treat pyoderma gangrenosum, acne and suppurative hidradenitis (PASH syndrome) following colectomy in ulcerative colitis. Int J Colorectal Dis. 2015;30:1139–40.
133. Ursani MA, Appleyard J, Whiteru O. Pyogenic arthritis, pyoderma gangrenosum, acne, suppurative hidradenitis (PA-PASH) syndrome: an atypical presentation of a rare syndrome. Am J Case Rep. 2016;17:587–91.
134. Wargo JJ, Emmer BT. Systemic inflammation gone awry: PASH syndrome and temporomandibular joint ankylosis. Am J Med. 2016;129:e1–3.
135. Staub J, Pfannschmidt N, Strohal R, et al. Successful treatment of PASH syndrome with infliximab, cyclosporine and dapsone. J Eur Acad Dermatol Venereol. 2015;29:2243–7.

Final Remarks

26

Angelo Valerio Marzano, Daniel Wallach, and Marie-Dominique Vignon-Pennamen

Neutrophils are essential players in inflammatory responses and are the first line of defence against harmful stimuli. However, dysregulation of neutrophil homeostasis can result in excessive inflammation and subsequent tissue damage. The neutrophilic dermatoses reviewed in this book are a spectrum of inflammatory disorders characterized by polymorphic cutaneous lesions resulting from a neutrophil-rich inflammatory infiltrate in the absence of infection.

In some cases, the neutrophilic inflammation is not limited to the skin but also involves other organs, leading to proposing the name of "neutrophilic disease" for this cutaneous and non-cutaneous neutrophilic inflammation.

Pyoderma gangrenosum is a rare chronic cutaneous and systemic disease regarded as the most severe and the prototype of the neutrophilic dermatoses. The study of syndromic pyoderma gangrenosum group which includes forms like pyogenic arthritis, acne, and pyoderma gangrenosum (PAPA), traditionally considered a monogenic autoinflammatory syndrome, and other more recently described autoinflammatory syndromes such as pyoderma gangrenosum, acne, and hidradenitis suppurativa (PASH) and pyogenic arthritis, acne, pyoderma gangrenosum, and hidradenitis suppurativa (PAPASH), provided insights also on the pathophysiology of the neutrophilic dermatoses.

A. V. Marzano (✉)
Dipartimento di Fisiopatologia Medico-Chirurgica e dei Trapianti, Universita' degli Studi di Milano, Unita' Operativa di Dermatologia, IRCCS Fondazione Ca' Granda, Ospedale Maggiore Policlinico, Milano, Italy
e-mail: angelo.marzano@unimi.it

D. Wallach
Physician (Hon.) of Paris Hospitals, Paris, France

M.-D. Vignon-Pennamen, M.D.
Pathology Department, APHP Hôpital Saint Louis, Paris, France
e-mail: dominique.vignon-pennamen@wanadoo.fr

D. Wallach et al. (eds.), *Neutrophilic Dermatoses*,
https://doi.org/10.1007/978-3-319-72649-6_26

Molecular mechanisms causing autoinflammatory monogenic diseases are also potentially relevant in neutrophilic dermatoses and their syndromic forms, which encompass a spectrum of polygenic autoinflammatory conditions. Indeed, mutations of proline-serine-threonine-phosphatase protein 1 (PSTPIP1), the gene of PAPA, as well as of a number of other genes involved in classic autoinflammatory diseases are likely to play a role in the pathogenesis of both isolated PG and its syndromic, non-monogenic form PASH. Both inherited autoinflammatory syndromes and neutrophilic dermatoses share the overactivation of the innate immune system leading to increased production of interleukin (IL)-1 family members and sterile neutrophil-rich inflammation, giving rise to consider them as "innate immune disorders". On the other hand, a possible contributing role of adaptive immunity is conceivable and thus needs to be evaluated.

Systemic corticosteroids are the first step in the therapeutic algorithm of the neutrophilic dermatoses.

As these distressing entities are all associated with the over-expression of IL-1 and tumour necrosis factor (TNF)-α, biological agents targeting these cytokines are currently the most specific and effective treatments for refractory cases of neutrophilic dermatoses. Given the emerging pathogenetic role of IL-17, IL-17 antagonists may represent the future management of these diseases.

Disease-based gene discovery and basic immunological research continue to go hand in hand in deciphering the molecular pathways that lead to excessive innate immune responses and cause the chronic autoinflammatory mechanisms underlying the neutrophilic dermatoses features. Growing insights into the pathogenesis of neutrophilic dermatoses will in turn provide us with novel therapeutic targets that will allow us to treat these challenging conditions with a "tailored" approach that is based on the genetic and cytokine expression profile of the single patient.

FSC
www.fsc.org
MIX
Papier aus verantwortungsvollen Quellen
Paper from responsible sources
FSC® C105338

If you have any concerns about our products, you can contact us on
ProductSafety@springernature.com

In case Publisher is established outside the EU, the EU authorized representative is:
Springer Nature Customer Service Center GmbH
Europaplatz 3, 69115 Heidelberg, Germany

Printed by Libri Plureos GmbH
in Hamburg, Germany